Surgical Instrumentation

AN INTERACTIVE APPROACH

Surgical Instrumentation

AN INTERACTIVE APPROACH

RENEE NEMITZ, CST, RN, AAS, FAST
Surgical Technology Program Director
Western Iowa Tech Community College

ELSEVIER

Elsevier
3251 Riverport Lane
St. Louis, Missouri 63043

Notice

Practitioners and researchers must always rely on their own experience and knowledge in evaluating and using any information, methods, compounds or experiments described herein. Because of rapid advances in the medical sciences, in particular, independent verification of diagnoses and drug dosages should be made. To the fullest extent of the law, no responsibility is assumed by Elsevier, authors, editors or contributors for any injury and/or damage to persons or property as a matter of products liability, negligence or otherwise, or from any use or operation of any methods, products, instructions, or ideas contained in the material herein.

Senior Content Strategist: Kelly Skelton
Senior Content Development Manager: Laurie Gower
Senior Content Development Specialist: Rebecca Leenhouts
Publishing Services Manager: Deepthi Unni
Project Manager: Nayagi Anandan
Design Direction: Brian Salisbury

Printed in China

Last digit is the print number: 9 8 7 6 5 4 3 2

Working together
to grow libraries in
developing countries

www.elsevier.com • www.bookaid.org

To all my students—past, present, and future.
You are the reason for the inception, development, and
completion of this project.

Acknowledgments

I discovered throughout this project how blessed I am to have such incredible people in my life. I would like to acknowledge and sincerely thank the following people for their help, contributions, effort, and time.

First, to my husband, Rollin. Thank you for believing in me. Without your support, this project would not be a reality. To my daughters, Madison, Miranda, and Melia, who truly believe this is the longest book ever, for all the sacrifices you each made to let Mom work. To my parents, Marilyn and Dick Kreisel, for raising me to believe that I could accomplish anything and for all the time you spent with the girls during the first edition.

To the fantastic editorial staff at Elsevier: Kelly Skelton, Laura Goodrich, Melissa Rawe, and Rebecca Leenouts, thanks for your support, patience, and guidance. Without you, this project would not be a reality. I am particularly grateful to Michael Ledbetter for seeing my vision and believing in this project. Thanks for all your encouragement and fortitude.

Special thanks to Marsha McArthur, who was the Product Manager of Surgical Instruments at Integra LifeSciences Corporation (JARIT, Padgett, Ruggles, and R&B) during the first edition, for allowing us to photograph countless images for this book. Without her trust and access to the instruments, this book would not have been possible!

Also thanks to the following companies for working with us to photograph their instruments for the project: Stryker Corporation, DePuy, Miltex, Autosuture, and ACMI.

I would also like to thank Frank Pronesti and Gary Deamer at Heirloom Studio in Newtown, Pennsylvania, for providing their beautiful, high-resolution photography for all the instruments and supplies in this book and all the editions. Also thank you to Fran Pronesti for assisting Frank with the onsite shoot for this edition. Thank you to Elizabeth Pronesti for her consulting during the many photoshoots we had for the first edition of this book.

To my friend, Chris Keegan CST, MS, FAST. I thank you for your friendship, encouragement, and wisdom; it was simply immeasurable. I would not have made it through this without you. To Clifford Smith, MSN, BSEd, ONC, CRNFA, for all the time you spent helping with revisions and your contributions to the Orthopedic chapter in the first edition of the book. I am so grateful to you, Karen Craig, CSTFA; thank you for your contributions to the Cardiovascular Thoracic chapter in the first edition.

Thanks to Master Key Consulting in St. Louis, Missouri, for your hard work developing the interactive portion of this project.

A special thanks to Sam Riordan, CST, Central Processing Manager, Mercyone Sioux City, who contributed to the basic sterilization chapter and graciously assisted me throughout this project. Your help was much appreciated. I couldn't have done it without you. Our thanks go out to the following facilities and surgical staff for allowing us to conduct on-site photoshoots for the first and second editions of this book: St. Luke's Hospital Operating Room, St. Louis, Missouri; Jane Spiller, RN, BS, Orthopedic Team Leader; Cynthia M. Clisham, RN, BSN, Associate Head Nurse-Clinical Educator; Virginia Babcock, RN, Head Nurse; Marsha Helms, RN, Associate Head Nurse; Brenda Kelly, RN, BA, Vice President; and Jerry Smith, Executive Assistant. Thanks also to Ruth E. Morse, RN, MSN, CEN, CNA, BC, Director of Nursing Resources at Christiana Hospital, Wilmington, Delaware; Peggy Maley, RN, BSN, CNOR, RNFA, and the entire Central Processing Department at Penn Presbyterian Medical Center in Philadelphia, Pennsylvania.

The willingness of all to work with our team was invaluable in developing this educational resource.

Preface

Instrumentation is one of the most important aspects of a surgical procedure. Surgical instruments can be considered an extension of the surgeon's hands. When the surgical team knows the proper name, handling, and use of each instrument, it enhances the quality of the surgical procedure. As a learner, this can be extremely overwhelming due to the multitude of instruments and their similarities. Learning instruments is much more than just recalling the name. The idea for this book came about after years of watching my students struggle with this. They could often recall the names, categories, and specialty area but could rarely explain what it was or how it was used. I saw a pressing need for a product that had not only clear, detailed photos but also addressed common uses, gave insights about instruments, and allowed for interaction. Whether you are a student, surgical technologist, first assistant, registered nurse, or physician's assistant working in surgery, central service technician, or product sales representative, this instrumentation book with interactive exercises will help you, the learner, gain vital core knowledge about instrumentation.

This book consists of 17 chapters, starting with the basic instruments. Chapter 1 is an introduction to surgical instruments, followed by Chapter 2, which introduces the learner to basic decontamination and sterilization of instruments. Chapter 3 is designed to introduce the learner to the fundamental instruments. These are the basic essential instruments that can be seen in any instrument set, regardless of specialty area. The book then moves through commonly used instruments in the 12 different surgical specialty areas. Keep in mind that instruments may vary according to facility, surgeon, and procedure. To conserve space, some instruments may be addressed in one specialty area and may be used by other specialties, but these will not be repeated. Within each chapter, the instruments are grouped according to their category: accessory, clamping and occluding, cutting and dissecting, grasping and holding, probing and dilating, retracting and exposing,

suctioning and aspirating, suturing and stapling, or viewing.

Each page contains one to two instrument monographs with a consistent presentation of each, including:

- **Large, clear, full photo with details.**
- **Instrument name:** states proper instrument name.
- **Other names:** states alternate name or names that the instrument may be called.
- **Category:** distinguishes the instrument according to the function.
- **Description:** briefly describes instrument characteristics.
- **Use(s):** lists common uses and/or areas of use.
- **Instrument insight:** explains key information about the instrument.
- **Caution:** explains the dangers that can happen when handling the instrument.

Chapter 16 is a new chapter that introduces the learner to basic operating room supplies and equipment. This chapter includes operating room attire, operating room furniture, and basic operating room supplies. Each page is similar to the instruments, with a large photo, name, other names, description, use, and insight.

The final chapter in the book focuses on procedural setups for nine common surgeries. This will give the learner examples, suggestions, and hints for setting up. This will include photos of the Mayostand and Backtable, definition of the procedure, reason performed, and tech tips. Enhanced Evolve resources include the invaluable interactive component of this product. Access to the Evolve site requires a pin code (found on the inside front cover). Once registered, the interactive activities will allow you to interact with the instruments, taking your knowledge to the next level. No other product on the market offers this type of interaction. Included are:

- **Digital image library:** includes photos from the book with the ability to zoom in and out, and rotating views of more than 100 instruments.

- **Audio pronunciation:** allows the learner to click on the audio icon and hear the proper name for each instrument.
- **Drag-and-drop exercise:** allows the learner to place instruments onto a Mayo tray from select procedures.
- **Timed audio identification exercises:** challenges the learner to identify the instrument in 5 seconds or less. The instrument is asked for, and the learner will choose the correct instrument from a set of images.
- **Flash card exercises:** the learner clicks the card image, and it "flips" to reveal its name, category, and discipline.
- **Small fragment fixation set:** allows the learner to explore a small fragment set. This exercise lets the user open the set and investigate each tray. The learner can view animation of the tray being opened; roll over any item in the instrument, screw, or plate trays; and click on it to view a close-up image and the name.
- **Large fragment fixation set:** allows the learner to explore a large fragment set. This exercise lets the user open each pan and investigate it; roll over any item in the instrument, screw, or plate pan; and click on it to view a close-up image and the name.
- **Other exercises:** allows the learner to fire a skin stapler; assemble the McIvor mouth gag and the bone cement system; and load a screwdriver, scalpel and clip, Stryker System 6 power, and TPS power (saws, drills, and reamers) and more.

To assist educators with course materials, all images in the book are downloadable for use in handouts and exams, and PowerPoint slides are provided for use in lectures. With the high-quality photographs and interactive exercises, your institution will not have to budget thousands of dollars for instrument sets used for demonstration only.

Table of Contents

1   Introduction to Surgical Instruments, *1*

2   Basic Sterilization, *6*

3   Basic Instruments, *21*

4   General Instruments, *52*

5   Laparoscopic Instruments, *66*

6   Robotic Instruments, *93*

7   Obstetrics and Gynecologic Instruments, *102*

8   Genitourinary Instruments, *121*

9   Ophthalmic Instruments, *140*

10   Otorhinolaryngology Instruments, *162*

11   Oral Instruments, *209*

12   Plastic and Reconstructive Instruments, *221*

13   Orthopedic Instruments, *234*

14   Neurosurgical Instruments, *283*

15   Cardiovascular Thoracic Instruments, *316*

16   Basic Operating Room Supplies and Equipment, *350*

17   Surgical Setups, *380*

Index, *390*

1 Introduction to Surgical Instruments

HISTORY

A surgical instrument is a specially designed device or apparatus used to carry out a specified task during a surgical procedure. Surgical instruments date back to prehistoric times when our early ancestors sharpened stones, flints, and animal teeth to perform surgery. Throughout history, surgical instruments have been created from a variety of materials, such as ivory, wood, bronze, iron, and silver. The discovery of anesthesia and asepsis in the 19th century and the development of stainless steel in the 20th century started the modern evolution of surgical instrumentation. The 20th century brought many changes with the development of electrocautery, ultrasonic, and endoscopic devices. New materials, such as titanium, vitallium, vanadium, carbides, and polymers, are being used in the manufacturing process of instruments. The 21st century has already seen advances in remote telesurgery, robotics, and image-guided systems, which have changed the way surgery is performed and how instruments are developed. The next generation of surgical systems and new materials will revolutionize the way surgical instruments are designed and created.

The vast majority of surgical instruments, however, are still manufactured from stainless steel. Stainless steel is a combination of carbon, chromium, iron, and other metals (alloys). This combination makes the instruments strong and resistant to wear and corrosion. During fabrication, one of the three types of finishes is used on stainless steel instruments. The mirror finish is highly polished and reflects light. This causes a glare, but the instrument is highly resistant to corrosion. Satin or matte is a dull finish that reduces glare and is the preferred finish. Ebony is a black chromium finish that completely eliminates reflection and glare; instruments with this finish are used during laser procedures to prevent light beam deflection.

Gold plating on an instrument designates that tungsten carbide was incorporated into the manufacturing process. Tungsten carbide is an extremely hard metal that is used to laminate scissor blades to increase and maintain sharpness and is inserted into the jaws of the needle holders to increase strength and gripping abilities. Black finger ringed scissors signifies that they are SuperCut scissors. These scissors have one razor-sharp blade for a clean precise cut and one microserrated blade that grips tissues and prevents slippage while cutting.

CARE AND HANDLING OF INSTRUMENTS

Surgical instruments are a large financial expense for medical facilities. Properly preparing, using, and processing instruments promotes patient safety, prolongs the life of the instrument, and decreases repair and replacement costs. All surgical instruments are designed for a specific use. Using them for any other purpose will damage or dull the instrument (e.g., using tissue scissors to cut drapes or dressings or using a hemostat to open a medication vial). Misuse of an instrument can also endanger patients. Simple steps can keep instruments in proper working order. Instruments should be handled individually or in small groups to prevent damage that might occur if they become entangled or are piled on top of one another. They should not be jostled around in the tray when setting up or looking for a certain item. Before, during, and after surgery, instruments should be placed onto the designated area. They should not be tossed or dropped. Heavy items and instruments should never be placed on top of smaller, more delicate instruments. These types of mishandlings cause misalignment and dull blades and can damage instrument tips. To ensure patient safety, instruments should be inspected and tested before each surgical procedure. Instruments should be clean and free of debris, properly aligned, damage free, and in good working order.

During surgery, instruments should be wiped or rinsed with sterile water as they become soiled with blood and tissue. This ensures removal from the box lock, serrations, jaws, and any crevice. Blood and tissue that is allowed to dry and harden can cause an instrument to become stiff and not work properly. This can also make the cleaning process difficult and interfere with the sterilization process. Nondisposable suction tips should be periodically irrigated with a syringe and sterile water or a sylet pushed through to remove trapped blood and debris. Saline should not be used to wipe, rinse, or soak instruments. Exposure to saline will cause corrosion and pitting.

After the surgical procedure, all disposable sharps and blades should be removed and discarded in a sharps container. Instruments should be opened, disassembled, and submerged in water or enzymatic solution. The instruments should be placed in the solution so that they do not become entangled or damaged. Heavy instruments should be placed first, and lighter, more delicate ones should be placed on top. Sharp edges or tips should be placed so that they do not endanger the personnel who will be cleaning them. Delicate instruments, rigid endoscopes, cameras, and fiberoptic light cords should be separated to prevent damage. All cords should be loosely coiled. Power saws and drills should never be immersed in solutions.

Microsurgical Instruments

Microsurgical instruments are delicate. Proper care and handling are essential to prevent damage. Generally, special storage containers are used to protect the instruments. These racks keep the instruments separate and help in identification by providing a place to label them. One should not drop these instruments, allow them to become entangled with each other, or place heavy items on top of them. All microsurgical instruments should be inspected for damage before use. Care should be exercised when handling these instruments. Many have sharp tips that can easily compromise the integrity of gloves and/or skin. When passing instruments, a surgeon should be able to remain focused and not have to move away from the microscope. Ringed forceps (cups, scissors, and nippers) are passed by holding the instrument just above the rings on the shaft and positioning against the palm of the surgeon's hand so he or she can easily place fingers into the loops. The instrument should be held in this position until the surgeon is allowed to adjust his or her fingers. Additional instruments (picks, knives, elevators, and suction tips) should be passed with the tips slightly downward and positioned into the surgeon's hand onto the web between the thumb and index finger (pencil style). Microsurgical instruments should be immediately retrieved from the surgeon to prevent unintentional dropping from the field. After each use, blood and debris should be removed from all instruments. Instrument tips wiped clean with a moistened instrument wipe or a sponge and suction tips should be irrigated often with water.

Powered Instruments

Powered surgical instruments have historically corresponded with surgical needs, predominantly in procedures involving bone. This progression has been important because their complexity has required the use of different types of implants. The use of power instruments has decreased the use of manual instruments, thereby reducing surgery time and improving overall outcomes. Powered surgical instruments are used to perform orthopedic, neurosurgical, ear, nose, and throat (ENT), and oral procedures as well as procedures on other bodily systems. These devices perform cutting, driving, drilling, and reaming and are driven by batteries, compressed gas, and electrical power. Each instrument consists of one or more handpieces and related accessories as well as disposable and limited reuse items, such as burrs, saw blades, drill bits, and reamers. Power instruments should not be submerged in fluid or placed on top of other instruments. Power sources to these instruments should be disconnected or removed before the cleaning process begins.

PARTS OF AN INSTRUMENT

The overall design of an instrument is dependent on what function it will perform. All instruments have a basic standard design and will be modified according to function and type.

Components of this basic design include handles, ratchets, shanks, joints, jaws or blades, and tips (Fig. 1.1).

Finger rings are on the proximal end; this is the handle area of the instrument. Above the rings are shanks that define the length of the instrument, which is determined by the depth of the wound. Above the rings and attached to the shank may be ratchets that allow for the jaws to be closed and locked on tissues. Between the shanks and the jaw is the joint, which is where the two halves of the instrument are joined to permit for opening and closing. These joints are either a box lock or a screw joint. Beyond the joint are the jaws, which are the working portion of the instrument. The inner jaws, tips, and shape determine how and on what tissues the instrument is used. Ringed instruments are placed in the palm of a surgeon's hand with the working end up.

Tissue forceps have a spring action joint at the distal end that holds the instrument open until compressed. The handle grip is where the surgeon's fingers are placed. The shanks determine the length of the forceps. The jaws and the tips are the working end of the forceps; these are determined by the type of tissue that is being grasped (Fig. 1.2). Tissue forceps are held between the thumb and index finger with the distal

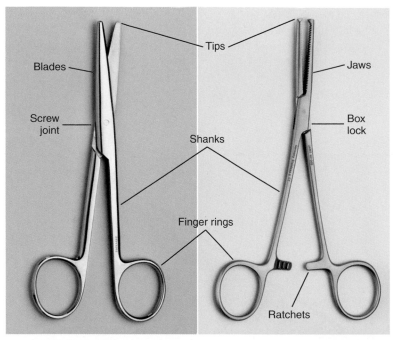

Figure 1.1 Mayo scissors and Kocher forceps illustrating the parts of a ringed instrument.

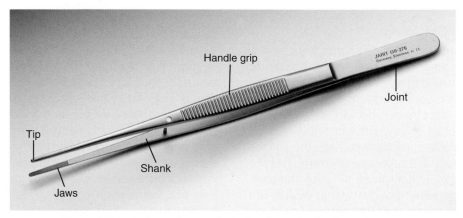

Figure 1.2 Plain tissue forceps illustrating the parts of a tissue forceps.

joint end resting on the top of the hand like a pencil.

Retractors are used to hold a surgical wound open to expose the site that is being worked on. A handheld retractor will be designed with a handle, a shank, a blade or blades, and tips. The handle is where the retractor is grasped; this may be on one end or in the middle. The shank is responsible for the length and runs from the handle to the blade. The blade determines the depth to which the retractor is placed into the wound. The tip is at the end of the blade and differs according to where and how the retractor is utilized. The retractor that is pictured in Fig. 1.3 is a double-ended retractor that has a blade on either end. The handle is positioned in the center of the two blades. The position of the handle determines how the retractor is handed to a surgeon.

INSTRUMENT CATEGORIZATION

Whether an instrument is curved or straight, long or short, wide or narrow, sharp or dull, it is designed for a particular task. An instrument is categorized according to its function. The nine categories include accessory, clamping and occluding, cutting and dissecting, grasping and holding, probing and dilating, retracting and exposing, suctioning and aspirating, suturing and stapling, and viewing.

Accessory

An accessory is an instrument that does not fall into any of the other categories but has a specific function and is an integral part of the surgical procedure. An example of an accessory item is a mallet, electrosurgical pencil, lens warmer, screwdriver, or harmonic scalpel.

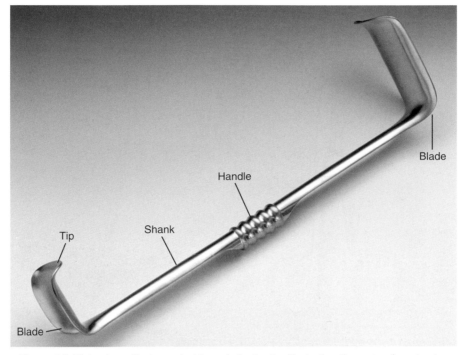

Figure 1.3 Richardson–Eastman double-ended retractor illustrating the parts of a retractor.

Clamping and Occluding

Clamping and occluding instruments are used to compress vessels and other tubular structures to impede or obstruct the flow of blood and other fluids. These clamps are atraumatic ratcheted instruments that are straight, curved, or angled and have a variety of inner jaw patterns. These clamps may totally occlude or partially occlude the tissues between the jaws. A total occlusion clamp has the ability to completely compress or close the jaws at the initial engagement of the ratchet device. The partial occlusion clamp is capable of varying levels of compression. The jaws gradually come together as each increment of the ratcheting is employed. The most common example of a clamping and occluding instrument is the Crile hemostatic forceps or hemostat. Other examples are the Kelly forceps, Glover bulldog, Satinsky clamp, Doyen intestinal clamp, and Mixter forceps.

Cutting and Dissecting

Cutting and dissecting instruments are used to incise, dissect, and excise tissues. Cutting instruments have single or double razor-sharp edges or blades, such as a scalpel, scissors, or osteotome. Dissecting instruments may have a cutting edge and come in a variety of designs. Examples include curettes, cone tip dissectors, and biopsy forceps.

Grasping and Holding

Grasping and holding instruments are designed to grip and manipulate body tissues. They are often used to stabilize tissue that is to be excised,

dissected, repaired, or sutured. Tissue forceps are the nonratcheted style and are often referred to as pickups or thumbs. The tips may be smooth or serrated and may have interlocking teeth. They vary in size and shape according to use. Common examples of tissue forceps are DeBakey, Adson, Cushing, Russian, and Ferris-Smith. The ratcheted type of grasping forceps can be curved or straight; the jaws may be smooth or serrated and have interlocking teeth or sharp prongs. Some examples are the Kocher forceps, Allis forceps, bone-holding forceps, and tenaculum.

Probing and Dilating

Probing instruments are used to explore a structure, opening, or tract. These are often blunt, malleable, and wire-like instruments. Dilating instruments are used to gradually enlarge an orifice or tubular structure, to open a stricture, or to introduce another instrument. They come in sets numbered from the smallest to the largest. A few examples of dilators are Hanks, Van Buren, Bakes, and Mahoney.

Retracting and Exposing

Retracting and exposing instruments are designed to hold back or pull aside wound edges, organs, vessels, nerves, and other tissues to gain access to the operative site. They are generally referred to as retractors and are either manual (handheld) or self-retaining (stay open on their own). Retractors have one or more blades. These blades are used for holding back tissues without causing trauma and should not be confused with a cutting blade.

Retractor blades are usually curved or angled and may be blunt or have sharp or dull prongs. The blades will vary in size according to the depth of the wound and the area of placement. Handheld retractors consist of a blade attached to some type of handle, which is pulled back or held in place by the user. Manual retractors are often used in pairs, one on each side of the wound. Some are double-ended, with a blade on each end and a slight variation in size or shape. Examples of handheld retractors are Parker, Joseph Skin Hook, Senn, Ragnell, and Richardson. Self-retaining retractors are holding devices with two or more blades that spread the wound apart or hold tissues back. A self-retaining retractor has a ratchet, crank, spring, or locking device that holds it open. Some will have permanent attached blades, whereas others will have interchangeable blades that come in a variety of shapes, lengths, and widths, depending on the operative location. Screws, hooks, wing nuts, or clamping devices secure the blades in place. Some retractors attach directly to the operating room table for stability. Examples of self-retaining retractors are the Balfour, Omni-Tract, Bookwalter, Burford, Finochietto, Weitlaner, and Gelpi.

Suctioning and Aspirating

Suctioning and aspirating devices are used to remove blood, fluid, and debris from operative sites. These suction tips may be disposable or nondisposable and come in a variety of shapes and sizes according to use. Some examples of these hollow tips include the Yankauer, Frazier, Poole, and Baron.

Suturing and Stapling

Suturing instruments are used to ligate, repair, and approximate tissues during a surgical procedure. This mainly includes needle holders, which are used to hold curved suture needles, but also includes other items such as a knot pusher, endo stitch, and endo loops. Stapling devices are used to ligate, anastomose, or approximate tissues. Stainless steel, titanium, and INSORB absorbable material are used for stapling. Staples are designed to be noncrushing when inserted into the tissues to promote healing. A nondisposable stapler uses disposable stapling cartridges that have to be assembled during setup. Disposable staplers are assembled, packaged, and sterilized by the manufacturer. They are designed to be reloaded with a new cartridge for multiple uses on the same patient. Some examples of stapling devices are skin staplers, ligating clips, linear cutters, and intraluminal staplers.

Viewing

Viewing instruments allow visualization of a structure or cavity. Various examples include the nasal speculum, ridged and flexible endoscopes, and endoscopic camera.

INSTRUMENT SETS

Instruments are generally placed into sets according to the type of procedures that are performed at the facility. These sets will vary from facility to facility. Typically, instruments from each category will be selected for the assembly of a set. These sets are then assembled, labeled, sterilized, and stored for later use. Instrument sets are often labeled according to the procedure, degree of the procedure (i.e., major or minor), or the specialty area. For instance, a hysterectomy set would be used to perform a hysterectomy, and an orthopedic basic set can be used for a number of orthopedic procedures.

2 Basic Sterilization

INTRODUCTION

Millions of invasive surgical procedures are performed each year. Surgical instruments come in contact with the tissues and organs of the patient during every procedure. It is essential that these instruments do not transmit pathogens that lead to infection in the patient. The processes of decontamination and Sterilization are imperative in preventing infection. Decontamination is a cleaning process which decreases the number of microorganisms on an item. Sterilization is the rendering of an item free of all microorganisms, including spores. All instruments and supplies used in the sterile field must be sterile. This chapter will focus on the basic processes of decontamination and sterilization that the instruments go through from point of use to storage.

POINT OF USE DECONTAMINATION

The process of cleaning instruments starts with the surgical technologist during the surgical procedure. The instruments should be kept as free of bioburden as possible. Organic materials such as blood, fluid, tissue, and debris that are allowed to dry or bake on the surfaces or inside a lumen become difficult to remove and can affect the decontamination and sterilization process. During the surgical procedure, when an instrument is returned to the Mayo stand, it should be quickly wiped clean with a water-moistened sponge. Instruments with lumens should be periodically irrigated with water, and instruments that are hard to wipe clean or used once should be placed in a basin of water to soak. Saline should not be used for cleaning or soaking instruments. The chloride ion is extremely corrosive and can cause pitting and deterioration of the instruments.

Following the procedure, the instruments are placed in a biohazard transport container (Fig. 2.1) that is puncture resistant, leak-proof, and latches closed. The container is filled with a ratio of enzymatic detergent and water. For a proper ratio, follow manufacturer's recommendations. An enzymatic presoak foam or gel may also be used. The surgical technologist will properly open, disassemble, separate, and place all instruments into the container. When placing instruments, heavy ones should go in on the bottom and lighter

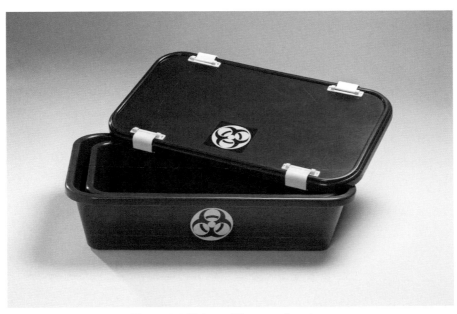

Figure 2.1 Biohazard Transport Container

ones on top. Instruments that are sharp, extremely heavy, or microscopic should be placed in a separate container. The instruments are then transported to the decontamination area on a closed or cover case cart.

STERILE PROCESSING DEPARTMENT

A sterile processing department/area is normally made up of three divided areas: decontamination, prep and pack, and clean holding. Decontamination is where the soiled instruments come after being used in the operating room. The prep and pack or assembly area is where the instruments are inspected, reassembled, and sterilized. The clean holding is where all the sterile instruments and supplies are stored until use.

Manual Cleaning

Once the instruments are received in the decontamination area, manual cleaning begins (Fig. 2.2).

During the decontamination process, there are several methods used to remove contaminants that have accumulated on the instruments to make them safe to handle. Personal protective equipment (PPE) must be worn by the personnel who will come in contact with these instruments. This should include eye protection, fluid-resistant facemask, fluid-resistant gown, gloves, and hair and shoe covers. The manufacturer's information of use (IFU) is referred to for proper cleaning and sterilization methods. The FDA requires manufacturers of medical instruments and devices to provide step-by-step instructions on how to properly clean, disinfect, and sterilize the item. Each patient care item has its own IFU, and the facility is expected to follow these instructions. These are kept in a database for every instrument.

The process of decontamination will start with manual cleaning. A three-sink method is preferred, the first sink is filled with warm water and a neutral pH detergent and/or enzymatic cleaner (Fig. 2.3). The temperature of the water should range between 80 and 100°F to activate the detergent. The ratio of detergent to water is determined by the manufacturer's instructions. The second sink is for rinsing and is filled with tap water, and the third sink is the final rinse and is filled with distilled deionizing water to prevent staining of the instruments. Facility policies determine how the cleaning process is done; this

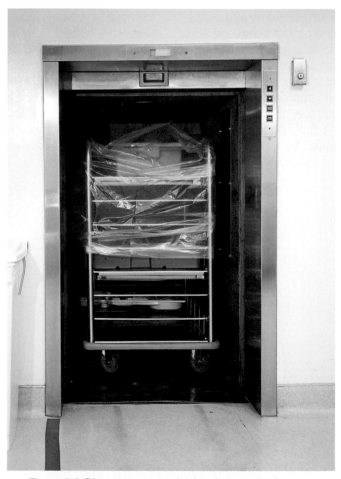

Figure 2.2 Dirty case cart received in decontamination area

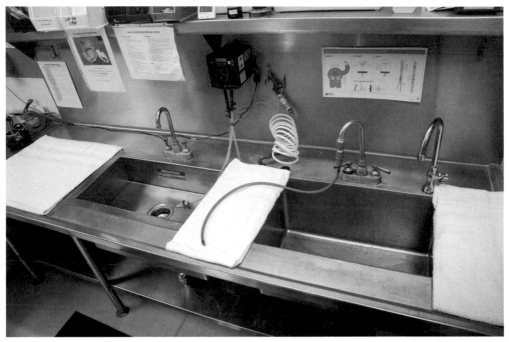

Figure 2.3 Manual cleaning sinks

process may vary. The pretreated contaminated instruments are moved from the transport container into the sink with detergent. Each instrument is manually cleaned with brushes and cloths using friction, concentrating on the serrations and teeth of the jaws, the lockbox and the ratchets, and any other hard-to-clean areas. When using a brush to clean instruments, the brush and instrument should be completely submerged under the water to prevent aerosolization of bioburden. Lumens are cleaned with a lumen/channel brush. The brush size is determined by the diameter of the lumen. If the brush is too small, the bristles will not adequately reach all surfaces. If it is too large, the bristles will bend and not allow adequate friction. Proper brush size can be found in the manufacturer's IFU. Once cleaning is complete, the lumen must be flushed with water to remove any remaining detergent and debris. This can be done using a syringe, or with a high-pressure flushing device. During the manual cleaning process, the instruments will be inspected and tested for proper working order, and that the bioburden is eliminated. Following the rinsing process, the instruments will go into a washer rack or ultrasonic cleaner.

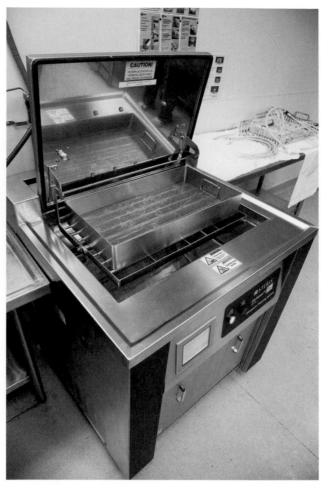

Figure 2.4 Ultrasonic cleaner

Ultrasonic Cleaner

Once manual cleaning is finished, some instruments will be run through an ultrasonic cleaner. An ultrasonic cleaner uses cavitation, which creates tiny bubbles that implode, creating a vacuum-like scrubbing action that removes the bioburden. This process reaches all the nooks, crannies, crevices, irregular surfaces, and passageways that are hard to reach without damaging the instrument. Before placing instruments into the ultrasonic cleaner, they should be cleaned, and lumens should be brushed and flushed. Common instruments that need ultrasonic cleaning are laparoscopic instruments that come apart, da Vinci robotic instruments, anything with lumens, instruments from total joints, and delicate microscopic instruments such as eyes. When placing the instruments in the ultrasonic tray, ratchets are opened, multiple parts are disassembled, and the tray should not be densely packed or stacked. The IFU should always be checked for compatibility. Some instruments and devices have adhesive on the optical system or rubber components that are not recommended for ultrasonic cleaning. Metals such as copper, brass, aluminum, and chrome plating may not be compatible and should not be placed with stainless steel instruments. Some new ultrasonic cleaners have channel adapters for lumened instruments, which allow them to be connected and flushed while running through a cycle. The water and ultrasonic cleaner should be changed every eight hours unless it becomes cloudy.

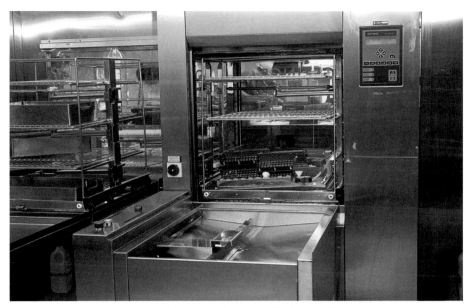

Figure 2.5 Automated washer (Washer Sterilizer)

Automated Washer (Washer Sterilizer)

Following manual decontamination, the majority of instruments are processed through the automated washer. Always refer to the IFU before sending instruments through the washer. Most automated washers have multiple racks. The instruments are placed in the open position, disassembled into a wire pan, and then placed on one of the racks. There are special trays that can be used for laparoscopic instruments. These hold the instruments up at an angle so water and detergent can be flushed through them during the cycles. The robotic instruments from the da Vinci system have a special tray that continuously flushes the instruments during the cycle. When the rack is fully loaded, it is pushed into the washer on the decontamination side and the cycle is started. There are five phases in the cycle: prewash, wash, rinse, sterilization, lubrication, and drying. The automated washer is essentially a modified dishwasher with heavy-duty spraying power and a sterilization cycle. The automated washer is a pass-through that separates the decontamination room from the prep and pack room (Fig. 2.6).

Once the cycle is finished, the door will open on the clean side and the instruments can be retrieved. These instruments are now considered safe to handle.

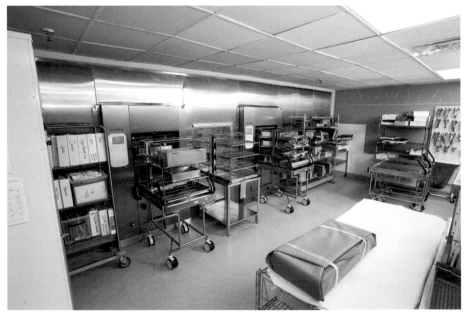

Figure 2.6 Automated washer pass through to the prep and pack room

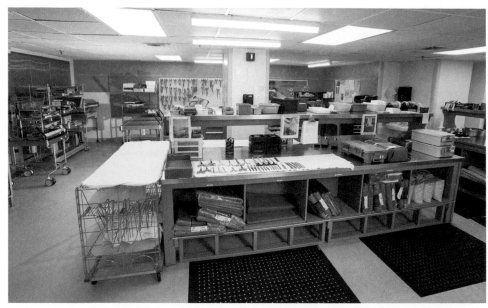

Figure 2.7 Prep and Pack Area

Perp and Pack

The instruments are retrieved from the washer rack and taken to a workstation. The instrument set is determined, and an instrument list will be used to assemble the set. This process can be done in many ways. Some facilities have instrument identification tape or tags on the instruments, which identify the set and the list. Other facilities have instrument-tracking systems consisting of barcodes and scanners. The barcode on the pan is scanned, and an instrument list is populated on a computer at the workstation. Regardless of which system is used, there is a list that identifies the instruments that belong in each set. As the set is being reassembled, the instruments are inspected for cleanliness and working quality. Examples of quality testing are making sure the laparoscopic instrument sheaths do not have defects in the insulation and checking the sharpness of scissors by cutting tissue paper. Once these checks are made, the instruments are sorted and placed into piles according to types (like instruments with like instruments [Fig. 2.8]). Ringed instruments are placed on a stringer or racks to keep them open. The instruments sets can be assembled into a pan or tray by following the list. A chemical indicator strip must be placed inside with the instruments. Once the indicators have been placed, the tray will be inserted into the rigid instrument container, external indicators are attached, and a locking device

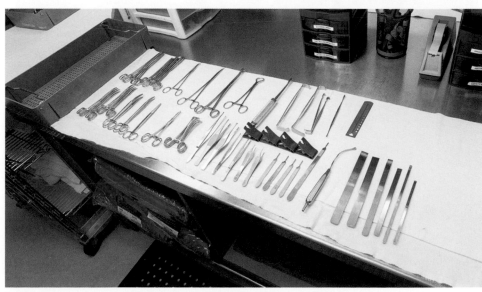

Figure 2.8 Sorted Instruments

is secured on the latch. If an instrument pan is used, it will be wrapped in CSR and indicator tape will be used to secure the wrap. CSR is a disposable nonwoven wrapping material used for sterilizing instruments and items. Individual instruments can be placed in a sterilization peel pouch, and large items can be wrapped in CSR (Figs. 2.9–2.10). All packaged items and instruments must be labeled with the name of the tray or item, sterilization date, load number, and the initials of the preparer. A load sticker is placed on each item being sterilized. These stickers normally have the date of sterilization, the sterilizer it was run in, and the load number. If there is a load or sterilizer failure, these items can be recalled by referencing the stickers.

Once the item has the sticker, it can be placed on the sterilization rack (Fig. 2.11). In a steam sterilizer, instruments sets will be arranged on the rack based on their weight/density and if they are in a sterilization hard container. The heavier, denser pans will be placed at the bottom. The lighter pans and peel packs will be placed at the top. Sterilization hard containers must be placed below items wrapped in CSR. A CSR-wrapped item has a greater chance of having wet packs when it is placed under a hard container due to condensation. A wet pack is the presence of moisture left inside or outside of an instrument set or item following sterilization. If there are two or more wet packs, it is considered a wet load, and the load should not be released. Wet packs and loads have to be completely reprocessed. A load card is used to document each load, which

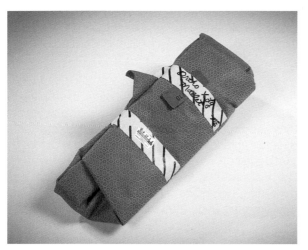

Figure 2.9 CSR Wrapped item

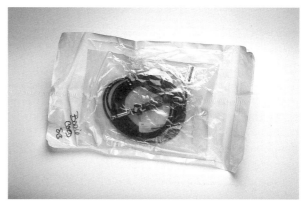

Figure 2.10 Peel Packed Item

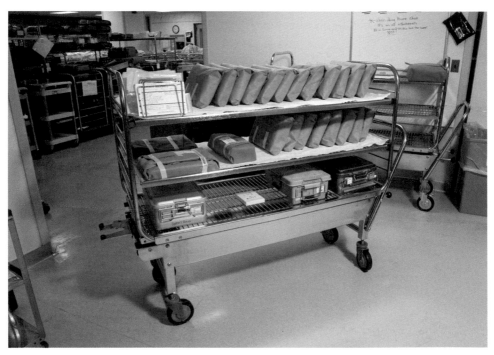

Figure 2.11 Loaded Steam Sterilizer Rack

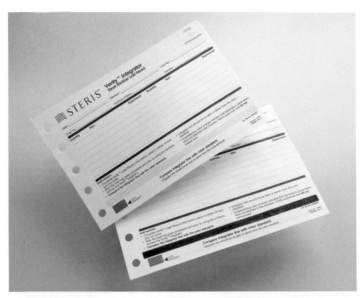

Figure 2.12 Load Card

includes information such as the sterilization date, sterilizer ID, load number, and the preparer's initials. Each card contains a chemical indicator and is processed with the load (Fig. 2.12).

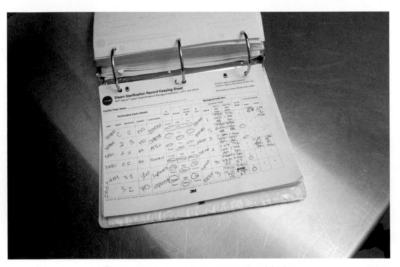

Figure 2.13 Load Documentation binder

STERILIZATION OF THE INSTRUMENTS

The next step in the process is sterilization. Sterilization renders an item free of all microorganisms including spores. Many methods can be used to sterilize instruments and items: steam, hydrogen peroxide gas plasma (Sterrad or V-PRO), peracetic acid (Steris), ETO, ozone, radiation. Methods of sterilization are constantly changing and improving. Most facilities do not have the capabilities or resources to use all these methods. Many facilities use steam sterilization and hydrogen peroxide. Regardless of the method of sterilization, certain parameters must be met for each type. These parameters can be found in the manufacturer's IFU. The IFU will state what method or methods of sterilization the instrument or item can be exposed to, the duration of exposure, and dry times.

Quality Assurance of the Sterilization Process

Several methods are used to ensure that the parameters of the sterilization processes are met. These parameters must be tested regularly and documented. Documentation of the sterilization process establishes accountability, ensures monitoring is occurring, and assures that the cycle parameters are being met. Depending on the facility policy and procedure, the documentation process may vary (Fig. 2.13). Most sterilizers have microprocessors that provide printouts of the parameters of each phase of the sterilization cycle. These are the easiest for personnel to read and provides early indication of load failure. Various devices are used to monitor sterilization, such as chemical indicators, biological indicators, and Bowie-Dick tests.

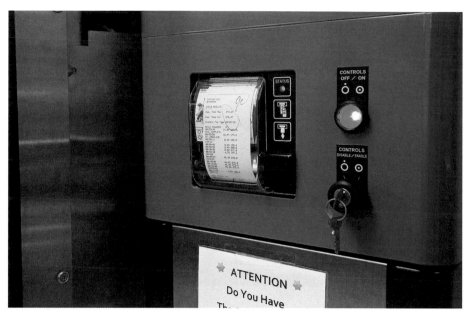

Figure 2.14 Sterilizer Printout

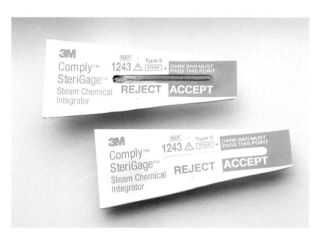

Figure 2.15 Indicator Strip

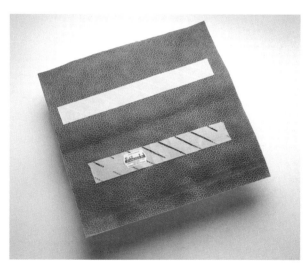

Figure 2.16 indicator tape

Chemical Indicators

A chemical indicator is used to ensure that sterilant has reached the items being sterilized. Depending on the sterilizer used, during the sterilization process the indicator will change color when one or more parameters are met. It is important to understand that a chemical indicator does not confirm sterility; it only indicates that sterilization parameters have been met. Chemical indicators are used both internally and externally. There are several types of chemical indicators including, but not limited to, strips, tapes, tags, labels, and locks. These indicators are used with every item and all methods of sterilization. The type of chemical indicator used will be determined by the type of sterilizer used. These chemical indicators are extremely important to the surgical technologist in the operating room, as they are a patient safety measure. These chemical indicators are checked and verified. If the indicator is missing or has not changed color, the item or set is considered unsterile and must not be used. This should be reported to the sterile processing department, so they can test the sterilizer and pull all items from that load.

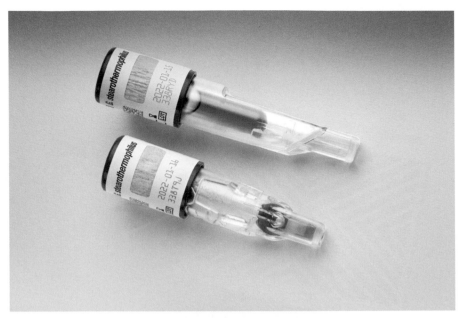

Figure 2.17 Biological indicators

Biological Indicators

A biological indicator is the only test that guarantees an item is sterile. The biological indicator is a small vial that contains highly resistant bacteria. When the parameters of the sterilization process are met, the bacteria are killed. These bacteria differ depending on the type of sterilization process being used. Steam sterilization and ozone use *Geobacillus stearothermophilus* biological indicators, while hydrogen peroxide gas plasma and ethylene oxide use *Bacillus subtilis*. Once an indicator has been run through the sterilization process, it is placed in an incubator for a set amount of time according to the manufacturer (Fig. 2.18). The time and other instructions can be found in the IFU. A negative test indicates the load is sterile, and a positive indicates the sterilization process has failed. Biological indicators should be run in the sterilizer daily and in every load that contains implants.

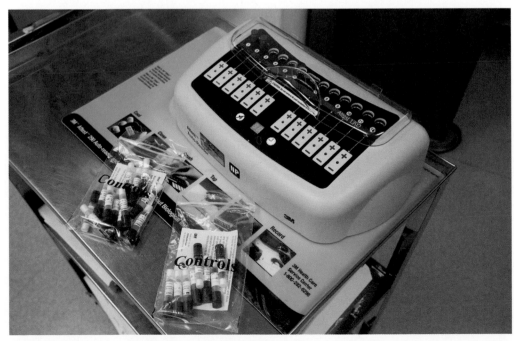

Figure 2.18 Biological Indicator Incubator

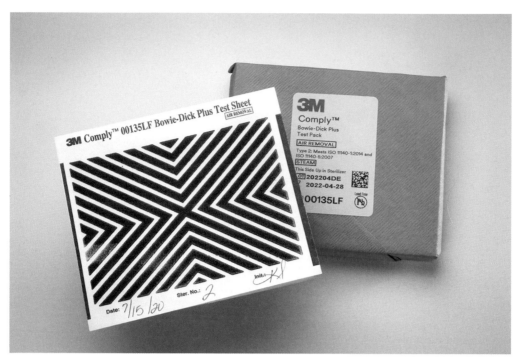

Figure 2.19 Bowie Dick Test

Bowie-Dick Test

This is an air test. A Bowie-Dick test is used in pre-vacuum steam sterilizers, not gravity-displacement sterilizers. The purpose of this test is to ensure that the air is removed from the chamber and there are no air leaks. This test needs to be run daily before the first load.

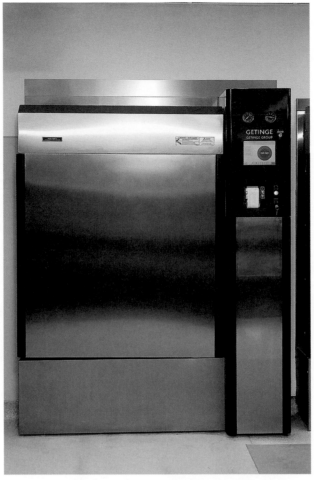

Figure 2.20 Larger steam sterilizer

Steam Sterilization (High Heat)

Steam sterilization is the most commonly used reliable, effective, and inexpensive method of sterilization for items that can tolerate high heat and moisture. Examples of items that can be steam sterilized are surgical instruments, implants, and linens. Any instrument or item being sterilized should be checked for compatibility with the IFU. Steam sterilization is accomplished in an autoclave by exposing the items to saturated steam under pressure, at a required temperature, and for a set length of time. Therefore, the three parameters of steam sterilization are pressure, temperature, and time. The two basic types of steam sterilizers (autoclaves) are the gravity displacement autoclave and the prevacuum sterilizer.

Gravity Displacement

Gravity displacement sterilization is accomplished by forcing steam into the chamber and pushing the air out through a drain in the bottom of the chamber. The absence of air allows the steam to penetrate the items in the load. Recommended cycle parameters for a wrapped load are 30 minutes at 250°F (121°C) with 25 psi and a drying time of 30 minutes.

Prevacuum

Prevacuum sterilization is a high-power vacuum that sucks the air out of the chamber while pulling steam in. This pull allows the steam to penetrate porous items that couldn't otherwise be reached. The absence of air within the chamber allows steam to penetrate the load almost instantly, resulting in a shorter cycle and reliable sterilization. The recommended cycle parameters for wrapped loads are 4 minutes at 270°F (132°C) with a 27 psi and a drying time of 30 minutes.

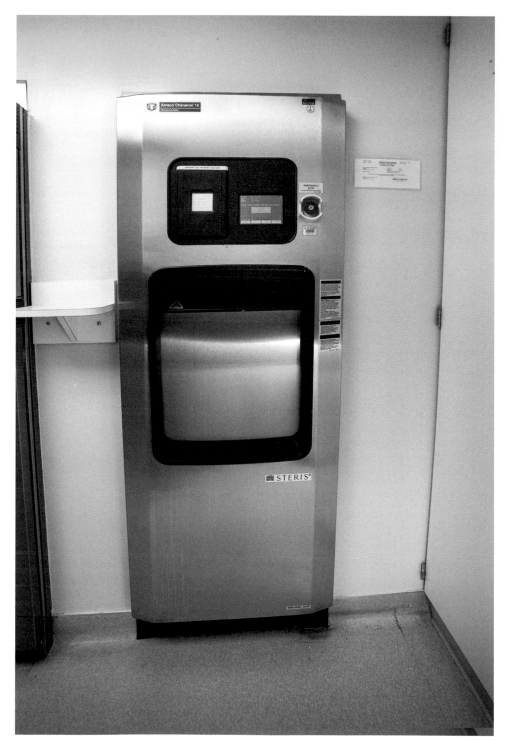

Figure 2.21 Immediate use steam sterilizer (Flash Sterilizer)

Immediate Use Steam Sterilizer (Flash Sterilizer)

This is a steam autoclave located near the operating room. It is used to quickly sterilize an unwrapped item that is needed for the procedure when time does not allow for regular sterilization methods. For example, when an instrument is dropped on the floor and there isn't another that has been packaged and sterilized, it can be placed in the immediate use sterilizer. The recommended parameters are 4 minutes at 270°F (132°C) then transferred to the operating room for use. Flash sterilization should only be used when there is no other option because of the potential for infection. Immediate use sterilization is not recommended for implantable devices. However, in certain circumstances such as an emergency, it may be unavoidable, and a biological indicator must be run with the load and confirmed negative.

Low-Heat Sterilizers

Low-temperature sterilizers are used to sterilize instruments and items that cannot tolerate the heat, moisture, and pressure of the steam sterilizer. Hydrogen peroxide plasma gas, ethylene oxide gas, and ozone are examples of low-temperature sterilizers commonly used. There are other types of low-temperature sterilizers on the market.

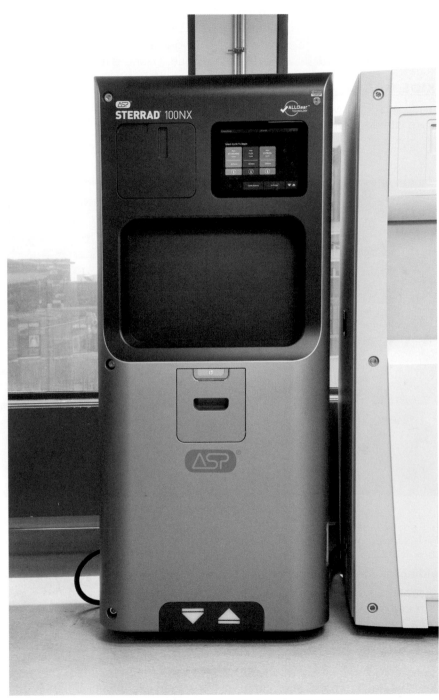

Figure 2.22 Hydrogen Peroxide Gas Plasma (STERRAD®)

Hydrogen Peroxide Gas Plasma (STERRAD)

Hydrogen Peroxide Gas Plasma (HPGP) has become one of the most widely used low-temperature sterilizers because of its shorter cycles and no aeration time. This is a self-contained unit that needs no plumbing or exhaust. Hydrogen peroxide vapors are pulled into the chamber, then radiofrequency energy causes it to ionize and create a plasma reaction that eliminates microorganisms. Sterilizer cycles take 28 to 55 minutes, depending on the model. The items must be completely dry before packaging or wrapping, and the chamber must never be overloaded; otherwise, the cycle will be terminated. Linens and paper should not be used; they absorb the gas and cause the cycle to terminate. Tyvek/Mylar pouches, nonwoven polypropylene wrap, and an approved container system are used for packaging. Certain lengths and diameters of lumens cannot be reprocessed with HPGP; always refer to the IFU.

ETHYLENE OXIDE GAS

Once ethylene oxide gas (EtO) was the standard for low-temperature sterilization, but it is being phased out by other low-temperature sterilizers with faster cycles. EtO is an alkylating agent that disrupts the DNA of microorganisms and prevents reproduction. EtO has a long cycle, which can be 12 hours or more with aeration. EtO is flammable, explosive, and poses health and environmental risks.

OZONE

Oxygen and electrical energy are utilized to create ozone. Ozone is a toxic gas that causes the oxidization of microorganisms. The ozone will convert back oxygen, leaving no chemical residue or exhaust. Although there is no cost for sterilant, the cycle time of 4.5 hours is a downside.

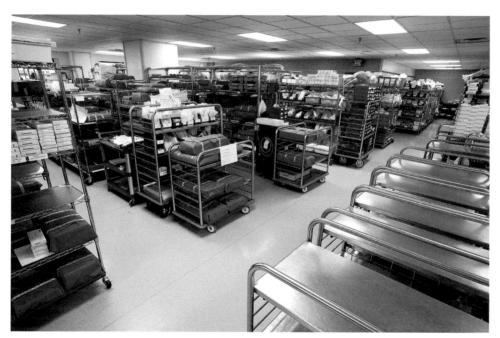

Figure 2.23 Sterile Storage and Holding Area

Storage and Holding of Sterile Instruments

Following the sterilization process, surgical instruments and items must be handled and stored in an aseptic manner. Closed cabinets are preferred for the storage of sterile items, but open shelving may also be used. Sterile items should be stored separately from nonsterile items, and they should be kept away from windows, vents, and drafts. Sterile items should also be stored 8 to 10 inches from the floor, 5 inches from the ceiling or 18 inches from the sprinkler head, and 2 inches away from the walls. This allows for cleaning, air circulation, and complies with fire codes. Sterile items should never be stored where they can come in contact with water. Heavy items should not be stacked, as this poses the risk of tearing the wrapper. Shelf life of the instruments are event related not time related. The length of time a device remains sterile depends on the events that affect its packaging. This is where instruments are kept until they are picked and placed on a case cart for their next use.

3

Basic Instruments

ACCESSORY INSTRUMENTS

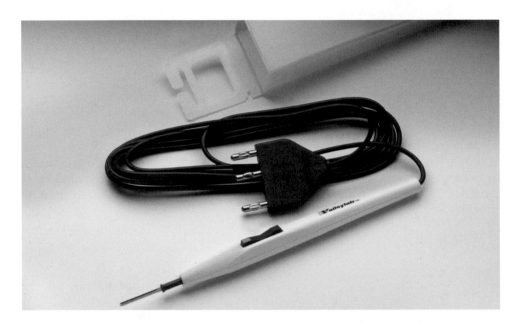

Instrument: ELECTROSURGICAL PENCIL
Other Names: Bovie, cautery, monopolar cautery, diathermy, electrocautery
Category: Accessory
Description: This is a disposable instrument that usually comes packaged with a blade tip and a holster. The current is activated by a switch or button on the pencil or with a foot pedal. There are several different types of interchangeable electrode tips that fit into the handpiece. Some of the common types of tips are blade, ball, needle, and extended-blade tips.
Use(s): Monopolar cautery uses electrical current to coagulate and cut blood vessels and tissues to provide homeostasis; it is also used for dissection.

Instrument Insight: All monopolar electrodes require a dispersive pad because the electricity enters the patient's body. Monopolar current travels from the generator to the active electrode and through the patient's body; the current is then captured by the dispersive pad, which channels it back to the generator, completing the closed circuit. A scratch pad is used to remove charred blood and tissue from the electrode tip. There are tips available with a Teflon coating, which can be easily wiped clean, and eliminates the need for a scratch pad.

⚠ **CAUTION:** The tip of the pencil becomes hot after extended use. When not in use, the pencil should be placed in the holster to prevent burning the drapes or the patient.

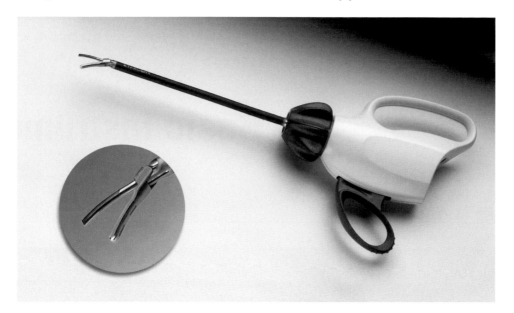

Instrument: HARMONIC SCALPEL
Other Names: Ultrasonic scalpel
Category: Accessory
Description: This device has a manufacturer-packaged disposable handpiece. A nondisposable cord and wrench are also needed. These two components need to be packaged and sterilized by the facility.

Use(s): The harmonic scalpel is a grasping instrument that delivers ultrasonic energy between the jaws to coagulate and divide tissue by low-temperature cavitation.
Instrument Insight: Blood and tissue can build up on the jaws and may need to be removed periodically with a moistened sponge.

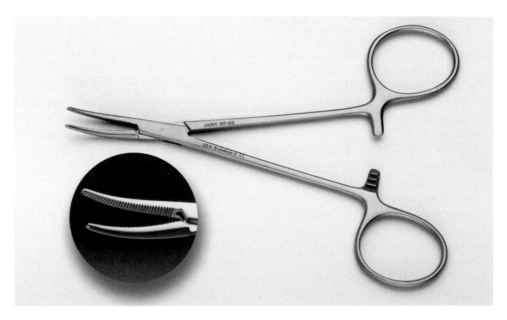

Instrument: HALSTEAD FORCEPS
Other Names: Mosquito forceps, Hartmann forceps
Category: Clamping and Occluding
Description: These are small curved or straight clamps with fine tips and horizontal serrations that run the length of the jaws.
Use(s): Halstead forceps are used for occluding bleeders in small or superficial wounds before

cauterization or ligation. These are used often for delicate or small confined procedures. Some examples are plastic, pediatric, thyroid, and hand procedures. Also used with suture boots to tag delicate Prolene sutures in vascular procedures.
Instrument Insight: These forceps are much smaller than a Crile or Kelly forceps.

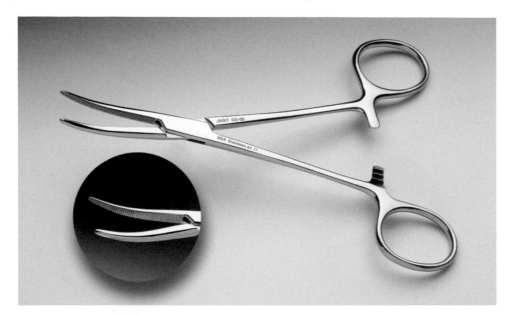

Instrument: CRILE FORCEPS
Other Names: Hemostat, snap, clamp, Kelly forceps, stat
Category: Clamping and Occluding
Description: These are curved or straight clamps with horizontal serrations that run the complete length of the jaws.

Use(s): Crile forceps are used for occluding bleeders before cauterization or ligation. These may also be used for blunt dissection when separating planes and tissues.
Instrument Insight: The curved Crile is the most widely used clamp in all specialty areas.

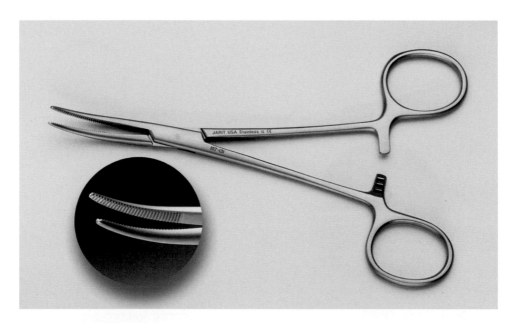

Instrument: KELLY FORCEPS
Other Names: Hemostat, Crile forceps, clamp
Category: Clamping and Occluding
Description: These are curved or straight clamps with horizontal serrations that run about half the length of the jaws.

Use(s): These are used for occluding bleeders before cauterization or ligation.

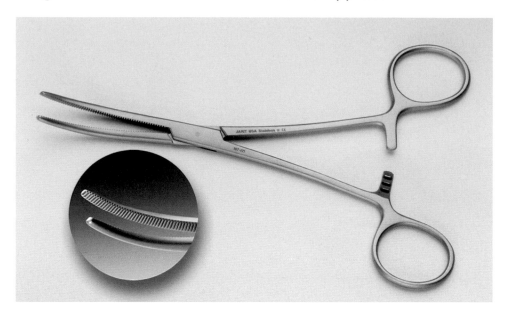

Instrument: ROCHESTER-PÉAN FORCEPS
Other Names: Péan, Mayo, Kelly-Péan forceps
Category: Clamping and Occluding
Description: These are curved or straight clamps that have heavier broader jaws with horizontal serrations that run the length of the jaws.

Use(s): These are used for occluding larger blood vessels and tissue before ligation, usually in a deeper wound or on heavier tissue.

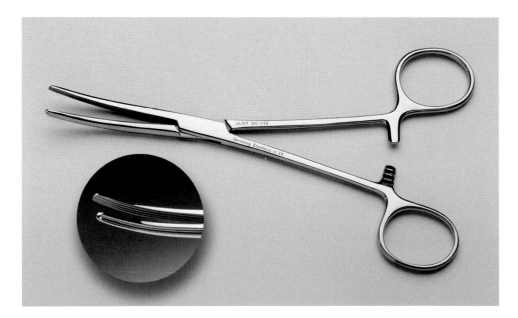

Instrument: CARMALT FORCEPS
Other Names: Carmalt, big curved forceps
Category: Clamping and Occluding
Description: These are curved or straight clamps with a crosshatch pattern at the tips that continues with vertical serrations that run the length of the jaws.

Use(s): Carmalt forceps are used for occluding larger blood vessels and tissue before ligation, usually in a deeper wound or on heavier tissue. These are often the forceps that the Kittner is loaded onto.

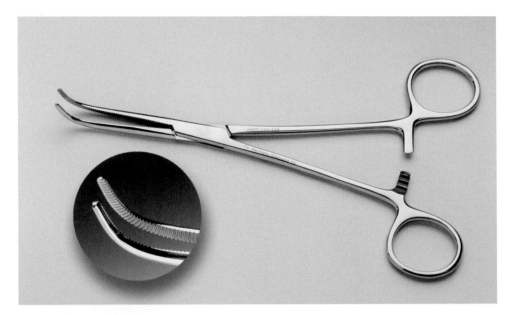

Instrument: MIXTER FORCEPS
Other Names: Right-angle forceps, Gemini forceps, Lahey forceps, obtuse clamp, ureter clamp
Category: Clamping and Occluding
Description: These are 45-degree angle clamps with horizontal serrations that run the length of the jaws.

Use(s): Mixter forceps are used to clamp, dissect, and occlude tissue. These are often used to place a tie or vessel loop under and around a tubular structure such as a vessel or a duct, enabling the surgeon to grasp the ligature or loop and pull it up and around the structure to either ligate or retract.

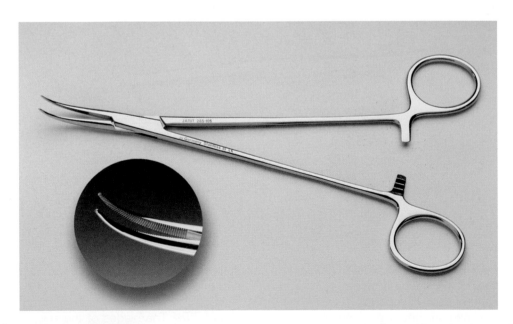

Instrument: ADSON FORCEPS
Other Names: Tonsil Schnidt forceps, fancy clamp, tonsil forceps, T and A
Category: Clamping and Occluding
Description: These are fine curved or straight clamps with horizontal serrations running

halfway down the jaws. The shanks are longer than those of a Crile or a Kelly forceps.
Use(s): Adson forceps clamp small vessels in a deep wound or hold tonsil sponges. Also these may be used to create a "tie on a passer."

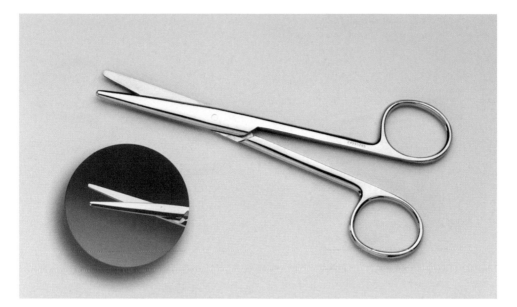

Instrument: STRAIGHT MAYO SCISSORS
Other Names: Suture scissors
Category: Cutting and Dissecting
Description: These are heavy scissors with straight blades.
Use(s): These are used for cutting sutures.
Instrument Insight: Use the very tips of the scissors when cutting sutures. Slightly rotate the scissors to visualize the knot or the appropriate length of the suture tail that will remain.

⚠ CAUTION: The blades of the scissors should be inspected for nicks, dents, or burrs, which will not allow for smooth cutting. It is important to always check the screw to ensure it is fully tightened to prevent it from dropping into the wound.

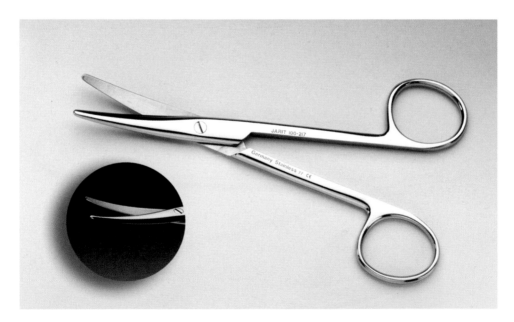

Instrument: CURVED MAYO SCISSORS
Other Names: Heavy tissue scissors
Category: Cutting and Dissecting
Description: These are heavy scissors with curved blades and blunt or sharp tips.
Use(s): These are used to dissect or undermine heavy fibrous tissues.
Instrument Insight: Tissue scissors are intended to cut tissue only and should never be used to cut other items. Inappropriate use of the scissors will cause the blades to become dull and not function properly.

⚠ CAUTION: The blades of the scissors should be inspected for nicks, dents, or burrs, which can cause damage to the tissues. It is important to always check the screw to ensure it is fully tightened to prevent it from dropping into the wound.

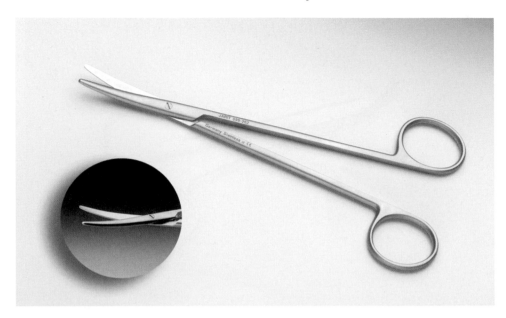

Instrument: CURVED METZENBAUM SCISSORS
Other Names: Metz scissors, tissue scissors
Category: Cutting and Dissecting
Description: These are longer thinner scissors with curved or straight blades that can have blunt or sharp tips.
Use(s): These are used to dissect and undermine delicate tissues.
Instrument Insight: Tissue scissors are intended to cut tissue only and should never be used to cut sutures or other items. Inappropriate use of the scissors will cause the blades to become dull and not function properly.

⚠ **CAUTION:** The blades of the scissors should be inspected for nicks, dents, or burrs, which can cause damage to the tissues. It is important to always check the screw to ensure it is fully tightened to prevent it from dropping into the wound.

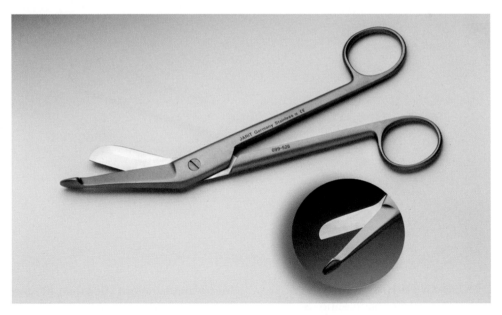

Instrument: LISTER BANDAGE SCISSORS
Other Names: Bandage scissors
Category: Cutting and Dissecting
Description: These are angled blunt scissors in which the lower blade has a smooth flattened tip.
Use(s): These are used to cut dressings, drapes, and other items and also used in a cesarean section to open the uterus without harm to the baby.

Instrument Insight: The flattened tip is designed to give these scissors the ability to get under dressings or drapes and cut the material without harming the patient.

⚠ **CAUTION:** It is important to always check the screw to ensure it is fully tightened to prevent it from dropping into the wound.

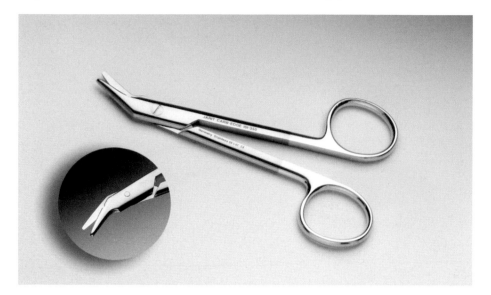

Instrument: WIRE SCISSORS
Other Names: Wire cutters
Category: Cutting and Dissecting
Description: These are angled scissors with fine serrations on the blades and a circular notch in the inner jaws.
Use(s): These are used to cut small-gauge wire and sutures.
Instrument Insight: The serrations are intended to facilitate grasping the item being cut. When the wire is placed inside the notch, it gives the scissors the ability to exert additional pressure to cut heavier gauged wire.

⚠ **CAUTION:** It is important to always check the screw to ensure it is fully tightened to prevent it from dropping into the wound.

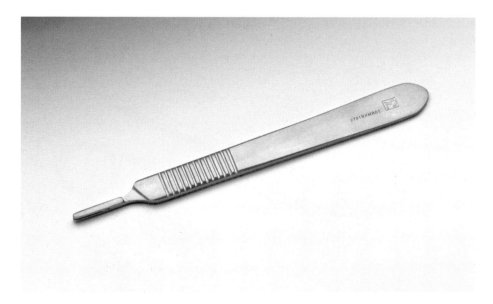

Instrument: NO. 3 KNIFE HANDLE
Other Names: No. 3 scalpel handle, no. 3 handle
Category: Cutting and Dissecting
Description: A no. 3 handle holds blades 10, 11, 12, and 15.
Use(s): No. 3 knife handles are used to hold various blades to create a scalpel. Scalpels are used to make skin incisions or whenever a fine precision cut is necessary.

Instrument Insight: Because the skin is not sterile, once the skin incision is made, the scalpel should be removed from the Mayo stand, isolated, and reused only to incise the skin.

⚠ **CAUTION:** Never retrieve the scalpel from the surgeon's hand after use; allow the surgeon to place it in the "neutral zone." Never use fingers to load or unload a knife blade from the handle. Always use a needle holder.

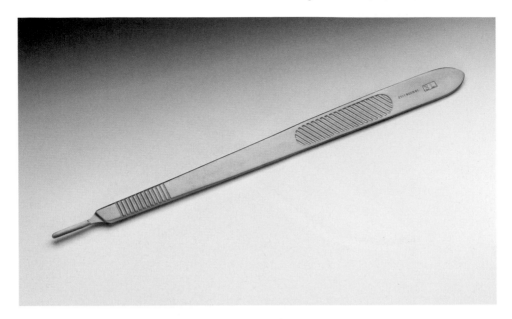

Instrument: NO. 3 LONG KNIFE HANDLE
Other Names: Long knife, long handle, long scalpel
Category: Cutting and Dissecting
Description: A no. 3 long knife handle holds blades no. 10, 11, 12, and 15.
Use(s): It is used for precision cutting deep within a wound.

⚠ **CAUTION:** Never retrieve the scalpel from the surgeon's hand after it is used; allow the surgeon to place it in the "neutral zone." Never use fingers to load or unload a knife blade from the handle. Always use a needle holder.

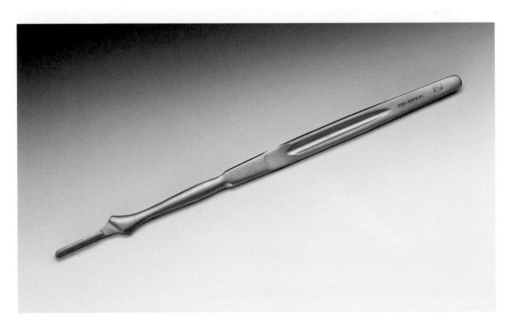

Instrument: NO. 7 KNIFE HANDLE
Other Names: No. 7 scalpel handle, no. 7 handle
Category: Cutting and Dissecting
Description: A no. 7 knife handle holds blades no. 10, 11, 12, and 15.
Use(s): It is used when precision cutting is needed in a confined space or a deep wound.

⚠ **CAUTION:** Never retrieve the scalpel from the surgeon after it is used; allow the surgeon to place it in the neutral zone. Never use fingers to load or unload a knife blade from the handle. Always use a needle holder.

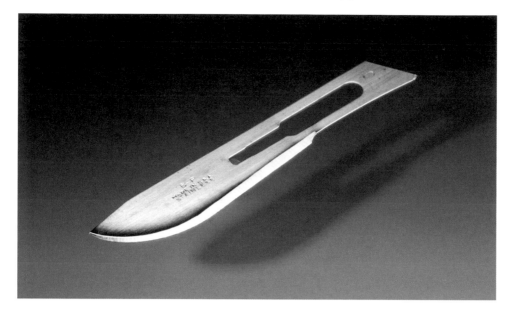

Instrument: NO. 10 BLADE
Category: Cutting and Dissecting
Description: It is an extensive body blade with a curved cutting edge to the tip.
Use(s): It is used for making skin incisions.
Instrument Insight: To load a scalpel blade onto a scalpel handle, grasp the blade with a needle holder just above the opening on the noncutting side. Line up the grooves on the handle with the opening on the blade. Make sure that the angle of the blade matches the angle of the handle. Advance the blade onto the handle until it clicks in place. A scalpel blade is a single-patient use item that comes prepackaged and sterilized from the manufacturer.

⚠ **CAUTION:** Never use fingers to load or unload a knife blade from the handle. Always use a needle holder.

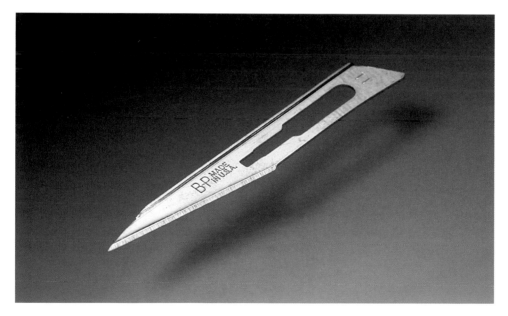

Instrument: NO. 11 BLADE
Category: Cutting and Dissecting
Description: It has an angled cutting edge that ascends to a sharp point.
Use(s): It is used for puncturing the skin or to initiate the opening of an artery.
Instrument Insight: The no. 11 blade is commonly loaded onto the no. 7 handle. A scalpel blade is a single-patient use item that comes prepackaged and sterilized from the manufacturer.

⚠ **CAUTION:** Never use fingers to load or unload a knife blade from the handle. Always use a needle holder.

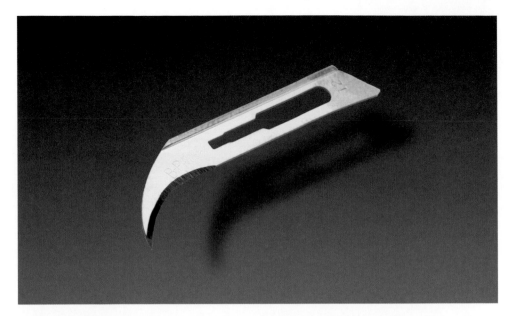

Instrument: NO. 12 BLADE
Other name: Sickle knife, tonsil blade
Category: Cutting and Dissecting
Description: A small crescent-shaped blade sharpened along the inside edge of the curve.
Use(s): A no. 12 blade is sometimes used during tonsillectomies, parotid surgeries, septoplasties, and cleft palate procedures. It can also be utilized for removal of calculi in the ureter and the kidney (ureterolithotomies and pyelolithotomies).

Instrument Insight: The no. 12 blade is commonly loaded onto the no. 7 handle but may also be used on a no. 3 regular or long handle. A scalpel blade is a single-patient use item that comes prepackaged and sterilized from the manufacturer.

⚠ **CAUTION:** Never use fingers to load or unload a knife blade from the handle. Always use a needle holder.

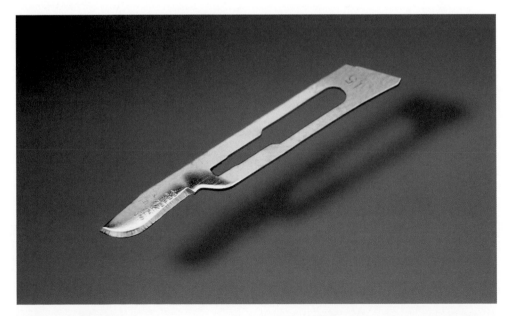

Instrument: NO. 15 BLADE
Category: Cutting and Dissecting
Description: It is a narrow blade that has a small, rounded cutting edge.
Use(s): It is used for creating small precise incisions.
Instrument Insight: It is commonly used for pediatric or plastic or reconstructive surgery. A scalpel blade is a single-patient use item that comes prepackaged and sterilized from the manufacturer.

⚠ **CAUTION:** Never use fingers to load or unload a knife blade from the handle. Always use a needle holder.

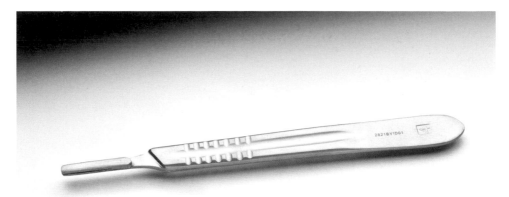

Instrument: NO. 4 KNIFE HANDLE
Other Names: No. 4 scalpel handle, no. 4 handle
Category: Cutting and Dissecting
Description: It has a larger tip to accommodate the larger blades.
Use(s): It is used with the no. 20 blade to create a larger and/or deeper incision in heavy tissue areas.

Instrument Insight: The no. 4 handle will hold blades no. 20, 21, 22, 23, 24, and 25.

⚠ CAUTION: Never use fingers to load or unload a knife blade from the handle. Always use a needle holder.

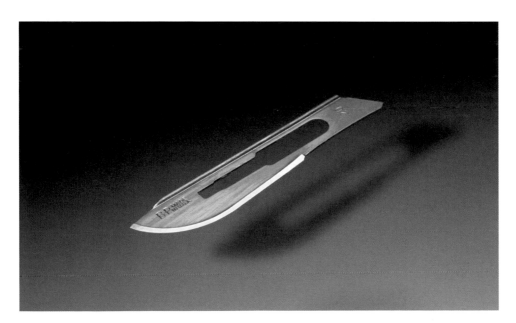

Instrument: NO. 20 BLADE
Category: Cutting and Dissecting
Description: It is a broader body blade with a curved cutting edge to the tip.
Use(s): It is used with the no. 4 handle to create a larger and/or deeper incision and on heavy tissues and bone.

Instrument Insight: Blades should never be loaded with your fingers.

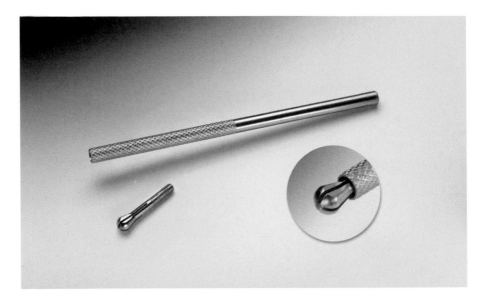

Instrument: BEAVER HANDLE
Other Names: Round handle
Category: Cutting and Dissecting
Description: It is a round handle with a ball tip that screws into the handle to tighten the blade in place.
Use(s): It is used when precision cutting is needed in a confined space or when incising a small structure. The beaver knife is commonly used in Otorhinolaryngology, ophthalmic, neurology, podiatry, and small orthopedic procedures.

The rounded tip has a slot that accepts the blade. As the tip is screwed into the handle, it tightens to hold the blade. There are a multitude of various blades available for specific purposes and procedures.
Instrument Insight: There are many types and shapes of blades that will fit on the Beaver handle depending on the surgeon's preference and procedure being performed.

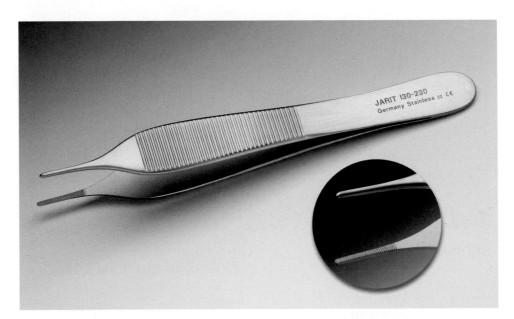

Instrument: PLAIN ADSON TISSUE FORCEPS
Other Names: Adson dressing forceps
Category: Grasping and Holding
Description: These have fine tips with horizontal serrations.

Use(s): These are used for grasping delicate tissue.
Instrument Insight: All of the Adson tissue forceps are the same size and shape. They are differentiated by the inner tips.

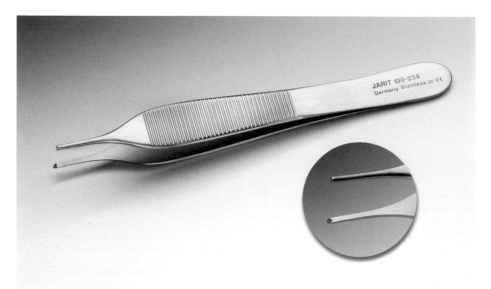

Instrument: TOOTHED ADSON TISSUE FORCEPS
Other Names: Adson with teeth, rat tooth
Category: Grasping and Holding
Description: The fine tips of these have two small teeth on one side and one small tooth on the other side that fit together when closed.
Use(s): These are used to align the edges of the wound during stapling of the skin; grasp superficial tissues so that Steri-Strips can be placed.

Instrument Insight: All of the Adson tissue forceps are the same size and shape. They are differentiated by the inner tips.

⚠ **CAUTION:** Exercise care when handling forceps with teeth. The sharp teeth can easily compromise the integrity of your gloves and skin and those of the surgeon.

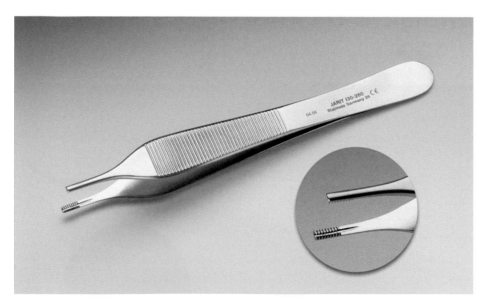

Instrument: BROWN-ADSON TISSUE FORCEPS
Other Names: Brown forceps
Category: Grasping and Holding
Description: On each side of the tip of these forceps, there are two rows of multiple teeth that interlock when closed.
Use(s): These are used for grasping superficial delicate tissues. Often used in plastic or hand surgery.

Instrument Insight: All Adson tissue forceps are the same size and shape. They are differentiated by the inner tips. It is important to ensure that the teeth are properly aligned and in working order before use.

⚠ **CAUTION:** Exercise care when handling forceps with teeth. The sharp teeth can easily compromise the integrity of your gloves and skin and those of the surgeon.

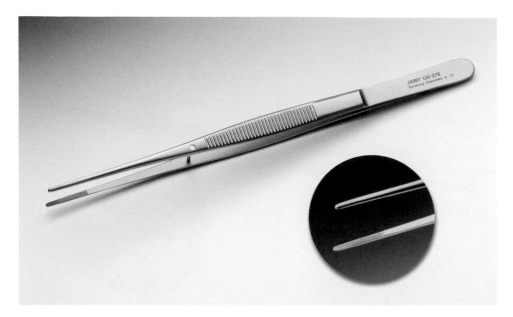

Instrument: PLAIN TISSUE FORCEPS
Other Names: Semken dressing forceps, Cushing tissue forceps without teeth, smooth forceps, tissue forceps without teeth
Category: Grasping and Holding

Description: These are atraumatic tissue forceps with horizontal serrated tips that vary from fine to heavy.
Use(s): These are used for grasping tissue and dressing application.

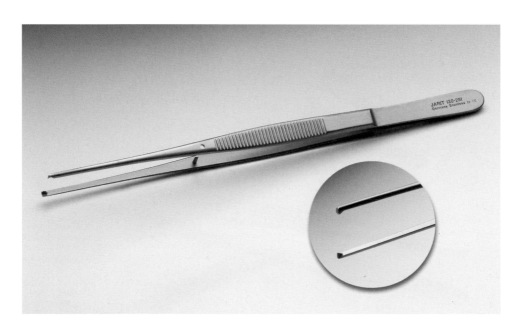

Instrument: TOOTHED TISSUE FORCEPS
Other Names: Semken tissue forceps, Cushing tissue forceps with teeth, rat tooth, tissue forceps with teeth
Category: Grasping and Holding
Description: The tips of these forceps have two teeth on one side and one tooth on the other side that fits between the opposite when closed.
Use(s): These are used for grasping moderate to heavy tissue and used during wound closure.

Instrument Insight: It is important to ensure the teeth are properly aligned and in working order before use.

⚠ **CAUTION:** Exercise care when handling forceps with teeth. The sharp teeth can easily compromise the integrity of your gloves and skin and those of the surgeon.

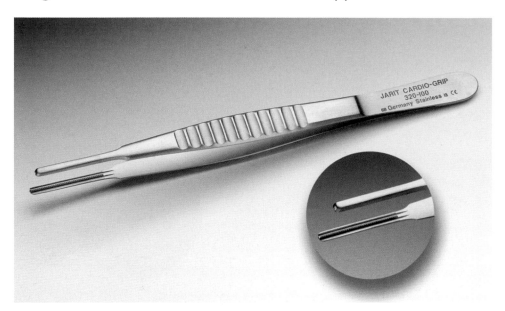

Instrument: DEBAKEY TISSUE FORCEPS
Other Names: DeBakey's, DeBakes
Category: Grasping and Holding
Description: There are atraumatic tissue forceps with an elongated, narrowed blunt tip. A set of parallel fine serrations runs the length of one jaw with a center row of serrations on the opposite side that interlocks to grip when closed.

Use(s): These are used to grasps numerous types of tissue; commonly used in cardiac, vascular surgery, and gastrointestinal procedures.
Instrument Insight: These are considered a vascular tissue forceps, but they are commonly used in all specialty areas because of the ability to securely grip without causing damage to the tissues.

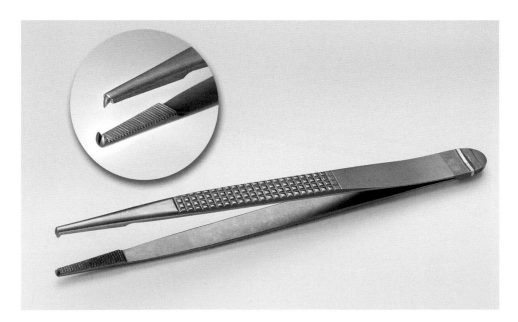

Instrument: BONNEY TISSUE FORCEPS
Other Names: Victor Bonney forceps, Victors
Category: Grasping and Holding
Description: This is always the same size and shape. The tips have 1×2 interlocking teeth followed by a horizontal serration.
Use(s): These are used to grasp heavy tissue, muscle, or bone; often used in obstetrics and orthopedics.

Instrument Insight: It is important to ensure that the teeth are properly aligned and in working order before use.

⚠ **CAUTION:** Exercise care when handling. The sharp teeth can easily compromise the integrity of your gloves and skin and those of the surgeon.

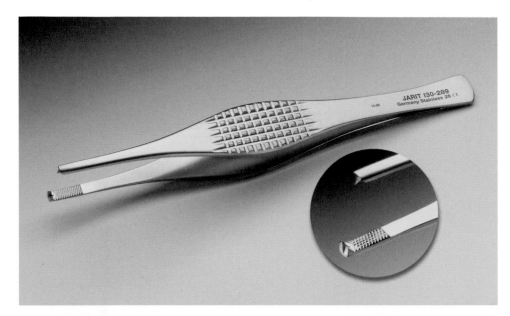

Instrument: FERRIS-SMITH TISSUE FORCEPS
Other Names: Big ugly's
Category: Grasping and Holding
Description: This is always the same size and shape. The tips have 1×2 interlocking large teeth followed by a crisscrossed pattern serration.
Use(s): These are used to grasp heavy tissue, muscle, and bone; often used in orthopedics, spinal, and obstetric surgery.

Instrument Insight: It is important to ensure that the teeth are properly aligned and in working order before use.

⚠ **CAUTION:** Exercise care when handling forceps with teeth. The sharp teeth can easily compromise the integrity of your gloves and skin and those of the surgeon.

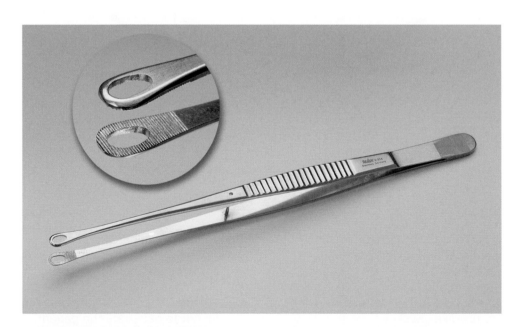

Instrument: SINGLEY TISSUE FORCEPS
Other Names: Tuttle thoracic tissue forceps
Category: Grasping and Holding
Description: These have oval-shaped tip with central fenestrated, horizontal serrated jaws.

Use(s): These are used for grasping intestinal tissue, delicate tissues, or dressings materials and sponges; often used in general, urology, thoracic, and OB/GYN surgeries.

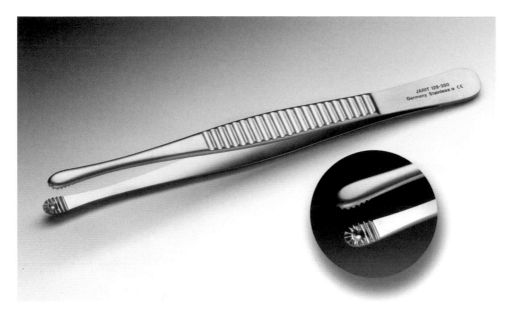

Instrument: **RUSSIAN TISSUE FORCEPS**
Other Names: Star forceps, Russian star forceps, Russians
Category: Grasping and Holding
Description: These have rounded tips with starburst pattern serrations.

Use(s): These are used for grasping dense tissues and used during wound closure.
Instrument Insight: Commonly used in OB/GYN procedures.

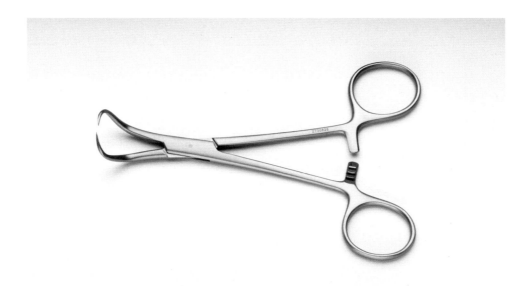

Instrument: **TOWEL CLIP (PENETRATING)**
Other Names: Backhaus towel clip, Roeder towel clip, Jones towel clip
Category: Grasping and Holding
Description: It is a ratcheted instrument with curved, sharp, tine-like jaws.
Use(s): It is used for holding towels in place when draping, when grasping tough tissue, and during reduction of small bone fractures.
Instrument Insight: It is used in all disciplines. Never use penetrating clips to attach the

electrosurgical unit (ESU), suction, or any other item to the drapes. This will perforate the drapes and compromise the sterile field.

⚠ **CAUTION:** When clipping towels together, be careful not to penetrate the patient's skin. Exercise care when handling penetrating forceps. The sharp tips can easily compromise the integrity of your gloves and skin and those of the surgeon.

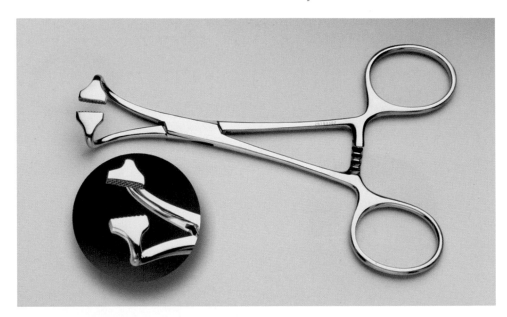

Instrument: NONPENETRATING TOWEL CLIP
Other Names: Atraumatic towel clamp
Category: Grasping and Holding
Description: There are many different types of towel clamps; they may be metal or plastic and may have a variety of nonpenetrating tips.

Use(s): It is used for attaching Bovie and suction to the drapes.

⚠ **CAUTION:** Care should be taken not to clamp the patient's skin between the jaws when attaching accessory devices to the drapes.

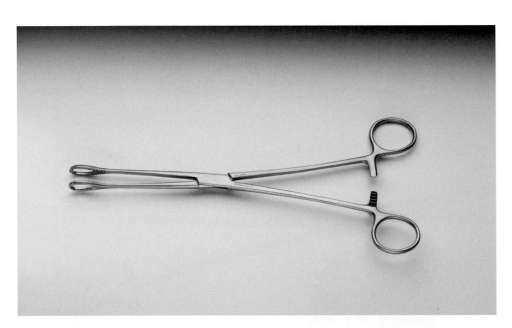

Instrument: FOERSTER SPONGE FORCEPS
Other Names: Fletcher sponge forceps, sponge stick forceps, ring forceps
Category: Grasping and Holding
Description: These can be curved or straight; the tips are oval fenestrated rings with horizontal serration.
Use(s): These are used for creating a sponge stick, for grasping tissues such as the lungs, or for removing uterine contents.

Instrument Insight: To assemble a sponge stick, fold a 4×4 Raytex in thirds and then in half and attach it to the ring forceps. A sponge stick can be used for the surgical preparation (painting) to absorb blood or for blunt dissection in deep wounds.

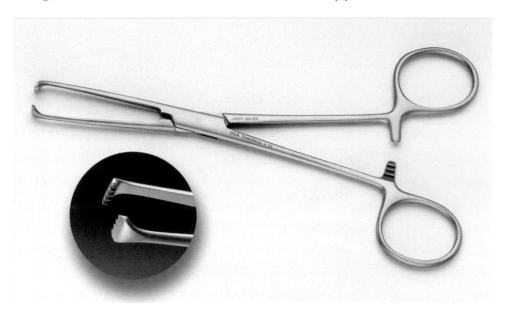

Instrument: ALLIS FORCEPS
Category: Grasping and Holding
Description: These are curved or straight with multiple, interlocking fine teeth at the tip that reduce injury to the tissues.
Use(s): These are used for lifting, holding, and retracting slippery dense tissue that is being removed. Also these are commonly used for tonsils; for vaginal, breast, and thyroid tissues; or for grasping bowel during a resection.
Instrument Insight: It is important to ensure the teeth are properly aligned and in working order before use.

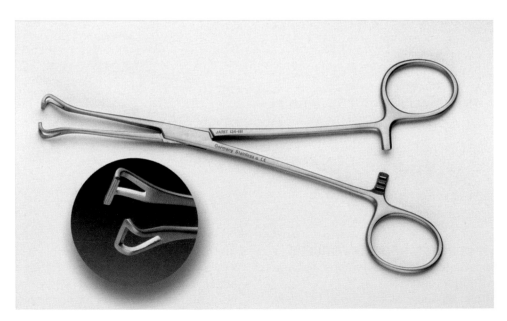

Instrument: BABCOCK FORCEPS
Category: Grasping and Holding
Description: These are atraumatic forceps with a flared, rounded, hollow end with smooth, flattened tips.
Use(s): These are used for grasping and encircling delicate structures such as the ureters, fallopian tubes, bowel, ovaries, and appendix.

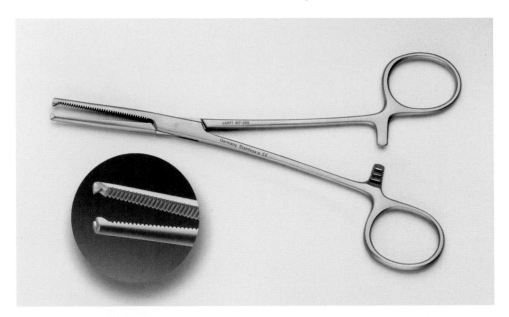

Instrument: KOCHER FORCEPS
Other Names: Koch forceps, Ochsner forceps
Category: Grasping and Holding
Description: The jaws of these forceps have horizontal serrations and 1×2 large interlocking teeth at the tip.
Use(s): These are used for grasping tough, fibrous, slippery tissues such as muscle and fascia.

Instrument Insight: It is important to ensure the teeth are properly aligned and in working order before use.

⚠ **CAUTION:** Exercise care when handling forceps with teeth. The sharp teeth can easily compromise the integrity of your skin and gloves and those of the surgeon.

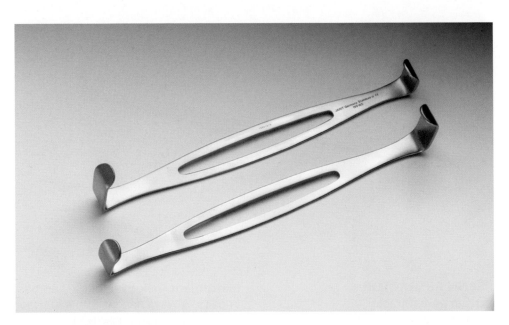

Instrument: ARMY-NAVY RETRACTOR
Other Names: Army's, Navy's, U.S. retractor
Category: Retracting and Exposing
Description: It is a handheld, double-ended retractor with an oval fenestration in the handle and a lateral curve to the blades on each end.

One end is longer than the other so that it can be placed deeper into the wound.
Use(s): It is used for retraction of small superficial incisions to allow better exposure.
Instrument Insight: It is often packaged in pairs.

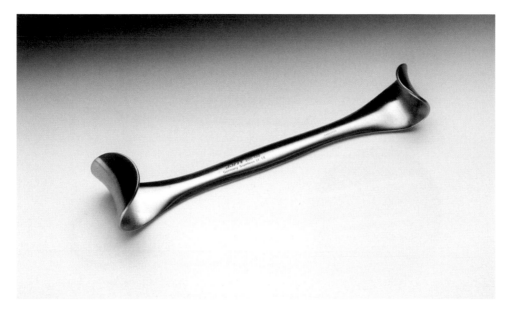

Instrument: GOELET RETRACTOR
Other Name: Bolt retractor
Category: Retracting and Exposing
Description: It is a handheld, double-ended retractor with smooth, cup-shaped curved blades with a crescent-shaped lip. One end is longer than the other so that it can be placed farther into the wound. The size and shape never change.
Use(s): It is used for retraction of small superficial incisions to allow better exposure.
Instrument Insight: It is usually packaged in pairs.

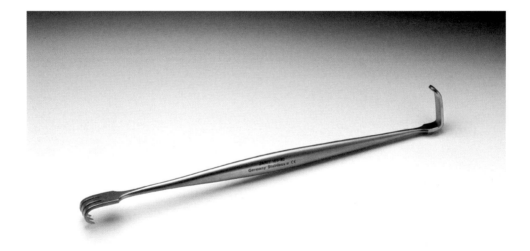

Instrument: SENN RETRACTOR
Other Names: Cat paw retractor
Category: Retracting and Exposing
Description: It is a double-ended, handheld retractor in which one end has three sharp or dull claws and the other end is a small, narrow, laterally bent blade.
Use(s): It is used for retraction of skin edges and deeper tissues of small incisions.

Instrument Insight: It usually comes packaged in pairs. Always hand it to the surgeon with the sharp claws facing downward.

⚠ **CAUTION:** Exercise care when handling retractors with sharp claws. The sharp claws can easily compromise the integrity of your gloves and skin.

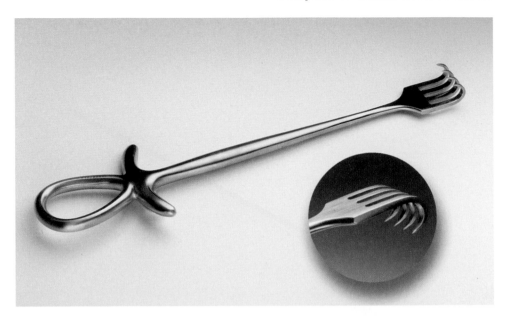

Instrument: MURPHY RETRACTOR
Other Names: Rake retractor
Category: Retracting and Exposing
Description: The retractor has four claws that may be blunt or sharp. The handle has a teardrop opening with two prongs on each side.
Use(s): It is used for superficial retraction of wound edges.

Instrument Insight: It usually comes packaged in pairs. Always hand this retractor to the surgeon with the sharp claws facing downward.

⚠ **CAUTION:** Be cognizant of the sharp claws. Sharp edges may puncture gloves and scratch the skin.

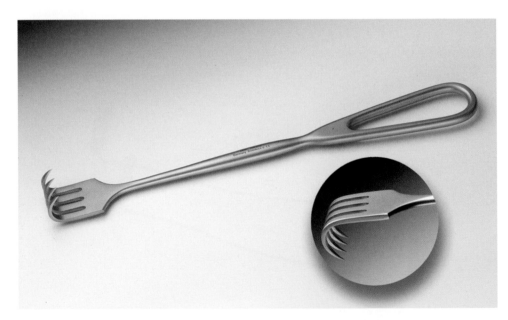

Instrument: VOLKMAN RETRACTOR
Other Names: Rake retractor, Israeli retractor
Category: Retracting and Exposing
Description: These may have two to six claws that may be blunt or sharp. The handle has a teardrop opening.
Use(s): It is used for superficial retraction of wound edges.

Instrument Insight: It usually comes packaged in pairs. Always hand this retractor to the surgeon with the sharp claws down.

⚠ **CAUTION:** Be aware of the sharp claws. Sharp edges may puncture gloves and scratch the skin.

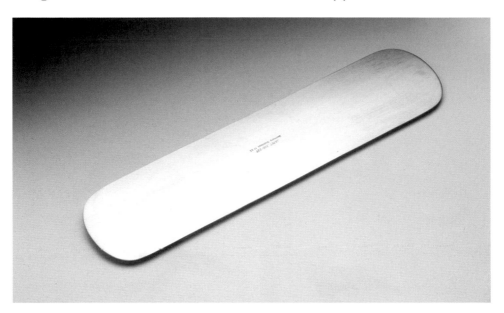

Instrument: RIBBON RETRACTOR
Other Names: Malleable retractor
Category: Retracting and Exposing
Description: It is a handheld, smooth, flat metal strip with rounded ends. These come in many different lengths and widths.

Use(s): It is used for retraction of organs and intestines in a wound.
Instrument Insight: It can be bent or molded as needed for use.

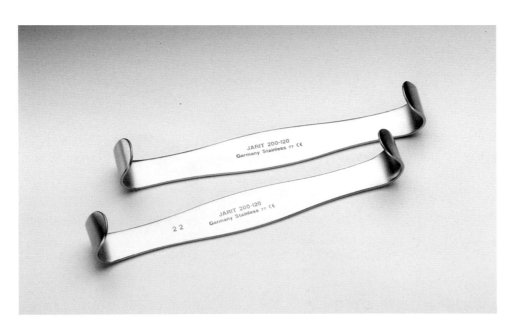

Instrument: PARKER RETRACTOR
Other Names: Park bench retractor, nested right angle retractor, double round retractor
Category: Retracting and Exposing
Description: It is handheld, double-ended with smooth rounded ends.

Use(s): It is used for retraction and exposure of a small or shallow wound.
Instrument Insight: It is usually packaged in pairs.

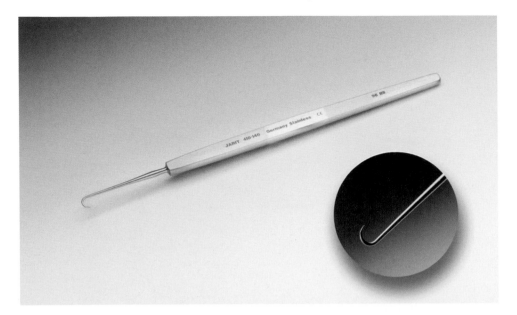

Instrument: SKIN HOOK
Other Names: Joseph hook, Gillies hook
Category: Retracting and Exposing
Description: It is a small handheld instrument with one or two sharp hooks at one end.
Use(s): It is used for retraction of the skin edges.

Instrument Insight: Always hand instrument to the surgeon with the hook(s) down.

⚠ **CAUTION:** The hooks are very sharp. Exercise care when handling sharp instruments to avoid puncture to gloves and/or skin.

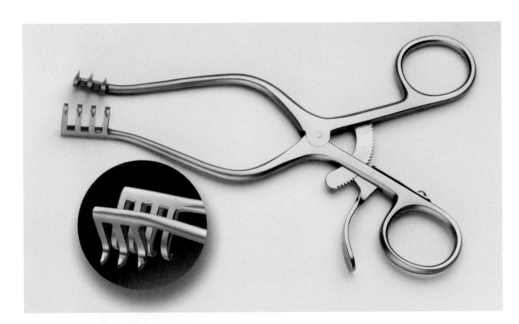

Instrument: WEITLANER RETRACTOR
Category: Retracting and Exposing
Description: It is a self-retaining, finger-ringed instrument with a ratchet release device on the shanks, which holds them open in the wound. The tip has three outward-curved prongs on one side and four on the other side that may be sharp or dull.

Use(s): It is used to hold wound edges open.
Instrument Insight: Always hand this retractor to the surgeon with the prongs down.

⚠ **CAUTION:** The prongs may be very sharp. Exercise care when handling sharp instruments to avoid puncture to gloves and/or skin.

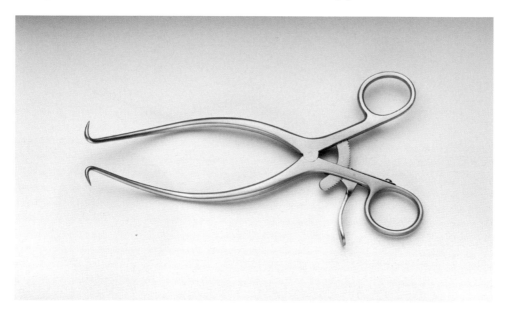

Instrument: GELPI RETRACTOR
Category: Retracting and Exposing
Description: It is a self-retaining, ringed instrument with a ratchet/release device on the shanks and two outward-turned sharp prongs, one on each side.
Use(s): It provides wound exposure, ranging from superficial to deep depending on the wound depth.

Instrument Insight: Always hand this retractor to the surgeon with the prongs down.

⚠ **CAUTION:** The prongs are sharp and can puncture gloves and skin.

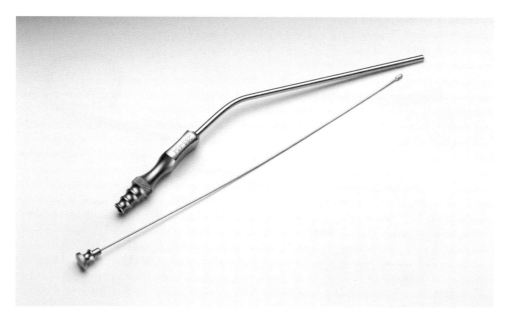

Instrument: FRAZIER SUCTION TIP
Category: Suctioning and Aspirating
Description: It is an angled cylindrical tube with a relief opening/hole on the handgrip. The diameter of the suction tube is measured on the French (F) scale and ranges from 3F to 15F.
Use(s): It is used for suctioning in confined spaces such as the nasal cavity, in lumbar and cervical procedures, or in craniotomies.

Instrument Insight: The Frazier suction tip is packaged with a thin wire stylet. This stylet fits inside the suction tip to push out any tissue, blood, or debris that gets trapped while suctioning. The suction is increased by covering the opening on the base of the tip.

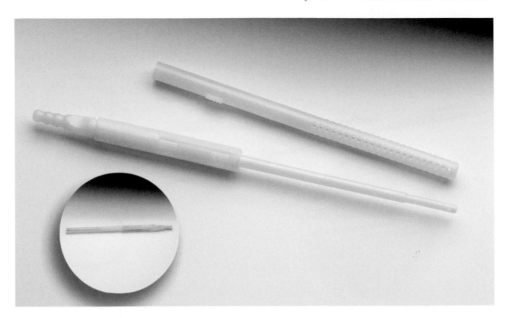

Instrument: POOLE SUCTION TIP
Other Names: Abdominal sucker
Category: Suctioning and Aspirating
Description: This can be disposable or reusable and has two components, an outer sheath and an inner cannula.
Use(s): It is used for suctioning large amounts of blood and/or fluids from a body cavity. The inner cannula of this suction tip can be used to suction down the shaft of the femur during a total hip replacement procedure.
Instrument Insight: Multiple fenestrations (holes) on the outer sheath of this Poole suction tip allow for more suction. If less suction power is desired, the surgeon may use the inner cannula only.

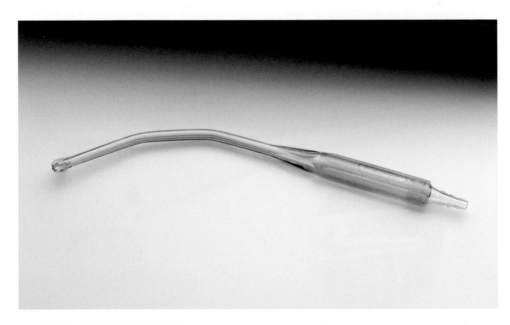

Instrument: YANKAUER SUCTION TIP
Other Names: Tonsil suction tip, oral suction tip
Category: Suctioning and Aspirating
Description: It is a hollow plastic tube with a grip handle and a slightly bent shaft that terminates with a bulbous tip and large opening.
Use(s): It is used for suctioning in all types of wounds. It allows for effective suctioning without aspiration damage to the surrounding tissue.
Instrument Insight: The disposable Yankauer is the most widely used suction tip. The reusable Yankauer has a detachable tip that screws on or off; make sure it is screwed down tightly.

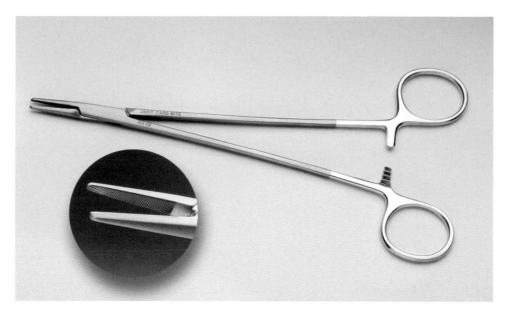

Instrument: CRILE-WOOD NEEDLE HOLDER
Other Names: Fine needle holder, fine needle driver
Category: Suturing and Stapling
Description: It is a narrow rounded tip with a crisscross gripping pattern in the inner jaws.

Use(s): It is used for holding delicate to intermediate-sized needles when suturing.
Instrument Insight: The type of procedure and depth of the wound will determine the type and size of needle holder.

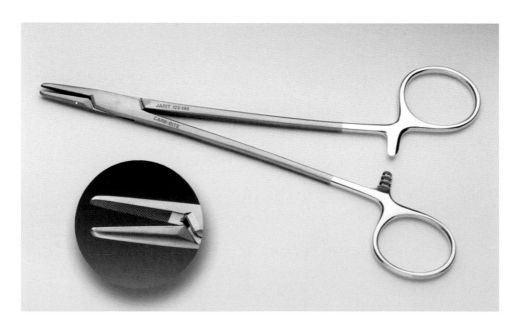

Instrument: MAYO-HEGAR NEEDLE HOLDER
Other Names: Heavy needle driver
Category: Suturing and Stapling
Description: It is a broader jaw that is rounded at the tip with crisscross pattern on the inner jaws.

Use(s): It is used for holding heavy needles when suturing.
Instrument Insight: The type of procedure and depth of the wound will determine the type and size of needle holder.

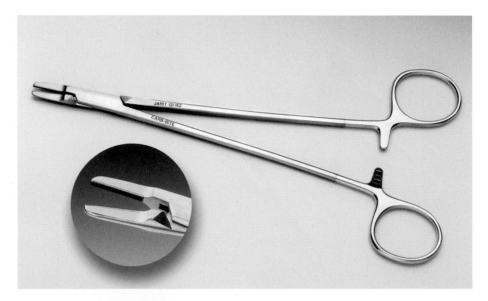

Instrument: RYDER NEEDLE HOLDER
Other Names: Ryder needle driver, fine needle driver
Category: Suturing and Stapling
Description: It has fine tapered jaws with carbide inserts.
Use(s): It is used for holding delicate to intermediate-sized needles when suturing. Often used for vascular procedures.

Instrument Insight: Never use it for grasping large heavy needles. The type and size of a needle holder to be used will be determined by the type of procedure and the depth of the wound.

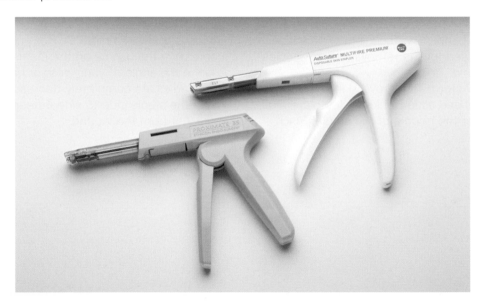

Instrument: SKIN STAPLER
Category: Suturing and Stapling
Description: It is a sterile, single-patient use instrument; it is preloaded with stainless steel rectangular staples that are used for approximation of the skin. There are many different manufacturers and models of staplers. It has a handle and a trigger that is squeezed to fire the staples; at the tip is an alignment arrow.
Use(s): It is used during wound closure for skin approximation.

Instrument Insight: The arrow at the tip of the device is to align the stapler with the approximated skin edges for proper staple placement. Two persons often perform skin stapling. The surgeon or assistant uses two Adson tissue forceps to grasp the skin edges and bring them together. The assistant or a surgical technologist positions the stapler over the wound, carefully aligning the arrow with the incision and squeezing the trigger until resistance is met. Once the staple is placed, remove the stapler and align it for the next firing until the wound is closed.

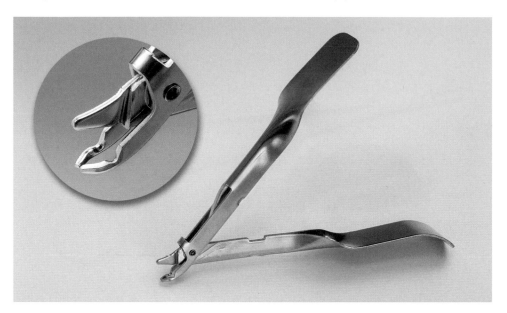

Instrument: STAPLE REMOVER

Other Names: Staple extractor

Category: Suturing and Stapling

Description: It is a disposable metal lever action device. The jaws consist of a small upper blunt blade and a lower fenestrated footplate that is thin enough to fit under a staple.

The functional part is a small blade; when pressure is exerted on the handles, it pushes down on the staple, pushes it through the fenestration in the footplate, and bends the staple into an M shape.

Use(s): It is used for the removal of skin staples from the wound.

Instrument Insight: To remove skin staples, open the jaws and slide the lower footplate of a remover under the middle of the staple. Pinch the handles of the staple remover together until they are fully closed. The upper blade of the staple remover will push down into the middle of the staple, causing the staple to bend and the two ends to pull outward and out of the wound. When both ends of the staple are visible, move the remover away from the wound and place the staple on sterile gauze.

⚠ **CAUTION:** Be careful not to pinch the skin in the jaws of the remover. Do not pull up while depressing the handle on the staple remover or change the angle of your wrist or hand. Once the handles are completely depressed, gently move the staple side to side if needed to release it from the wound.

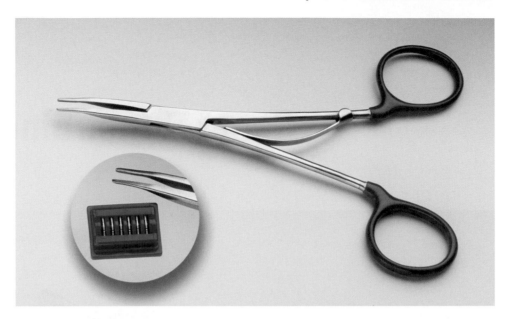

Instrument: HEMOCLIP APPLIER
Other Names: Clip applier, Weck clip, ligaclip
Category: Suturing and Stapling
Description: These have angled tips with fine grooves in the inner jaws that slide over the clip to pick it up. These are manufactured in various clip sizes and lengths in a color-coded cartridge for easy identification of clip size.
Use(s): It is used for occluding vessels or other tubular structures.
Instrument Insight: The size and type of clip have to match the appropriate clip applier.

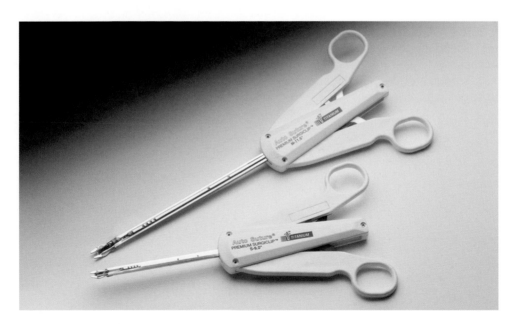

Instrument: SURGICLIP APPLIER
Other Names: Hemoclip, ligaclip
Category: Suturing and Stapling
Description: It is a sterile, single-patient use instrument, preloaded with clips. These are manufactured in various clip sizes and lengths.
Use(s): It is used for occluding vessels or other tubular structures.

4 General Instruments

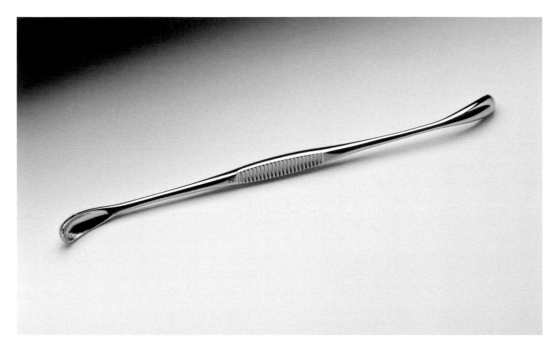

Instrument: FERGUSON GALLSTONE SCOOP
Other Names: Scoop, spoon
Category: Accessory
Description: It is double-ended, spoon-shaped, with one end larger than the other.

Use(s): It is used for removing stones from the gallbladder.
Instrument Insight: It is usually small, medium, and large scoops in the set.

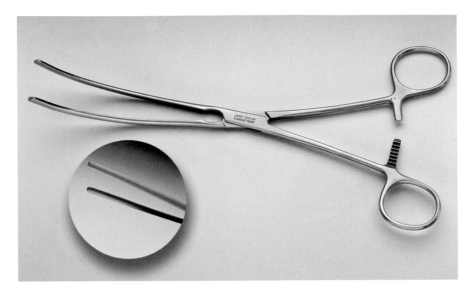

Instrument: CARTER-GLASSMAN INTESTINAL CLAMP
Other Names: Glassman intestinal clamp
Category: Clamping and Occluding

Description: It can be straight or curved and has cardio-grip inner jaws that grasp but are atraumatic.
Use(s): It is used for clamping bowel during a resection.

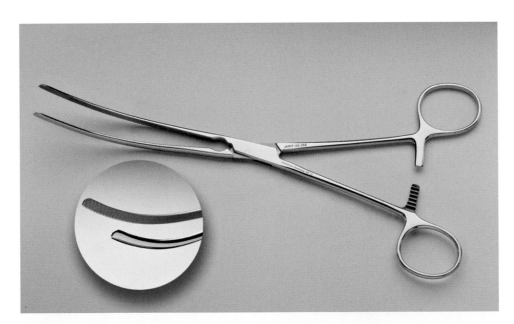

Instrument: DOYEN INTESTINAL CLAMP
Other Names: Doyen clamp
Category: Clamping and Occluding
Description: It can be curved or straight; has smooth inner jaws.
Use(s): It is used for clamping bowel during a resection.

Instrument Insight: The jaws of the Doyen clamp are covered with rubber shods or shoelaces. Shoelaces are tubular woven cotton that slips over the entire jaws. Shods are rubber tubing that slides over the jaws. These help grip the intestine without causing trauma.

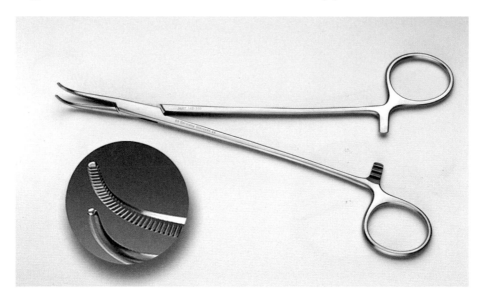

Instrument: GEMINI FORCEPS
Other Names: Right angle forceps, Lahey forceps, Mixter forceps
Category: Clamping and Occluding
Description: It is a 90-degree-angle clamp with horizontal serrations that run the length of the jaws.
Use(s): It is used for dissecting tissue planes, clamping vessels, and placing a tie or vessel loop under and around a tubular structure, such as a vessel or duct. This enables the surgeon to grasp the ligature or loop and pull it up and around the structure to either ligate or apply traction.
Instrument Insight: The Gemini, right angle, Lahey, and Mixter forceps are often referred to as the same instrument depending on the region of the country where they are being used, but they are in fact differentiated by the inner jaws.

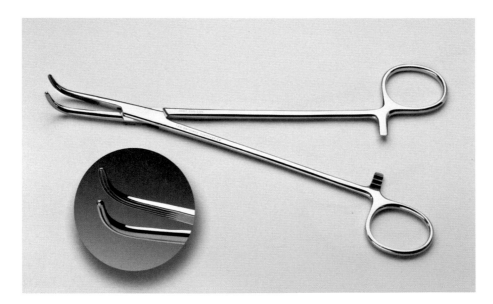

Instrument: LAHEY GALL DUCT FORCEPS
Other Names: Right angle forceps, Gemini forceps, Mixter forceps
Category: Clamping and Occluding
Description: These are 90-degree-angle clamps with vertical serrations that run the length of the jaws.
Use(s): These are used for dissecting tissue planes, clamping vessels, and placing a tie or vessel loop under and around a tubular structure, such as a vessel or duct.
Instrument Insight: The Gemini, right angle, Lahey, and Mixter forceps are often referred to as the same instrument depending on the region of the country where they are being used, but they are in fact differentiated by the inner jaws.

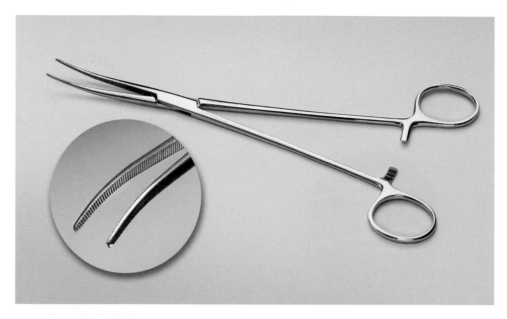

Instrument: SAROT FORCEPS
Other Names: Long curved forceps
Category: Clamping and Occluding
Description: These are long, ringed forceps with long, narrow jaws with horizontal serration running the length of the instrument.

Use(s): These are used for dissecting planes and clamping vessels deep in the wound.
Instrument Insight: Be sure to keep the tips free of blood and debris so the surgeon.

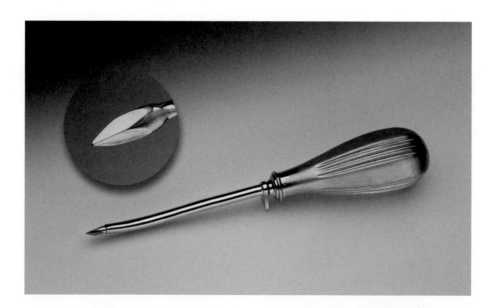

Instrument: GALLBLADDER TROCAR
Category: Cutting and Dissecting
Description: It is a two-pieced instrument that consists of an outer sheath and a sharp obturator. The obturator fits inside the sheath.

Drainage is facilitated by pushing the sharp trocar into the gallbladder and then removing the obturator and attaching a syringe to aspirate the bile.

Use(s): It is used for draining the gallbladder of bile during an open cholecystectomy procedure.
Instrument Insight: The obturator and sheath should be taken apart during the sterilization process. If it is inadvertently left together as one piece, the inside of the sheath and obturator would be considered unsterile and should be handed off the field as one piece. Do not separate the two pieces.

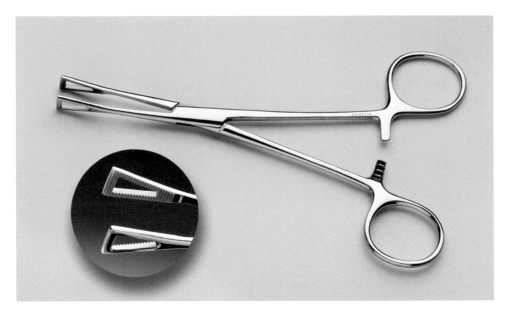

Instrument: PENNINGTON FORCEPS
Other Names: Duval forceps, triangle forceps, lung clamp forceps
Category: Grasping and Holding
Description: These have triangular tips with horizontal serrations.

Use(s): These are used for grasping tissue and organs during general procedures. Commonly used during intestinal and rectal procedures. Also used for grasping the uterine layers during closure of a cesarean section.

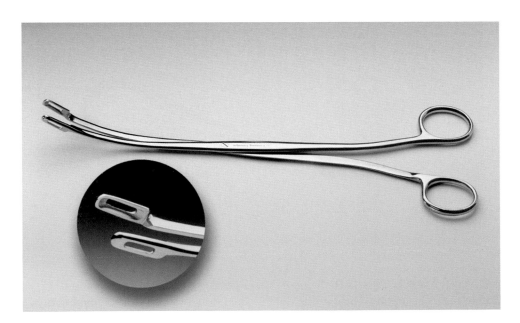

Instrument: DESJARDIN GALLSTONE FORCEPS
Other Names: Randall stone forceps
Category: Grasping and Holding
Description: These are curved instruments with no ratchets, and the jaws work like scissors. The tips are oval and cup-shaped with fenestrations.
Use(s): These are used for grasping polyps and stones in the common bile duct and gallbladder.

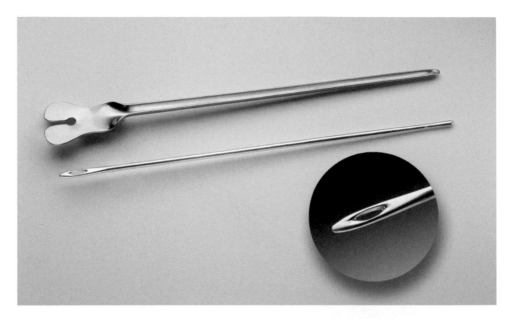

Instrument: PROBE AND GROOVED DIRECTOR
Category: Probing and Dilating
Description: The probe resembles a French-eye blunt needle. The grooved director has a tongue-shaped handle and a concave channel, which guides the probe into the opening.
Use(s): It is used to detect an obstruction in a tubular structure or determine the path and the extent of a fistula tract.

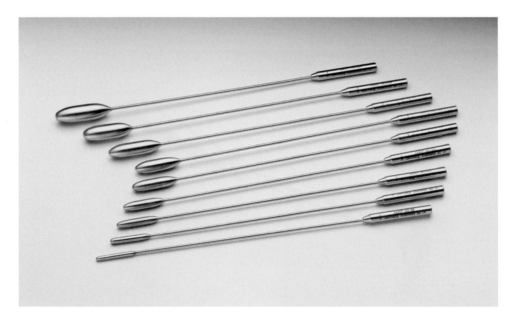

Instrument: BAKES COMMON DUCT DILATORS
Other Names: Common duct dilators
Category: Probing and Dilating
Description: It has an oval, solid stainless steel tip that attaches to a narrowed stem, which extends to a solid, smooth handle.
Use(s): These are used to open and expand the common bile duct to allow passage of bile from the liver.
Instrument Insight: These are packaged as a set in which each dilator graduates up in size. The stem is malleable and is often bent to allow passage into the duct.

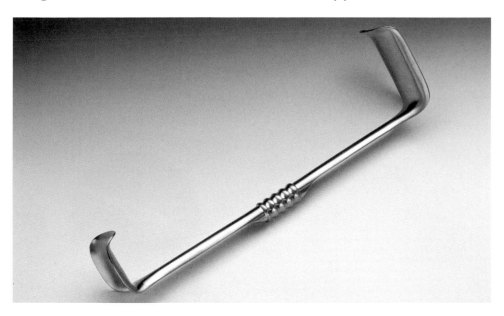

Instrument: RICHARDSON-EASTMAN RETRACTOR
Other Names: Double-ended Rich retractor, Eastman retractor, big Rich retractor
Category: Retracting and Exposing
Description: It is a handheld double-ended retractor with a lateral curvature of the blades.

The bodies of the blades are concave with crescent-shaped lips that are laterally bent.
Use(s): It is used for retracting the wound edges.
Instrument Insight: At initiation of the incision, the superficial end of the retractor is used; as the incision is deepened, the longer blade is used.

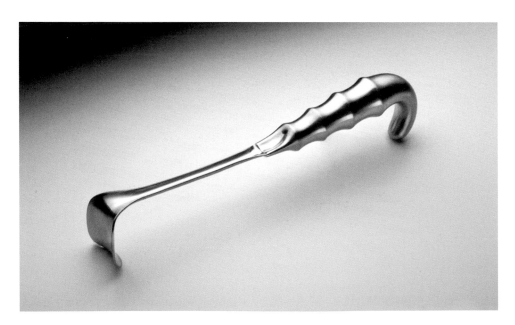

Instrument: RICHARDSON RETRACTOR
Other Names: Rich retractor
Category: Retracting and Exposing
Description: It has a hollow grip handle with a lateral curve to the blade. The body of the blade

is concave with a crescent-shaped lip that is laterally bent.
Use(s): It is used for retracting the wound edges.
Instrument Insight: These are often packaged in a set of three: small, medium, and large.

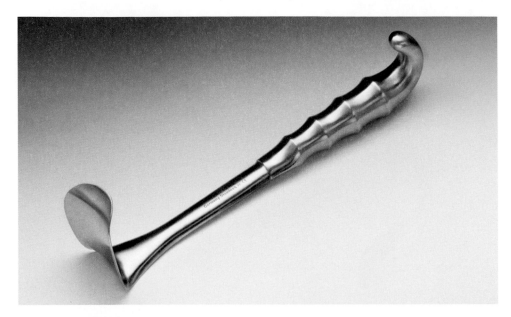

Instrument: KELLY RETRACTOR
Category: Retracting and Exposing
Description: It has a hollow grip handle with a lateral right-angle curvature of the blade. The body of the blade is slightly dipped with a crescent-shaped lip that is slightly bent.

Use(s): It is used for retracting the wound edges.
Instrument Insight: It is often confused with a Richardson retractor, but the blades are distinctly different.

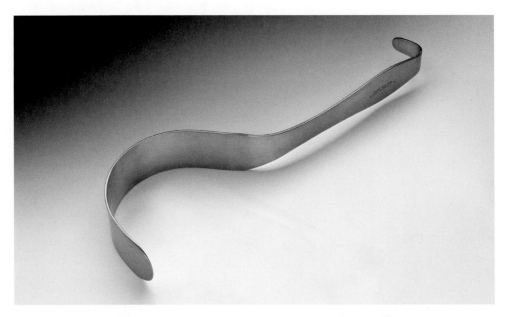

Instrument: DEAVER RETRACTOR
Category: Retracting and Exposing
Description: It is a flat stainless steel strip that resembles a question mark. The width and length vary according to need.
Use(s): It is used for deep retraction of organs and viscera.

Instrument Insight: Retraction with a Deaver sometimes can be awkward because of the flat shape of the handle. To aid in maintaining a grip, the handle should be placed in the palm of the hand and the hook should be placed over the top of the hand.

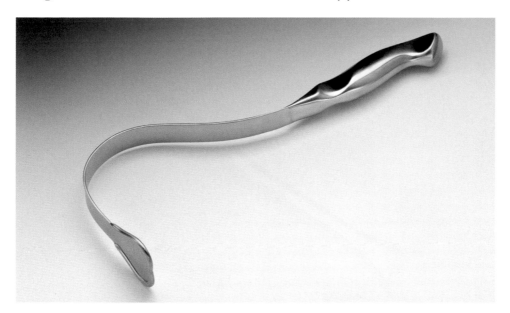

Instrument: HARRINGTON RETRACTOR
Other Names: Sweetheart retractor, Harrington heart retractor
Category: Retracting and Exposing
Description: It has a grip handle that extends into a curved, flat, stainless steel strip. The end of the blade enlarges into a heart shape. The heart-shaped portion is overlaid with a smooth ridge to decrease the chance of injury to an organ.
Use(s): It is used for retraction deep in an abdominal wound; often used to retract the liver and intestine.

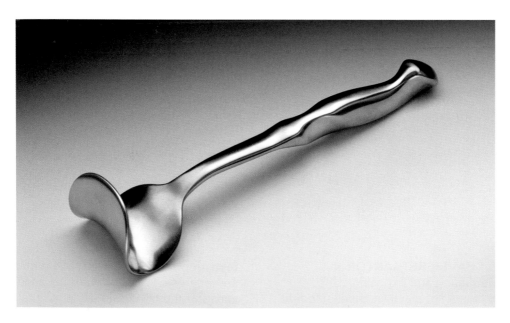

Instrument: MAYO ABDOMINAL RETRACTOR
Other Names: Abdominal wall retractor
Category: Retracting and Exposing
Description: The blade has a smooth, cup-shaped curve with a crescent-shaped lip.
Use(s): It is used for retraction of the abdominal wall.

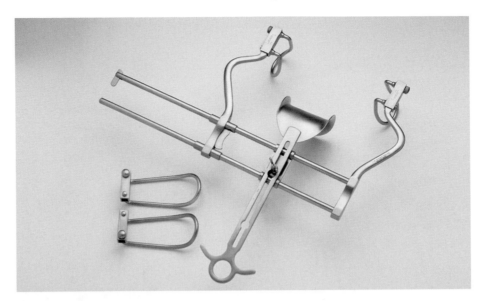

Instrument: BALFOUR RETRACTOR
Other Names: Self-retaining retractor
Category: Retracting and Exposing
Description: It is a self-retaining retractor with lateral wire blades and a wide center blade. A Balfour set includes the frame, four lateral sides, and two center blades, which are interchangeable according to the depth needed. The lateral blades may be solid, fenestrated, interchangeable, or fixed.

Use(s): It is used for retraction of a large abdominal wound.
Instrument Insight: All the interchangeable pieces have to be counted separately (e.g., one frame, four sides, and two blades). If the frame has any other removable parts, such as screws or wing nuts, these also need to be counted.

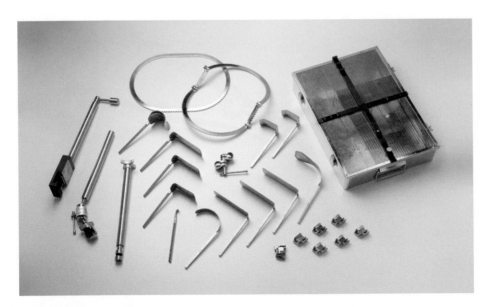

Instrument: BOOKWALTER RETRACTOR
Other Names: Jaritrack retractor
Category: Retracting and Exposing
Description: It is a large, self-retaining abdominal retractor that attaches to the operating table. It has blades in various sizes and shapes that attach to a frame to enhance visualization during the surgical procedure.
Use(s): It is used for retraction of large abdominal wounds.
Instrument Insight: Each individual piece has to be counted.

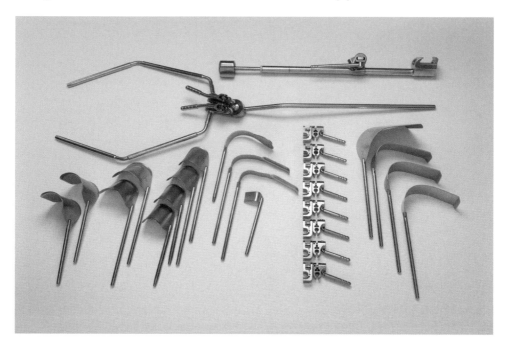

Instrument: OMNI RETRACTOR
Other Names: Omni tract retractor, upper arm retractor
Category: Retracting and Exposing
Description: It is a large, self-retaining abdominal retractor that attaches to the operating table. It has blades in various sizes and shapes that attach to a frame to enhance visualization during the surgical procedure.
Use(s): It is used for retraction of large abdominal wounds.
Instrument Insight: Each individual piece of the retractor must be counted.

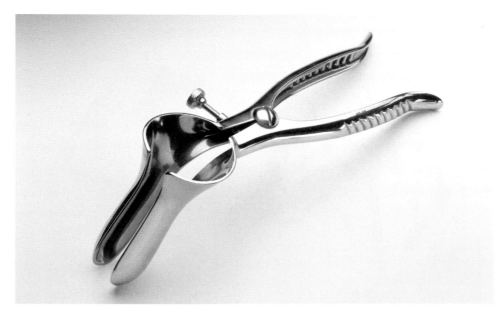

Instrument: PRATT RECTAL SPECULUM
Category: Retracting and Exposing
Description: It is a self-retaining speculum with rounded blades that open by squeezing the handles together. Turning the screw on the side will hold the blades open.
Use(s): It is used for providing exposure for visualization of the anus and rectum.
Instrument Insight: Apply copious amounts of lubrication to the blades to prevent tissue damage.

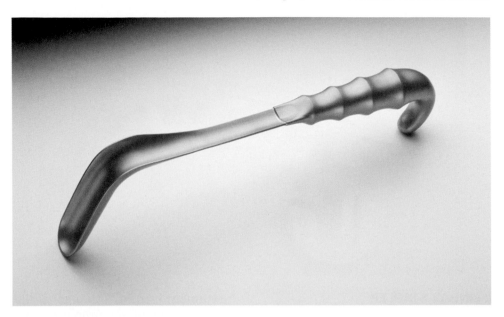

Instrument: SAWYER RECTAL RETRACTOR
Category: Retracting and Exposing
Description: It is a handheld retractor with a right-angle convex blade that extends to a hollow grip handle.

Use(s): It is used for providing exposure for visualization of the anus and rectum.
Instrument Insight: Apply copious amounts of lubrication to the blade to prevent tissue damage.

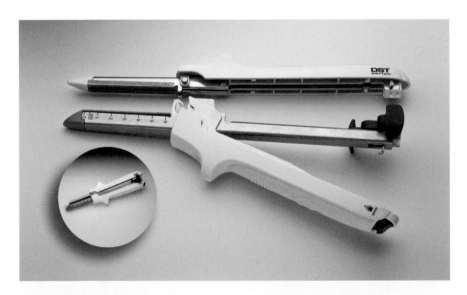

Instrument: LINEAR CUTTER-STAPLER
Other Names: GIA stapler
Category: Suturing and Stapling
Description: It is a disposable reloadable stapler that distributes two double-staggered rows of titanium staples while cutting the tissues between the rows. The length is determined by the tissue to be excised. This stapler comes in 60-, 80-, and 100-mm lengths.
Use(s): It is often used during gastric or bowel surgery for resection and reanastomosis. Also used to transect tissues in thoracic, gynecologic, and pediatric procedures.

Instrument Insight: Activation of linear cutter-stapler is accomplished by sliding the firing knob on the sides of the stapler forward until it stops completely. The manufacturer recommends that the stapler can be reloaded seven times for a total of eight firings. When reloading the stapler, make sure to wipe off the opposite side of the stapler to ensure that any staples left from the first firing are removed. Any staples left behind can cause the stapler to misfire or not to fire at all.

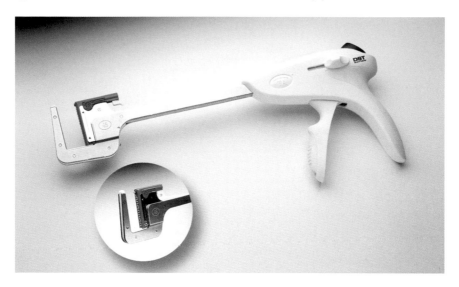

Instrument: LINEAR STAPLER
Other Names: TA stapler
Category: Suturing and Stapling
Description: It is a disposable reloadable stapler that distributes a double or triple (depending on model of stapler) staggered row of titanium staples. A scalpel is used to excise the tissue along the length of the staple line.
Use(s): It is used for transection and resection of tissues during abdominal, gynecologic, pediatric, and thoracic surgeries.

Instrument Insight: Activation of the linear stapler is done by squeezing the handles together, which compresses the tissues between the jaws and engages the staples. The manufacturer recommends that the stapler can be reloaded seven times for a total of eight firings.

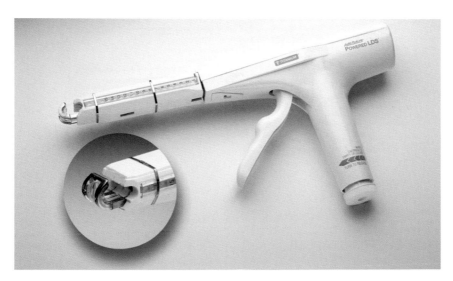

Instrument: LIGATING AND DIVIDING STAPLER
Other Names: LDS stapler
Category: Suturing and Stapling
Description: It is a disposable single-use stapler that distributes two titanium staples within the jaw for ligation. A scalpel divides the tissue between the staples.
Use(s): It is used for ligation and division of blood vessels and other tissues during abdominal, gynecologic, and thoracic procedures. The LDS stapler is often used in gastrointestinal surgery to ligate and divide the greater omentum and the mesentery.
Instrument Insight: Activation of ligating and dividing stapler is done by gripping the handles together. The stapler cartridge contains 15 pairs of staples. The remaining number of staples after each firing is indicated on the side panel of the cartridge.

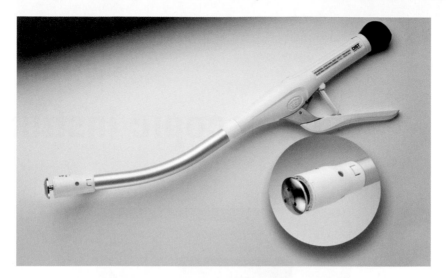

Instrument: INTRALUMINAL STAPLER
Other Names: CEEA stapler, EEA stapler, circular stapler
Category: Suturing and Stapling
Description: It is a disposable, single-use intraluminal stapler that places a circular, double-staggered row of titanium staples. Simultaneously following the staple formation, a circular knife blade cuts the excess tissue, creating a circular anastomosis.
Use(s): It is used for creation of end-to-end, end-to-side, or side-to-side anastomoses throughout the gastrointestinal tract. The stapler is used in open abdominal and laparoscopic procedures.
Instrument Insight: The stapler is activated by compressing the handles together as far as they will allow. After the anastomosis, excess tissue that is transected needs to be inspected for completeness. There should be two complete circular rings of tissue, often called donuts. This is accomplished by turning the wing nut at the bottom of the handle counterclockwise, which causes the shaft to extend, allowing removal of the specimen.

5 Laparoscopic Instruments

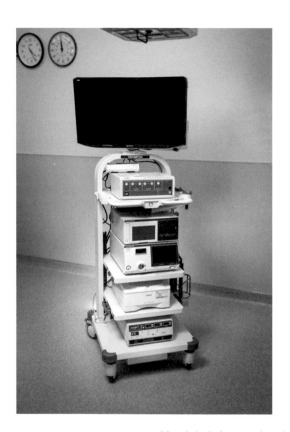

LAPAROSCOPIC CART

Other Names: Laparoscopic tower, laparoscopic trolly, video cart

Description: It is a rolling cart with a monitor mounted on the top and individual shelves that hold the camera unit, light source, insufflator, and printer and/or digital recorder.

Use(s): It is used to house, protect, and transport endoscopic video equipment.

Instrument Insight: An alternative to the cart is an overhead boom suspended from the ceiling.

TROCARS: Rapid change continues to occur in the development and improvement of trocars. These pictured represent a few manufacturer variations.

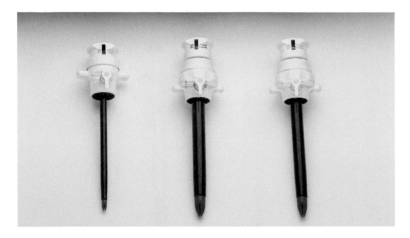

Instrument: VERSA PORT TROCARS
Category: Cutting and Dissecting
Description: It is a single-use, V-shaped, scalpel-bladed trocar with a spring-locking shield and a trocar cannula with a three-way stopcock. Versa port trocar sizes are 5 mm, 5–11 mm, and 5–12 mm.
Use(s): These are used to create an instrument port in which the endoscope and instruments can be introduced and exchanged through the cannula.

Instrument Insight: Upon entrance into a cavity, the shield advances to cover the blade, reducing the potential for injury to internal structures. The trocar cannula has a self-adjusting seal that prevents pneumoperitoneal loss when exchanging instruments and a three-way stopcock for gas insufflation and rapid desufflation. The self-adjusting seal accommodates from 5–12 mm as appropriate.

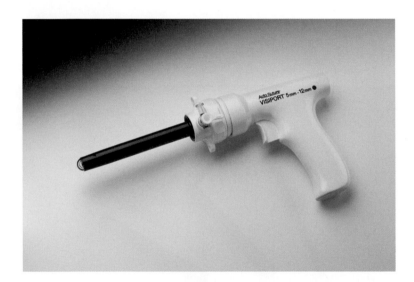

Instrument: VISIPORT
Other Names: Optical trocar
Category: Cutting and Dissecting
Description: It is a single-use, gun-like optical trocar that consists of a sheath with a blunt clear dome at the distal end that encases a crescent-shaped knife blade. The pistol-grip handle includes a trigger and an opening at the top that accommodates a 10-mm laparoscope, which allows visualization through the clear dome as the sheath passes through the abdominal or thoracic body wall. When the trigger is squeezed, the blade extends approximately 1 mm beyond the dome and instantaneously retracts. This action allows for a controlled sharp dissection through the tissue layers. The Visiport is available in 5–11-mm or 5–12-mm diameters.
Use(s): It is used to create an instrument port in which the endoscope and instruments can be introduced and exchanged through the cannula.
Instrument Insight: When entering a cavity, the clear dome shields the blade, reducing the potential for injury to internal structures. The trocar cannula has a self-adjusting seal that prevents pneumoperitoneal loss when exchanging instruments, and a three-way stopcock for gas insufflation and rapid desufflation. The self-adjusting seal accommodates 5–12 mm as appropriate.

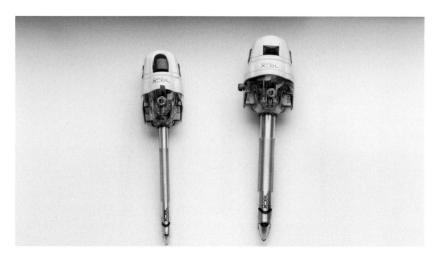

Instrument: XCEL TROCARS
Category: Probing and Dilating Instruments
Description: It is an optic tip bladeless trocar with a universal sealed sheath and a three-way stopcock.
Use(s): These are used to create an instrument port in which the endoscope and instruments can be introduced and exchanged through the cannula.

Instrument Insight: After the creation of a pneumoperitoneum, a small skin incision is made at the port site. A downward twisting motion causes the tissue to separate, eliminating the need for the tissue to be cut. The optic tip allows the surgeon to place the laparoscope inside the trocar to view the tissue layer during insertion.

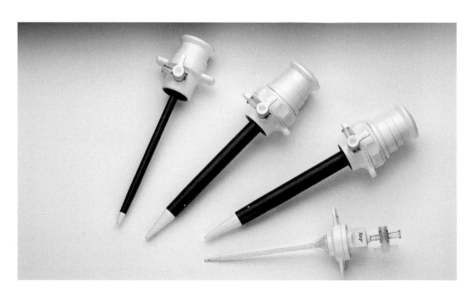

Instrument: VERSA STEP TROCARS
Category: Probing and Dilating Instruments
Description: It is a radial-dilating trocar system that includes an expandable mesh sleeve, an insufflation/access needle, a blunt-tipped fascial obturator and sheath, and a three-way stopcock. Rapid change continues to occur in the development and improvement of trocars. Those pictured represent a few manufacturer variations.
Use(s): These are used to create an instrument port in which the endoscope and instruments can be introduced and exchanged through the sheath or cannula.

Instrument Insight: After the creation of a pneumoperitoneum, a small skin incision is made at the port site. The expandable mesh sleeve is loaded over the access needle and introduced into the peritoneum. After removing the needle, the blunt-tipped obturator loaded into the sheath is passed through the mesh sleeve and into the peritoneum. The obturator is removed, and the sheath is left for the introduction of instruments.

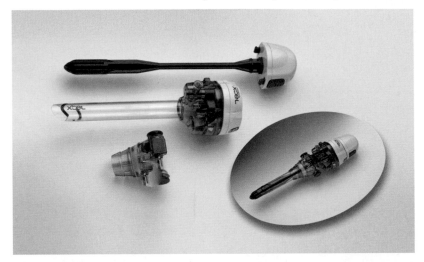

Instrument: BLUNT TROCAR

Other Names: Hasson trocar, Xcel blunt port trocar, blunt tip trocar

Category: Probing and Dilating Instruments

Description: It is a 5–12-mm trocar with a blunt obturator, self-sealing sheath, or cannula with a three-way stopcock, and a grip-anchoring device to secure it in place.

Use(s): It is used in the umbilical area first to create the pneumoperitoneum; this port is often used for the laparoscope and specimen retrieval.

Instrument Insight: The blunt trocar is used for the open or Hasson technique. This is accomplished by making a small incision at the umbilical area into the peritoneum. The blunt trocar is then placed and anchored down (usually with suture), and insufflation takes place. This is another technique to first visualize the abdominal cavity before placing a sharp trocar, preventing tissue or organ damage.

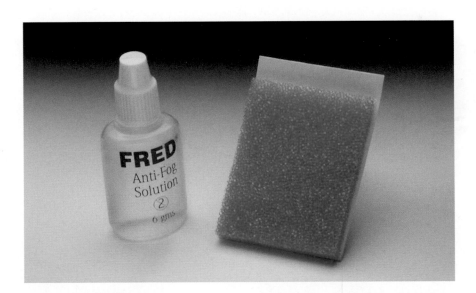

Instrument: ANTIFOG SOLUTION

Other Names: Endo fog, Fred, Dr. Fog solution

Category: Accessory

Description: It is packaged with a bottle of solution and a sponge.

Use(s): It is used to prevent the lens from fogging up during endoscopic procedures.

Instrument Insight: To use antifog solution, remove the paper backing over the adhesive on the sponge and stick it to the Mayo stand or on patient drape. Remove the solution cap and place 5 or 6 drops of antifog solution onto the sponge, then rub the end of the lens over the moistened sponge and blot with a sterile 4 × 4 sponge (do not wipe dry).

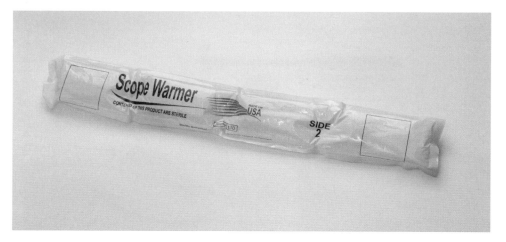

Instrument: LENS WARMER
Category: Accessory
Description: The lens warmer pictured is disposable and comes in a sterile package. To activate the warmer, squeeze the metal disc at the end of the bag. This mixes the chemicals and causes warming.

Use(s): It is used to warm the lens to body temperature to prevent condensation and fogging of the lens when entering the body cavity.
Instrument Insight: There are many types of lens warmers and methods for warming a lens.

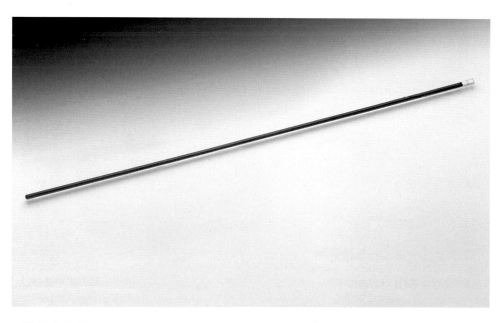

Instrument: ENDO KITTNER
Other Names: Endo kit, pusher, dissector, endo KD, Endo peanut
Category: Accessory
Description: It is a 3-mm-long cylinder rod with a cotton gauze tip.

Use(s): It is used for blunt dissection of tissue planes during laparoscopic procedures. The tip may be used to apply direct pressure to bleeders.
Instrument Insight: It can be inserted through a 5-mm or larger trocar.

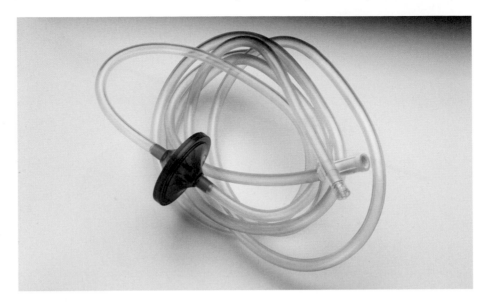

Instrument: INSUFFLATION TUBING
Category: Accessory
Description: It is a synthetic tubing 10–12-feet long with a Luer-Lok connector at the proximal end and a micron filter approximately 16–24 inches from the distal standard connection end. The micron filter is designed to prevent cross-contamination between the patient and the insufflator.

Use(s): It is used for creating and maintaining a pneumoperitoneum; delivers carbon dioxide from the insufflator to the abdominal cavity.
Instrument Insight: The distal filter end is handed off the sterile field to be connected to the insufflator. Air should be purged from the tubing before it is connected to the abdominal cavity.

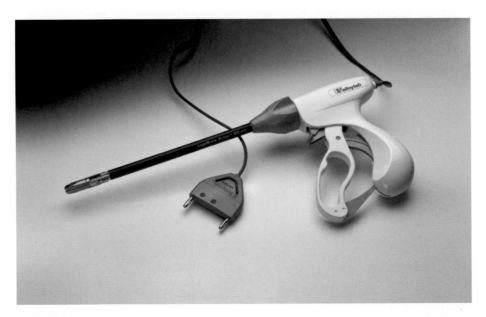

Instrument: LIGASURE
Category: Accessory
Description: The LigaSure system consists of a bipolar radio-frequency generator and forceps. The instruments are designed to mimic standard surgical clamps. They are available in a 7-inch Pean-style clamp (LigaSure Standard), a 9-inch Heaney-style clamp (LigaSure Max), and a 5-mm laparoscopic Maryland-style grasper/dissector (LigaSure Lap).

Use(s): LigaSure works by applying a precise amount of bipolar energy and pressure to change the nature of the vessel walls. The collagen and elastin within the vessel walls fuse and reform into a single structure, obliterating the lumen and creating a permanent seal.
Instrument Insight: Blood and tissue can build up on the jaws and may need to be removed periodically with a moistened sponge.

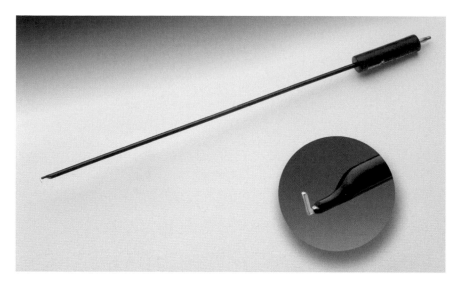

Instrument: L HOOK

Description: It is a long cylinder-insulated rod with an L-shaped monopolar tip. Depending on the model and manufacturer, the electrode can be reusable or disposable and attach to a monopolar cord or directly to the electrosurgical (ESU) pencil.

Use(s): It is used for ESU dissection of tissues and cauterizing vessels.

Instrument Insight: The electrode is insulated at the tip to ensure the current is directed to the targeted tissue. All monopolar electrodes require a dispersive pad on the patient, because the electrical current passes through the patient's body. Before use, carefully inspect the instrument for any breaks in the insulation. Monopolar current travels from the generator to the active electrode, through the patient's body, is captured by the dispersive pad, and is returned the generator.

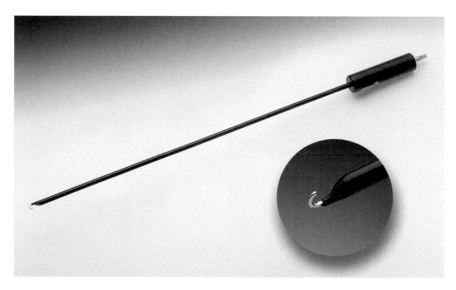

Instrument: J HOOK

Category: Accessory

Description: It is a long cylinder-insulated rod with a J-shaped monopolar tip. Depending on the model and manufacturer, the electrode can be reusable or disposable, and will attach to a monopolar cord or directly to the ESU pencil.

Use(s): It is used for ESU dissection of tissues and cauterizing vessels during laparoscopic procedures.

Instrument Insight: The electrode is insulated at the tip to ensure the current is directed to the targeted tissue. All monopolar electrodes require a dispersive pad placed on the patient, because the electrical current passes through the patient's body. Before use, carefully inspect the instrument for any breaks in the insulation. Monopolar current travels from the generator to the active electrode and through the patient's body; it is captured by the dispersive pad, which channels it back to the generator.

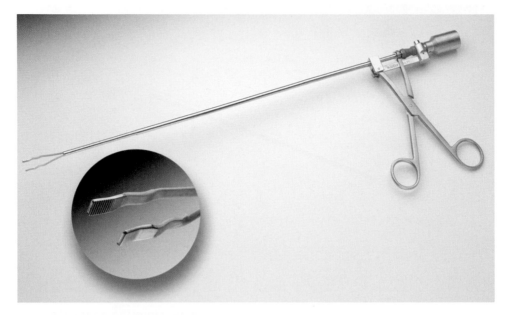

Instrument: KLEPPINGER BIPOLAR FORCEPS
Category: Accessory
Description: Paddle-tip forceps that attach to a bipolar cord. The bipolar energy is activated by grasping the targeted tissues between the jaws and stepping on the foot pedal.
Use(s): It is used for coagulation of tissues and vessels during laparoscopic procedures.

Instrument Insight: Bipolar forceps deliver current from one tip, through the tissue grasped, to the opposite tip. The electrical current does not pass through the patient's body; therefore, no dispersive pad is required.

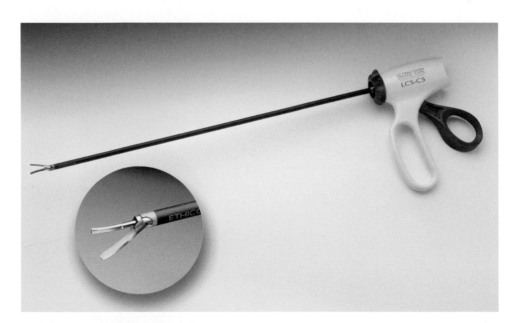

Instrument: ENDO HARMONIC SCALPEL
Other Names: Ultrasonic scalpel
Category: Accessory
Description: This device has a manufacturer-packaged disposable handpiece. A nondisposable cord and wrench are also needed. These are packaged and sterilized by the facility.

Use(s): The harmonic scalpel is a coagulating instrument that delivers ultrasonic energy between the jaws to coagulate and divide tissue through low-temperature cavitation.
Instrument Insight: Blood and tissue can build up on the jaws and may need to be removed periodically with a moist sponge.

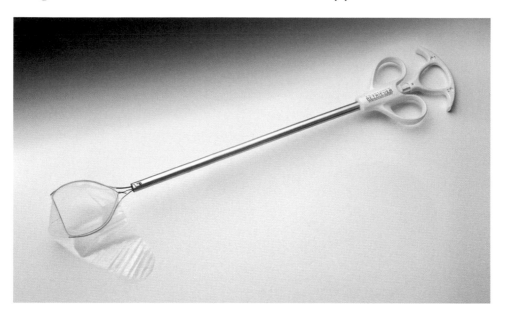

Instrument: ENDO CATCH
Other Names: Endo pouch, Endosac
Category: Accessory
Description: It is a single-use specimen pouch that consists of a long cylindrical tube and a polyurethane pouch. The small pouch has a 2.5-inch opening and is 6 inches in depth; the large pouch has a 5-inch opening and a 9-inch depth.
Use(s): It is used to retrieve and contain specimens while minimizing spillage of contaminates into the abdominal cavity during endoscopic procedures.
Instrument Insight: The small pouch is ideal for the removal of tissues such as the gallbladder, appendix, ectopic pregnancies, ovaries, lymph nodes, other structures, and lung resections. The larger specimen retrieval bag is generally used for advanced procedures including, but not limited to, laparoscopic bowel resections, splenectomies, and nephrectomies.

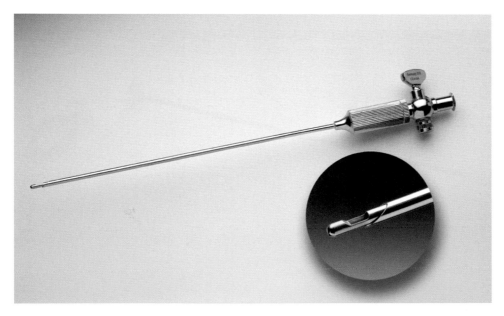

Instrument: VERESS NEEDLE
Other Names: Insufflation needle
Category: Cutting and Dissecting
Description: It is a hollow bore with a spring-loaded, retractable blunt stylet that extends beyond the tip of the needle. A stopcock at the proximal end is the connection site for the insufflation tubing.
Use(s): It is used to enter the peritoneum and deliver carbon dioxide into the abdominal cavity to create a pneumoperitoneum.
Instrument Insight: The stylet retracts as the needle is pushed against tissues, and will automatically advance to cover the needle upon entrance into the peritoneum.

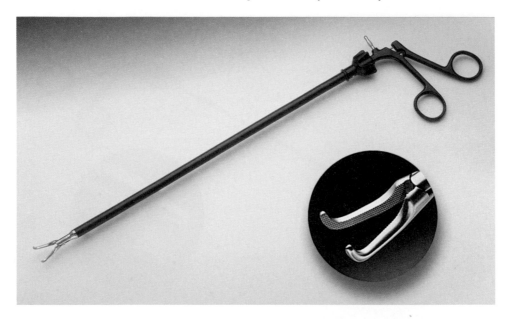

Instrument: ENDO RIGHT-ANGLE DISSECTOR
Other Names: Mixter forceps
Category: Cutting and Dissecting
Description: It has a curved, right-angle tip with cross-hatch serration running the length of the inner jaws.
Use(s): These are used for separating tissue planes and dissecting around tubular structures.

Instrument Insight: As a general rule, dissectors do not have ratchet handles, but graspers do. Often dissectors have monopolar capabilities. The connection site for the cable is the gold stem at the handle end, and the current is activated with a foot pedal.

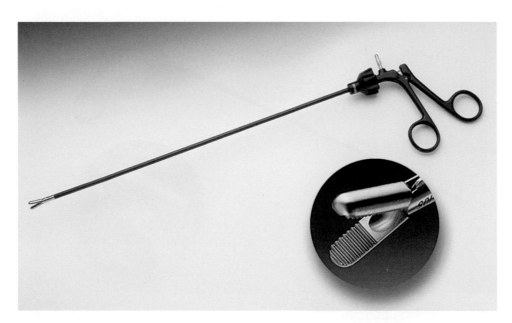

Instrument: BLUNT DISSECTOR
Category: Cutting and Dissecting
Description: It is a straight rounded tip with horizontal serrations and a proximal recess.
Use(s): It is used for blunt dissection and separation of tissue planes.

Instrument Insight: As a general rule, dissectors do not have ratchet handles, but graspers do. Often dissectors have monopolar capabilities. The connection site for the cable is the gold stem at the handle end, and the current is activated with a foot pedal.

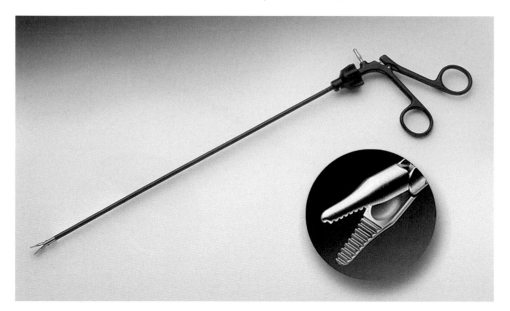

Instrument: DOLPHIN NOSE DISSECTOR
Description: It has straight jaws that taper to a fine point with horizontal serrations and a proximal recess.
Use(s): It is used for fine dissection and separation of thin adventitial tissue.

Instrument Insight: Often dissectors have monopolar capabilities. The connection site for the cable is the gold stem at the handle end, and the current is activated with a foot pedal. As a general rule, dissectors do not have ratchet handles, but graspers do.

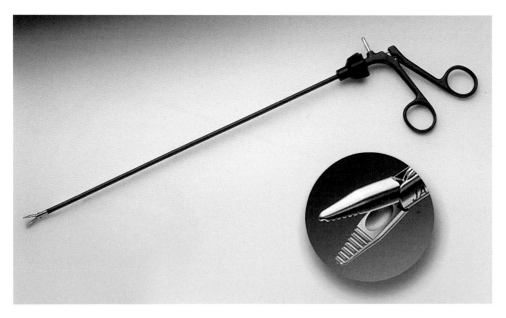

Instrument: CONE TIP DISSECTOR
Other Names: Bullet nose dissector
Category: Cutting and Dissecting
Description: It has bullet-shaped tapered jaws with horizontal serrations and a proximal recess.
Use(s): It is used for blunt dissection and separation of tissue planes.

Instrument Insight: Often dissectors have monopolar capabilities. The connection site for the cable is the gold stem at the handle end, and the current is activated with a foot pedal. As a general rule, dissectors do not have ratchet handles, but graspers do.

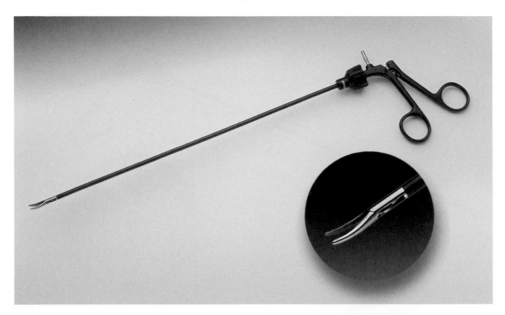

Instrument: MARYLAND DISSECTOR
Category: Cutting and Dissecting
Description: It has curved, fine-tapered jaws with horizontal serrations running the length of the jaws.
Use(s): It is used for fine dissection and separation of thin adventitial tissue.

Instrument Insight: Often dissectors have monopolar capabilities. The connection site for the cable is the gold stem at the handle end, and the current is activated with a foot pedal. As a general rule, dissectors do not have ratchet handles, but graspers do.

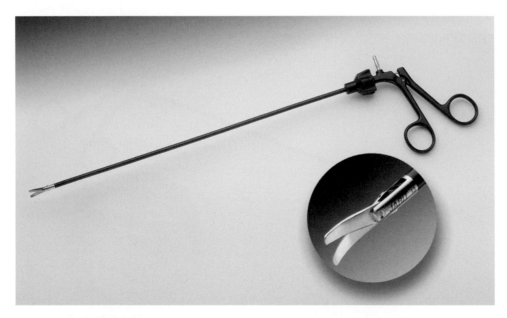

Instrument: ENDOSCOPIC SCISSORS
Other Names: Endo shears, coag scissors
Category: Cutting and Dissecting
Description: I has rounded, blunt tip with curved blades.
Use(s): It is used to cut and dissect tissues, ducts, vessels, and suture material.

Instrument Insight: Generally endo scissors have monopolar capabilities. The connection site for the cable is the gold stem at the handle end, and the current is activated with a foot pedal.

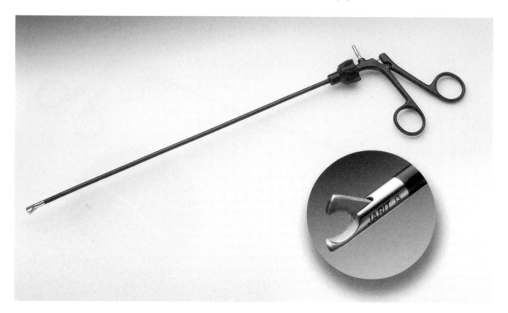

Instrument: **ENDOSCOPIC HOOK SCISSORS**
Category: Cutting and Dissecting
Description: It has straight, squared-off blunt tip with concave arching of the inner cutting blades.
Use(s): It is used to lift, isolate, and transect tissues such as ducts and vessels.

Instrument Insight: Generally endo scissors have monopolar capabilities. The connection site for the cable is the gold stem at the handle end, and the current is activated with a foot pedal.

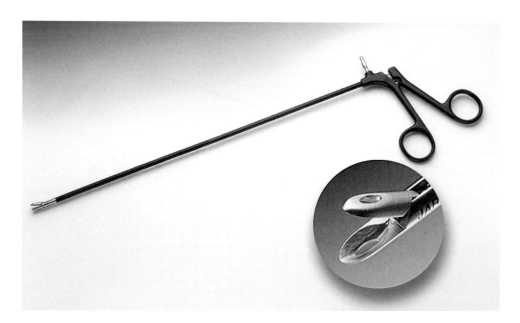

Instrument: **ENDOSCOPIC BIOPSY FORCEPS**
Category: Cutting and Dissecting
Description: It has sharp, oval cup-shaped jaws that are fenestrated.
Use(s): These are used for excision of small pieces of tissue for examination.

Instrument Insight: To prevent crushing or damaging the biopsy tissue, it can be swished in saline or pushed out with a fine needle through the fenestration in the jaws.

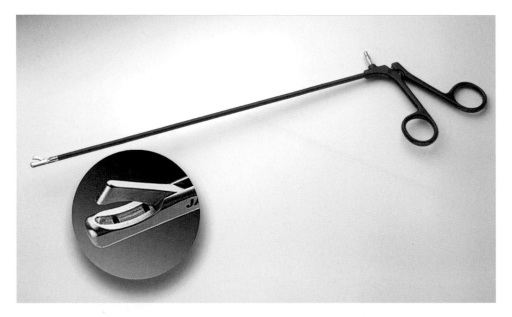

Instrument: ENDOSCOPIC BIOPSY PUNCH
Category: Cutting and Dissecting
Description: It has rectangular-shaped hollow jaws; the upper jaw has a sharp rim that fits inside the serrated edge of the lower jaw when closed.

Use(s): It is used for excision of small pieces of heavy tissue for examination.
Instrument Insight: To prevent crushing or damaging the biopsy tissue, it can be swished in saline or pushed out with a fine needle.

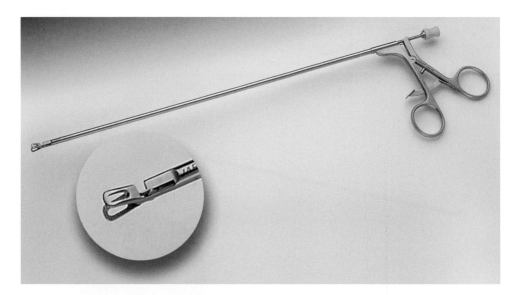

Instrument: ENDOSCOPIC CHOLANGIOGRAM FORCEPS
Other Names: Olsen clamp
Category: Grasping and Holding
Description: These are long grasping forceps with a proximal port that leads to rounded fenestrated and horizontally serrated jaws.
Use(s): These forceps are used to grasp the cholangiogram catheter and guide it into the

common bile duct for injection of the contrast medium.
Instrument Insight: The cholangiogram catheter is fed through the proximal port until the tip extends just beyond the jaws of the forceps. The forceps are then closed, holding the catheter in place.

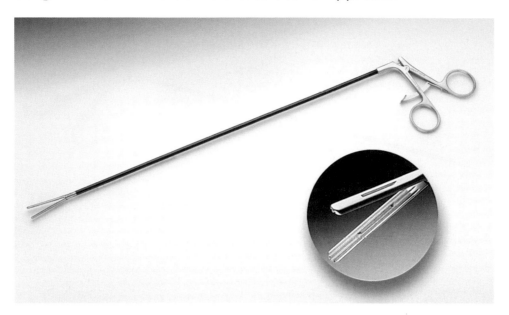

Instrument: ENDOSCOPIC DEBAKEY FORCEPS
Category: Grasping and Holding
Description: These have fenestrated elongated jaws with a blunt tip and two parallel rows of fine serrations running the length of one jaw and one row of serrations in the center on the other. These interlock when the instrument is closed.
Use(s): These are used for grasping tissues and organs without causing trauma.

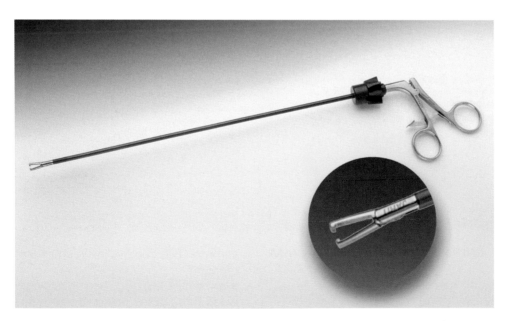

Instrument: ENDOSCOPIC ALLIS FORCEPS
Category: Grasping and Holding
Description: These have straight jaws with multiple, intertwining fine teeth at the tip.

Use(s): These are used for grasping, holding, and retracting slippery dense tissue.

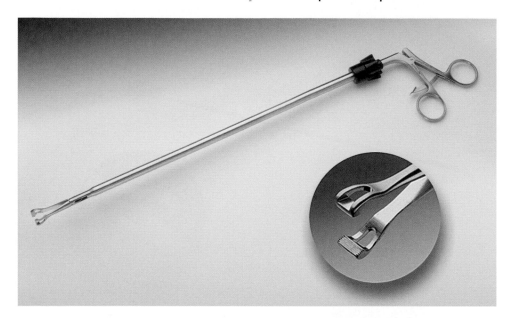

Instrument: ENDOSCOPIC BABCOCK FORCEPS
Category: Grasping and Holding
Description: It has a flared, rounded end with smooth, flattened tips. It comes in 5- and 10-mm and can be either disposable or nondisposable.

Use(s): These are used for grasping and encircling delicate structures such as the ureters, fallopian tubes, ovaries, appendix, or bowel.

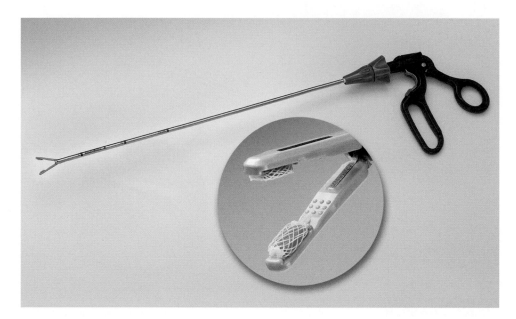

Instrument: ATRAC GRASPER
Other Names: Direct drive grasper, atraumatic grasper
Category: Grasping and Holding
Description: The working tip of Atrac grasper has a padded jaw with a mesh grip overlay. These are manufactured in completely disposable, or disposable inserts with a reusable handle.

Use(s): It is used to grasp bowel and other delicate structures.
Instrument Insight: The one pictured is a two-piece grasper in which the jaw inserts screw into the handle. The jaw insert is a single-patient use (disposable), and the handle is reprocessed to be used again.

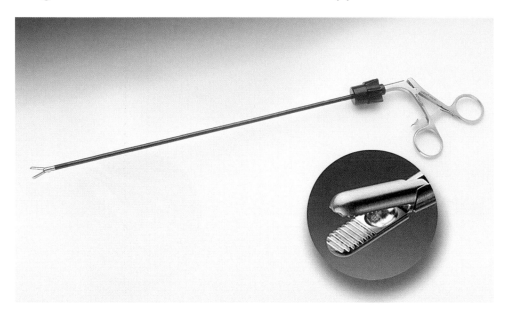

Instrument: BLUNT GRASPER
Category: Grasping and Holding
Description: It has a straight rounded tip with horizontal serrations and a proximal recess.

Use(s): It is used for grasping and manipulating tissues and organs, causing minimal trauma. These graspers are often used on tissue that is to be removed.

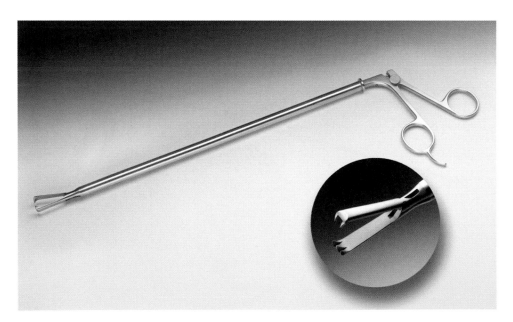

Instrument: CLAW GRASPER
Other Names: Mother-in-law grasper
Category: Grasping and Holding
Description: It has wide, elongated spring-loaded jaws with 2 × 3 heavy interlocking teeth.
Use(s): It is used for penetrating and holding excised organs and tissues for extraction from the abdominal cavity.

Instrument Insight: As a general rule, graspers have ratcheted handles, but dissectors do not.

⚠ **CAUTION:** Exercise care when handling penetrating forceps. The sharp tips can easily comprise the integrity of gloves or skin.

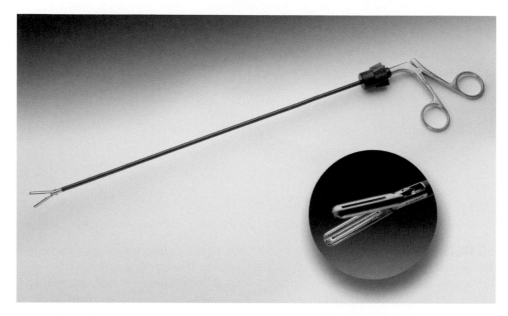

Instrument: HUNTER BOWEL GRASPER
Category: Grasping and Holding
Description: It has fine, long jaws with rounded tips and DeBakey-style serrations.

Use(s): It is used for atraumatic grasping and manipulating delicate tissues, such as the bowel and stomach.

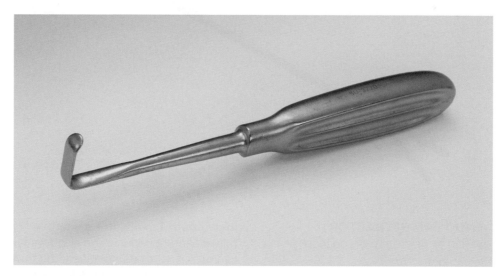

Instrument: POLE RETRACTOR
Other Names: Lahey retractor
Category: Retracting and Exposing
Description: It is a handheld retractor with a thin right-angle blade and a thick oval handle.

Use(s): It is often used for exposure when placing the umbilical trocar when using the Hasson technique in laparoscopic and robotics procedures. May also be used during thyroid and radical neck surgeries.

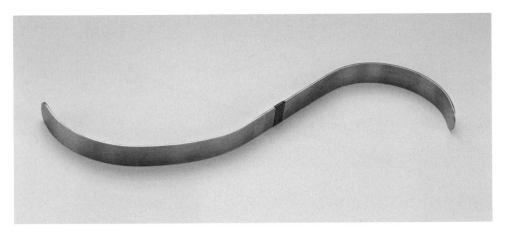

Instrument: S RETRACTOR
Other Names: Snake retractor
Category: Retracting and Exposing
Description: This is a double-ended thin metal ribbon formed in an S shape. One end has less of a curve than the other.

Use(s): It is often used for exposure when placing the umbilical trocar when using the Hasson technique in laparoscopic and robotic procedures. It may also be used on small wounds such as breast biopsies.

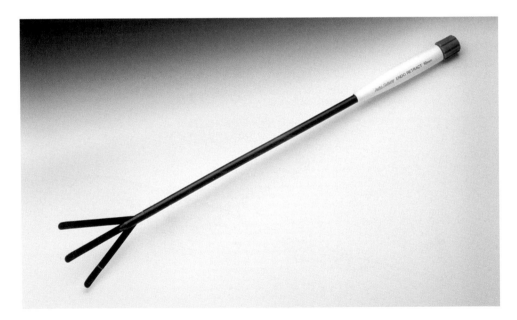

Instrument: ENDO FAN RETRACTOR
Other Names: Fan finger retractor, peacock retractor
Category: Retracting and Exposing
Description: It is a single-use retractor with three or five telescoping atraumatic blades.
Use(s): It is used for elevation, retraction, and mobilization of organs and tissues, providing optimal visualization of the surgical field.

Instrument Insight: The finger blades should be fully closed upon insertion and removal from the cannula. The blades are closed by turning the proximal teal knob counterclockwise and are deployed by turning the knob clockwise.

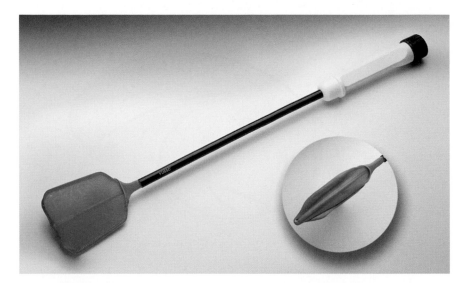

Instrument: ENDO PADDLE RETRACTOR
Category: Retracting and Exposing
Description: It is a single-use retractor with a nylon-covered paddle frame, introducer sheath with seal housing, and black rotation knob.
Use(s): Used for elevation, retraction, and mobilization of organs and tissues, providing optimal visualization of the surgical field.
Instrument Insight: To retract the paddle, turn the rotation knob clockwise until the paddle is fully closed. Push the white seal housing forward until the paddle is completely housed inside the introducer sheath. Grasp the seal housing, and insert the retractor through the trocar cannula. After it is inserted through the cannula, pull the seal housing back completely, exposing the paddle. Turn the rotation knob counterclockwise to deploy the paddle within the body cavity. The paddle must be fully retracted and housed in the introducer sheath before removal.

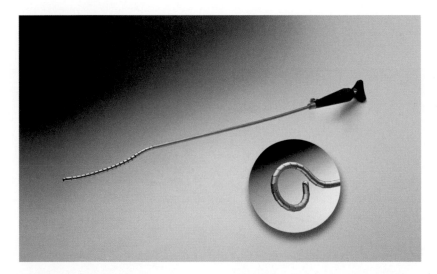

Instrument: ENDOFLEX RETRACTOR
Other Name: Snake retractor, Diamond-flex retractor
Category: Retracting and Exposing
Description: The device originates as snake-like, malleable, hollow, 5-mm metal tubes with small individual sections at the working end that are threaded over internal tension cables affixed at the tip. Each tubular section is cut obliquely so that when the inner metal cables are tightened by turning the knob on the handle, the retractors conform to its designated shape.
Use(s): It is used for elevation, retraction, and mobilization of abdominal organs, providing optimal visualization during endoscopic procedures. Commonly used for retraction of the liver in complex upper gastrointestinal procedures, such as fundoplication and gastric bypass.
Instrument Insight: Normally, the retractor is inserted loose and flexible through a 5-mm port and articulated after being placed within the abdominal cavity to form the retractor.

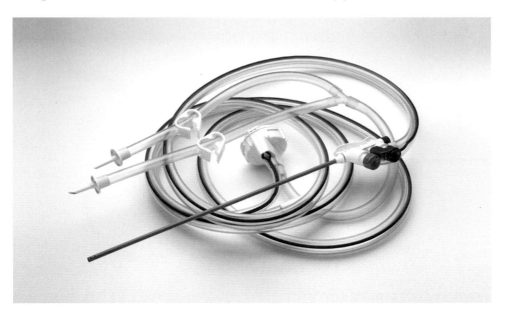

Instrument: SUCTION IRRIGATOR
Category: Suctioning and Aspirating
Description: It is a long, straight, and hollow suction tube attached to a combination tubing that has a suction valve and an irrigation valve.

Use(s): It is used to irrigate and aspirate fluid and debris from the surgical site.
Instrument Insight: There are many types and manufacturers of suction irrigators, such as gravity, pump, or battery operated.

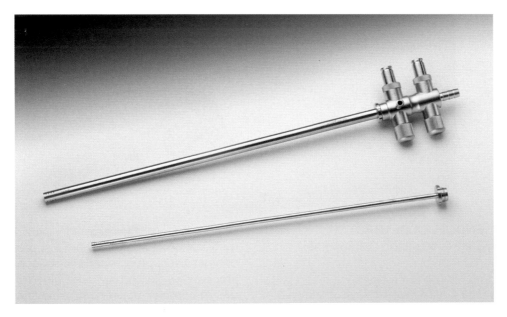

Instrument: NEZHAT-DORSEY SUCTION TIPS
Category: Suctioning and Aspirating
Description: It is a long, hollow suction tip with a bivalve. One is for suction and the other for irrigation.

Use(s): This suction tip is used for irrigating and aspirating fluid and debris from the surgical site.

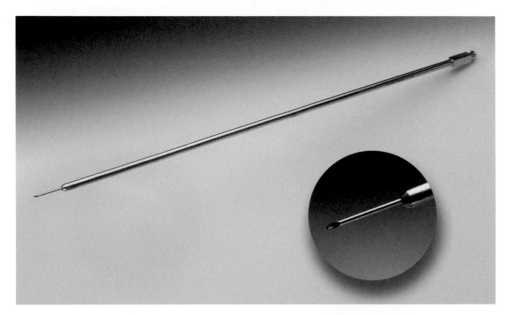

Instrument: ENDOSCOPIC ASPIRATING NEEDLE
Category: Retracting and Exposing
Description: The proximal end of this is a Luer-Lok fitting that is attached to a long 5-mm hollow tube with a 19-gauge needle tip.
Use(s): This needle is used for the aspiration of body fluids and cysts.

⚠ **CAUTION:** The tip should be within the vision of the operator at all times when in the abdominal cavity. The aspiration is accomplished by attaching a syringe or suction.

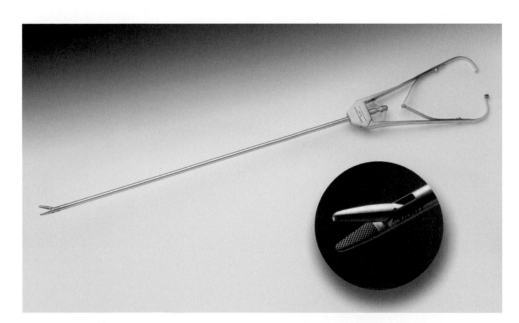

Instrument: APPLE NEEDLE HOLDER
Category: Suturing and Stapling
Description: It is tapered straight, curved, or angled tip with cross-hatch carbon-bite inner jaws and a leaf-spring mechanism handle for ease in release and closure.

Use(s): It is used to securely grasp the needle during suturing.
Instrument Insight: The apple needle holder is designed for grasping 5–0 and smaller needles.

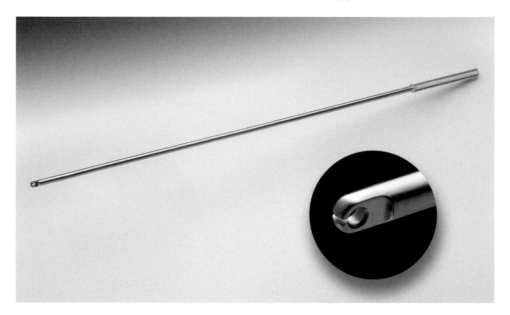

Instrument: **KNOT PUSHER**
Category: Suctioning and Aspirating
Description: It is a long cylindrical rod with a round hole toward the end and a transverse slot at the very tip.
Use(s): It guides knots from outside of the trocar cannula to the suture site. This technique is known as extracorporeal suturing.

Instrument Insight: The throw of the suture is placed into the open slot and slid into the round hole; it is then guided through the cannula to the suture site, which sets the knot. This action is repeated until the knot is secure.

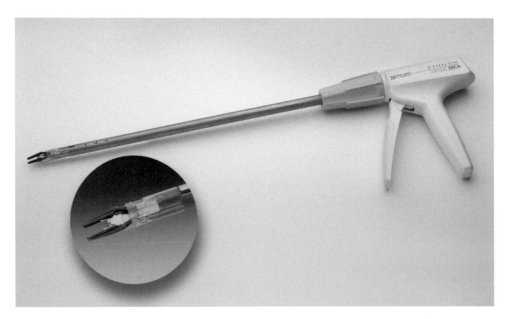

Instrument: **ENDO CLIP APPLIER**
Other Names: Hemoclip applier, clip applier
Category: Suturing and Stapling
Description: A sterile, single-patient-use instrument, preloaded with clips. These are

manufactured in various titanium clip sizes from 5–10 mm and different lengths.
Use(s): It is used for occluding vessels or other tubular structures.

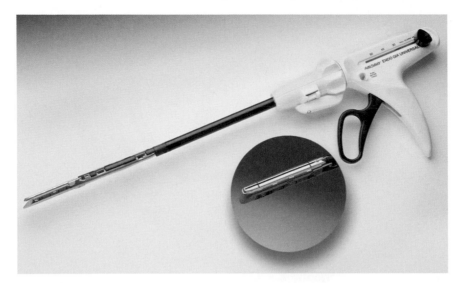

Instrument: ENDO GIA STAPLER
Category: Suturing and Stapling
Description: It is a single-patient-use, reloadable articulating and rotating stapler that distributes two triple staggered rows of titanium staples while cutting the tissues between the rows. The length is determined by the tissue to be excised. This stapler is available in 30-mm, 45-mm, and 60-mm sizes.
Use(s): It is often used during laparoscopic appendectomy and gastric and bowel resections.

It is also used to transect tissues in endoscopic thoracic or gynecologic procedures.
Instrument Insight: The stapler loads come packaged with a bright-colored plastic safety guard over the row of staples that need to be removed before handing it to the surgeon. Activation is accomplished by sliding forward the firing knob on the side of the stapler until it stops completely. The manufacturer recommends that the stapler can be reloaded up to 25 times for a total of 25 applications.

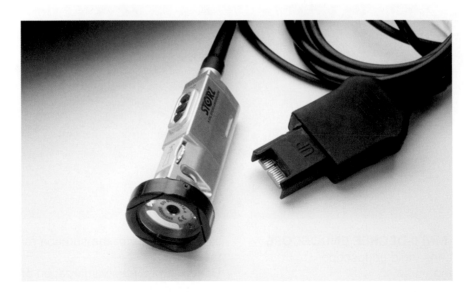

Instrument: ENDOSCOPIC CAMERA
Category: Viewing
Description: At the distal end of the endoscopic camera is the coupler that attaches the camera to the eyepiece of the rigid scope. The coupler is attached to the camera head, which provides the image quality. Attached to the camera head is a cord, which relays the images back to the video system.

Use(s): It is used for the transmission of images from the rigid or flexible endoscope to the video monitor.
Instrument Insight: Most camera failures are related to a damaged cord. Care should be taken when handling the camera and cord. They should never be placed under a heavy object or dropped, twisted, or kinked. Also, keep the distal end covered until it is ready to be plugged into the unit.

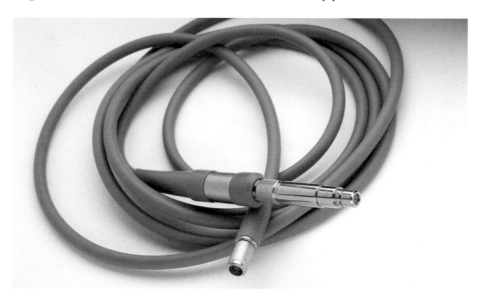

Instrument: **FIBEROPTIC LIGHT CORD**
Other Names: Light cord
Description: It is a 10-foot-long fiber optic cable with an endoscope adapter at the proximal end and a light source adapter at the distal end.
Use(s): It is used for illumination during endoscopic procedures; delivers high-intensity light through the endoscope.
Instrument Insight: Exercise care when handling a fiber optic cord; it should never be placed under a heavy object, dropped, twisted, or kinked, because the tiny fibers inside can be easily damaged.

⚠ CAUTION: When not in use, the light source must be placed on standby or turned off. The intense heat from the beam can cause the patient's drapes or any flammable vapors around the patient to ignite.

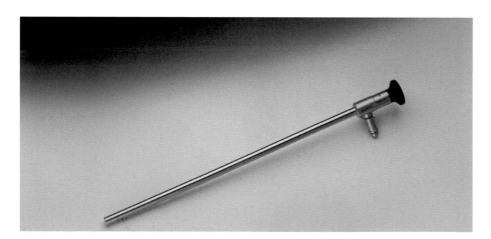

Instrument: **10-MM 0-DEGREE ENDOSCOPE**
Other Names: Lens, rigid endoscope
Category: Viewing
Description: It is a rigid, stainless steel, 10-mm endoscope containing an optical chain of precisely aligned glass lenses and spacers. The objective lens is located at the distal tip of the scope. This determines the viewing angle. The stainless steel cylinder rod is called the optical element of the telescope, providing both images and light. The light connector allows the attachment of the light cord to the telescope. At the proximal end is the eyepiece or ocular lens; this attaches to the camera coupler, or the surgeon may directly view the cavity.
Use(s): It provides visualization of body cavities and contents, which may include internal organs and structures, through an orifice or surgical opening.
Instrument Insight: The 10 mm indicates the diameter of the scope, and 0 degrees is the forward angle in which the objective lens views. Endoscopes are expensive and fragile. When handling an endoscope, grip it by the eyepiece and not the shaft, and it should not be dropped. Heavy objects should not be placed on top of it.

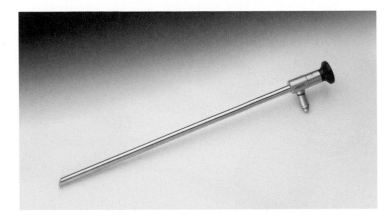

Instrument: 10-MM 30-DEGREE ENDOSCOPE
Other Names: Lens, rigid endoscope
Category: Viewing
Description: It is a nonflexible, stainless steel, 10-mm endoscope containing an optical chain of precisely aligned glass lenses and spacers. The objective lens is located at the distal tip of the scope. This determines the viewing angle. The stainless steel cylinder rod is called the optical element of the telescope, providing both images and light. The light connector allows the attachment of the light cord to the telescope. At the proximal end is the eyepiece or ocular lens; this attaches to the camera coupler, or the surgeon may directly view the cavity.

Use(s): It is used for visualization of body cavities, internal organs, and structures through an orifice or surgical opening.
Instrument Insight: The 10 mm indicates the diameter of the scope, and 30 degrees is the oblique angle in which the objective lens views.

⚠ **CAUTION:** Endoscopes are expensive and fragile.
 When handling an endoscope, grip it by the eyepiece and not the shaft, and it should not be dropped. Heavy objects should not be placed on top of it.

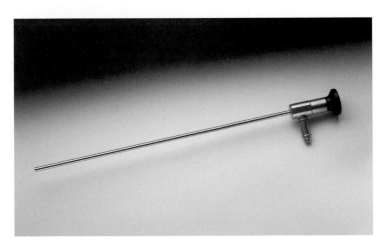

Instrument: 5-MM 0-DEGREE ENDOSCOPE
Other Names: Lens, rigid endoscope
Category: Viewing
Description: It is a nonflexible, stainless steel, 5-mm endoscope containing an optical chain of precisely aligned glass lenses and spacers. The objective lens is located at the distal tip of the scope. This determines the viewing angle. The stainless steel cylinder rod is called the optical element of the telescope, providing both images and light. The light connector allows the attachment of the light cord to the telescope. At the proximal end is the eyepiece or ocular lens; this attaches to the camera coupler, or the surgeon may directly view the cavity.
Use(s): It is used for visualization of body cavities, internal organs, and structures through an orifice or surgical opening.
Instrument Insight: The 5 mm indicates the diameter of the scope, and 0 degrees is the forward angle in which the objective lens views.

⚠ **CAUTION:** Endoscopes are expensive and fragile.
 When handling an endoscope, grip it by the eyepiece and not the shaft, and it should not be dropped. Heavy objects should not be placed on top of it.

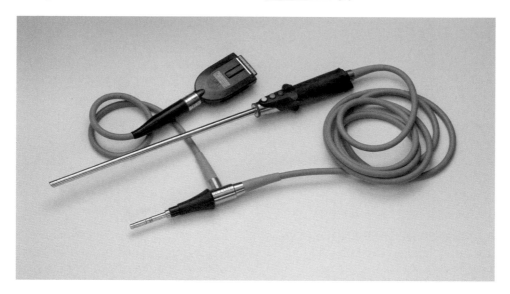

Instrument: ENDOEYE
Other Names: Scope, endoscope
Category: Viewing
Description: This is an all-in-one endoscope with a camera, endoscope, and light cord combined. The ENDOEYE diameter is either 10 or 5 mm with a directional view of 0 or 30 degrees.

Instrument Insight: The ENDOEYE is fully autoclavable.
Use(s): It is used for the visualization of body cavities, internal organs, and other structures through an instrument port in laparoscopic procedures.

6

Robotic Instruments

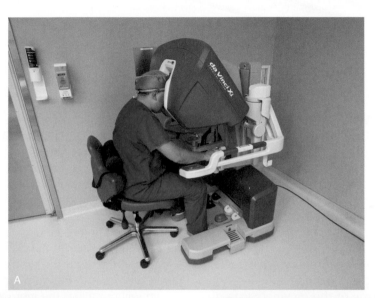

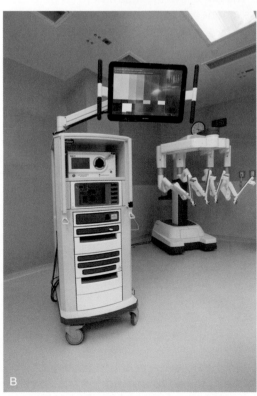

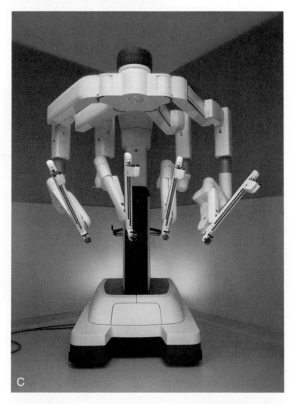

The da Vinci System consists of a console where the surgeon sits while operating, a patient side cart with interactive robotic arms that is docked over the patient during the procedure, a three-dimensional (3D) high-density (HD) vision system, and EndoWrist instruments.

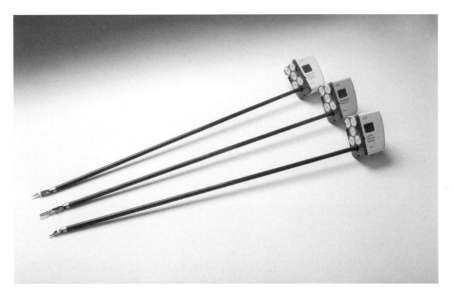

Instrument: ENDOWRIST TIPS

Description: The EndoWrist tips are characterized by instruments that are commonly used by the surgeons in open and minimally invasive surgeries; these include scissors, forceps, retractors, scalpels, electrocautery, and others that are commonly used devices. These are approximately 5 to 8 mm in diameter and between 49 and 51 cm in length.

Use(s): The EndoWrist instruments are modeled after the human wrist and fasten to the electromechanical arms of the da Vinci System. These instruments offer full range of motion and natural dexterity that represents the surgeon's right and left hands when performing intricate tissue manipulation and dissection through minute ports. The da Vinci System is commonly used for, but not limited to, gynecologic, urologic, general, cardiovascular, thoracic, and otorhinolaryngologic specialties.

Instrument Insight: EndoWrist instruments are called "smart disposables" because they are resterilized and reused for a distinct number of procedures. An internal computer chip confirms the manufacturer, the type and function of the instrument, and the number of past uses. The chip will not allow the instrument to be used if it has exceeded the approved number of procedures. This ensures proper performance of the instrument during every procedure.

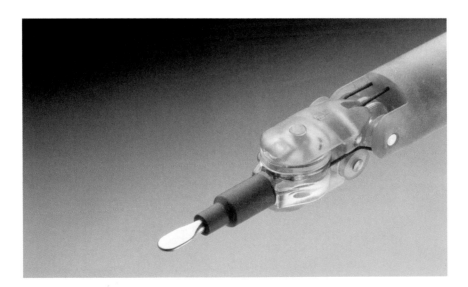

Instrument: PERMANENT CAUTERY SPATULA

Other Names: Bovie spatula, cautery spatula
Category: Accessory
Description: It is a monopolar cautery device with a long paddle blade.

Use(s): It is used to coagulate tissues and maintain hemostasis and aid in blunt dissection.
Instrument Insight: All of the EndoWrist instruments that have electrosurgical capabilities have amber-colored insulation at the wrist joint.

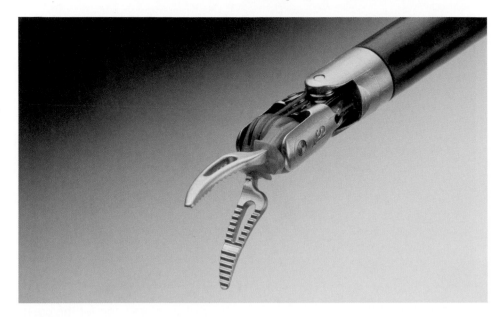

Instrument: MARYLAND BIPOLAR FORCEPS
Other Names: Bipolar forceps, Maryland forceps
Category: Accessory
Description: It is a bipolar device with curved tapered jaws and triangular fenestration at the base.

Use(s): It is used for grasping, dissecting, and coagulating tissues.
Instrument Insight: All of the EndoWrist instruments that have electrosurgical capabilities have amber-colored insulation at the wrist joint.

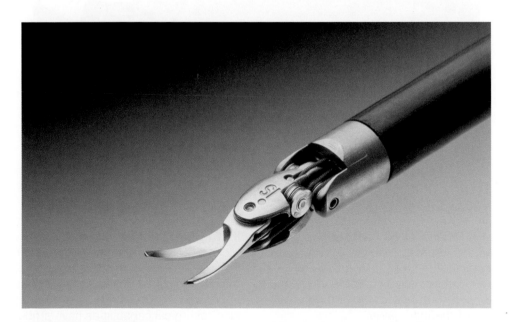

Instrument: CURVED SCISSORS
Other Names: Shears
Category: Cutting and Dissecting
Description: These are curved, beveled blades with tapered atraumatic tips.

Use(s): These are used for precision cutting and sharp and blunt dissection of tissue.

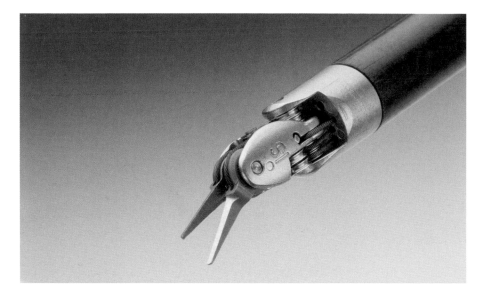

Instrument: POTTS SCISSORS
Category: Cutting and Dissecting
Description: These are straight, fine, tapered, beveled blades.

Use(s): These are used for the creation of an arteriotomy for coronary anastomosis.

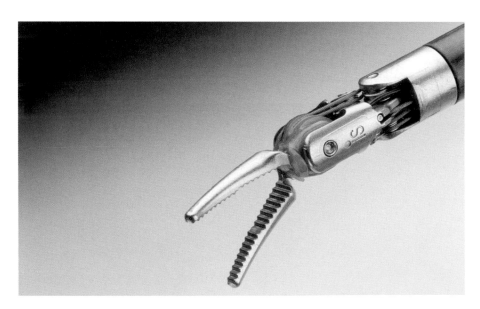

Instrument: PK DISSECTING FORCEPS
Other Names: PK forceps
Category: Accessory
Description: PK forceps have curved and tapering outer jaws with horizontal serration that runs the length of the inner jaws.
Use(s): This is used for grasping, coagulating, and cutting tissues.

Instrument Insight: The PK forceps provide radiofrequency energy to seal, transect, and mobilize tissues at a low temperature, which minimizes tissue sticking, charring, and plume.

All of the EndoWrist instruments that have electrosurgical capabilities have amber-colored insulation at the wrist joint.

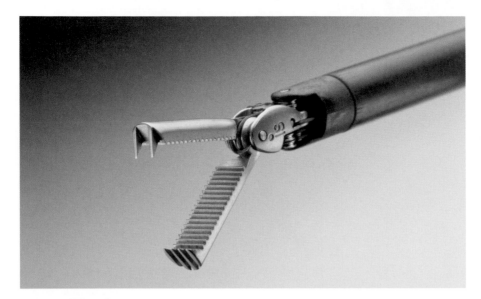

Instrument: COBRA GRASPER
Other Names: Biter, toothed grasper
Category: Grasping and Holding
Description: It has straight jaws with horizontal serration running the length. At the tip, one jaw has two sharp teeth and the other has four, and when closed, they interlock.

Use(s): The cobra grasper is used for grasping and retracting dense tissues. Commonly used for grasping the pelvic fascial layers during cuff closure in a hysterectomy.

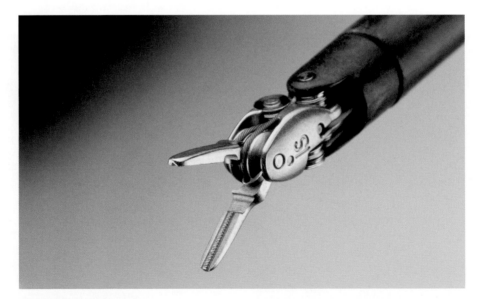

Instrument: DEBAKEY FORCEPS
Category: Grasping and Holding
Description: These are straight, smooth forceps with an elongated, narrowed blunt tip. A set of parallel fine serrations runs the length of one jaw with a center row of serrations on the opposite side that interlocks to grip when closed.

Use(s): These are used to facilitate atraumatic tissue handling.
Instrument Insight: Debakey forceps are considered to be vascular tissue forceps, but are commonly used in all specialty areas because of their ability to securely grip without causing damage to tissues.

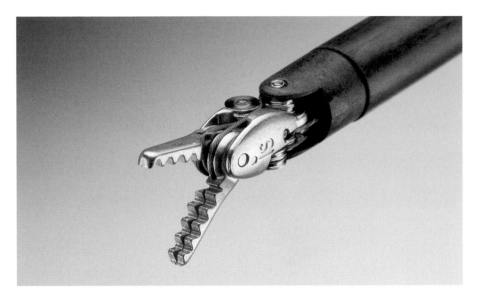

Instrument: RESANO FORCEPS
Other Names: Shark forceps
Category: Grasping and Holding
Description: These have smooth, straight outer jaws with blunt triangular serrations that interlock when closed.

Use(s): These facilitate firm but atraumatic handling of valve and arterial tissues.

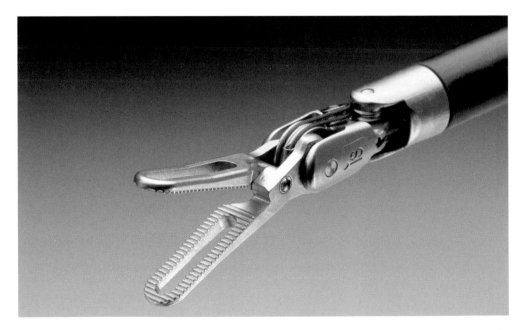

Instrument: PROGRASP FORCEPS
Other Names: Delicate grasper, fenestrated forceps
Category: Grasping and Holding
Description: These have smooth, flattened wide outer jaws with an oval fenestration in the middle and horizontal serrations running the length of the inner jaws.
Use(s): These are used to grasp and retract delicate tissues. Also these are commonly used to grasp and retract bowel during abdominal procedures.

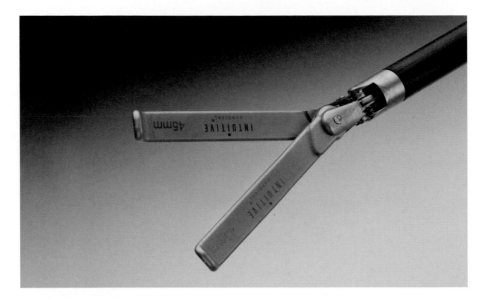

Instrument: ATRIAL RETRACTOR
Other Names: Fan retractor, finger retractor
Category: Retracting and Exposing
Description: It has two straight atraumatic blades with a slight curve at the end.
Use(s): The atrial retractor provides exposure of the mitral valve and atrial retraction. It is often used during a mitral valve repair.

Instrument Insight: The two blades of the atrial retractor draw in on one another to resemble one blade, which facilitates insertion into a tiny port.

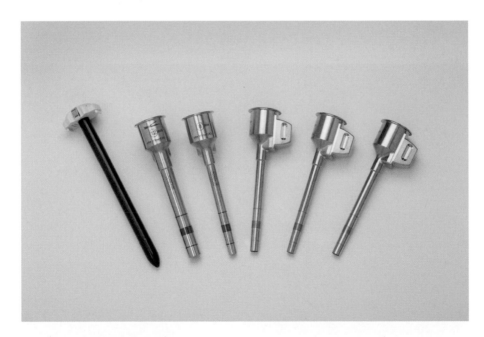

Instrument: DA VINCI ROBOTIC PORTS
Other Names: Nondisposable ports
Category: Probing and Dilating
Description: Da Vinci provides 8-mm and 12-mm reusable steel cannulas with disposable seals for the robotic arms. They come with a bladeless obturator for insertion. These come in two lengths, short (11-cm cannula) and long (16-cm cannula), for high body mass index (BMI) patients.

Use(s): These are used to create a port through which the robotic endoscope and instruments can be introduced and exchanged.
Instrument Insight: The port positions are determined by size of patient, procedure, surgeon, and target anatomy. Placements of the trocars are framed to maximize endoscopic view, instrument reach, and to minimize external arm clashing.

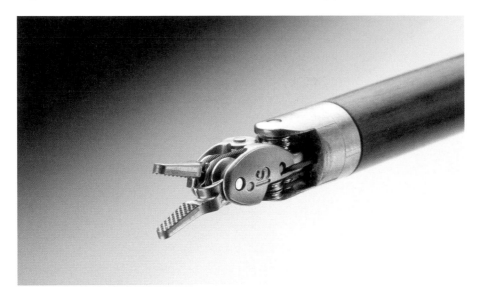

Instrument: SUTURECUT NEEDLE DRIVER
Category: Suturing and Stapling
Description: It has tapered, smooth outer jaws with cross-hatch serrations on the inner jaws and scissor blades at the base.
Use(s): It is used for grasping needles and cutting sutures. It is often used when placing interrupted sutures; also used when closing the vaginal cuff during a hysterectomy.
Instrument Insight: Suturing and cutting with one instrument reduces instrument exchange and saves time.

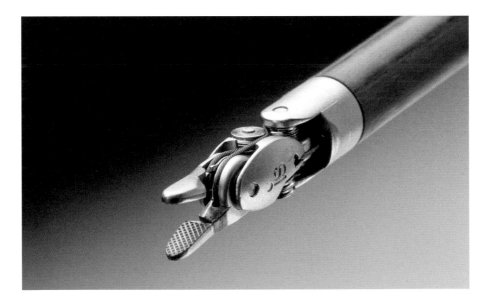

Instrument: LARGE NEEDLE DRIVER
Other Names: Large needle holder
Category: Suturing and Stapling
Description: It has a straight, smooth, tapering outer jaw with diamond pattern carbide inserts in the inner jaw.
Use(s): It is used for securing the needle while suturing tissues.
Instrument Insight: The carbide inserts give the needle holder better gripping properties to secure the needle.

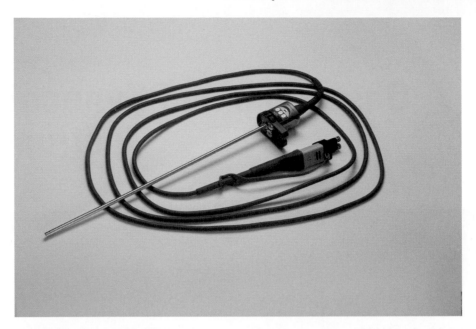

Instrument: DA VINCI ENDOSCOPE
Category: Viewing
Description: This is an all-in-one endoscope with camera, endoscope, and light cord combined. There are two sizes of endoscopes, 8.5- and 12-mm; both have a 0-degree directional view.

Use(s): It is used for the visualization of body cavities, internal organs, and other structures through an instrument port in robotic surgery.
Instrument Insight: These endoscopes are created with crystal clear 3D HD optics.

This allows surgeons to see anatomic structures with heightened clarity and in natural color.

7

Obstetrics and Gynecologic Instruments

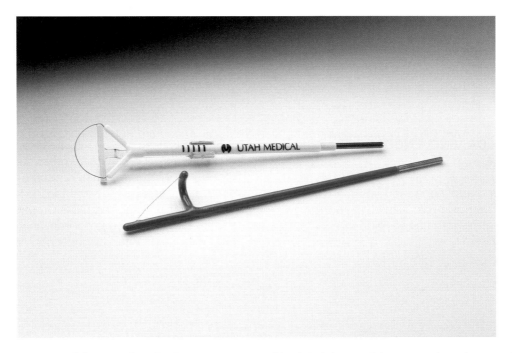

Instrument: LEEP LOOP ELECTRODE
Other Names: Loop
Category: Accessory
Description: Loops come in different shapes and sizes. Most loops have an insulated shaft and crossbar to prevent accidental thermal injury with the stainless-steel or tungsten wire of the loop that is approximately 0.2-mm thick.

Use(s): It is used for removing abnormal cervical cells electrosurgically for further pathologic examination. This procedure is often called a hot-cone biopsy.
Instrument Insight: The size and shape of the loop will be determined by the amount of cervical dysplasia and surgeon preference.

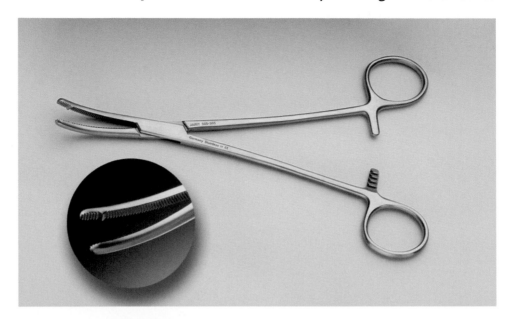

Instrument: HEANEY HYSTERECTOMY FORCEPS
Other Names: Hyster clamp, Heaney clamp
Category: Clamping and Occluding
Description: It has a heavy clamp with horizontal serrations running the length of the jaws and with a single tooth on the inner jaws.

Use(s): These are used for clamping vessels and uterine ligaments during a hysterectomy.
Instrument Insight: The tooth or teeth are not sharp but provide greater gripping capabilities.

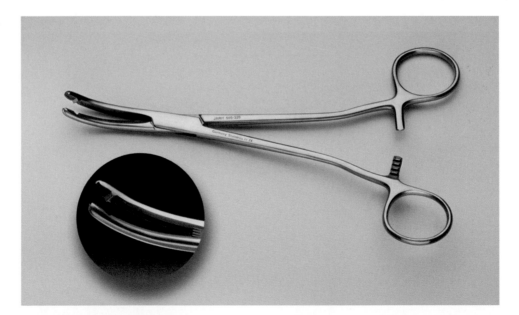

Instrument: HEANEY-BALLENTINE HYSTERECTOMY FORCEPS
Other Names: Heaney clamp, Masterson clamp
Category: Clamping and Occluding
Description: It has a heavy clamp with vertical serrations running the length of the jaws and with a single or double tooth on the inner jaws; it can have either straight or curved jaws.
Use(s): These are used for clamping vessels and ligaments during a hysterectomy.
Instrument Insight: The tooth or teeth are not sharp but provide greater gripping capabilities.

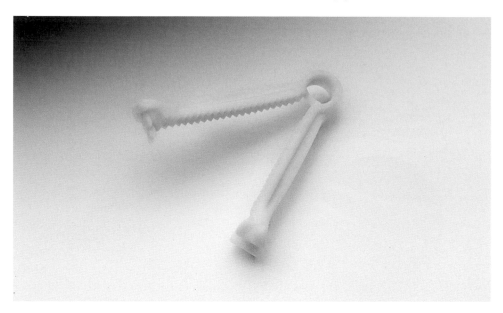

Instrument: CORD CLAMP
Category: Clamping and Occluding
Description: It has a plastic disposable clamp with horizontal serrations running the length of the jaws.
Use(s): It is used to clamp the umbilical cord of the neonate; the cord remains attached to the newborn following separation from the placenta.
Instrument Insight: The cord clamp is a single-use device and should not be closed before use because this can damage its reliability.

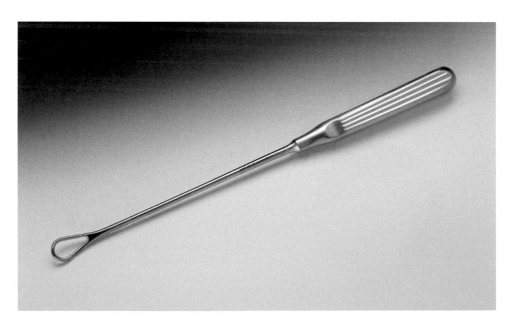

Instrument: THOMAS UTERINE CURETTE
Other Names: Blunt curette
Category: Cutting and Dissecting
Description: It has a hollow grip handle that extends to a malleable shaft and a blunt looped tip.
Use(s): It is used for bluntly removing uterine contents after sharp curetting.

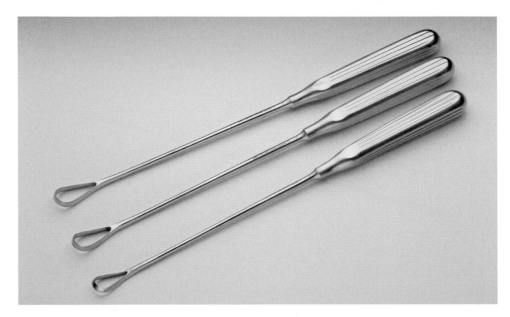

Instrument: **SHARP UTERINE CURETTE**
Other Names: Sharp curette
Category: Cutting and Dissecting
Description: It has a hollow grip handle that extends to a malleable shaft and a sharp looped tip.

Use(s): It is used for scraping the endocervical and endometrial lining of the uterus during a dilation and curettage (D&C) procedure.
Instrument Insight: The shaft is malleable so that the surgeon can bend it to the angle needed to scrape the uterus.

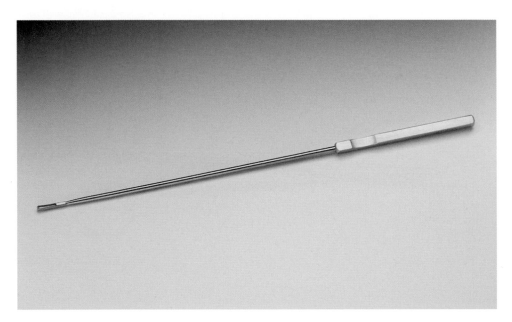

Instrument: **KEVORKIAN-YOUNGE ENDOCERVICAL CURETTE**
Other Names: Kevorkian curette, endocervical curette, box curette
Category: Cutting and Dissecting

Description: It has a grip handle that extends to a narrow and sharp rectangular tip.
Use(s): It is used for obtaining cervical scrapings or biopsies.

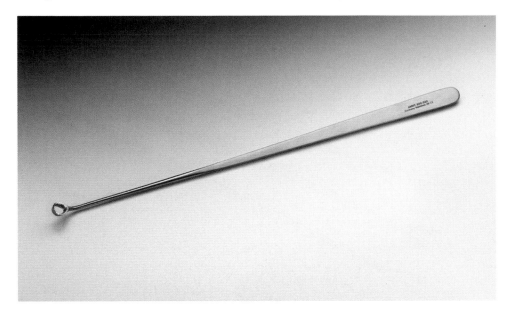

Instrument: HEANEY UTERINE BIOPSY CURETTE
Category: Cutting and Dissecting
Description: It has a flattened handle that extends to a sharp, serrated looped tip.

Use(s): It is used for obtaining uterine scrapings.

⚠ **CAUTION:** The serrations are sharp and can easily compromise the integrity of your gloves and skin, and those of the surgeon.

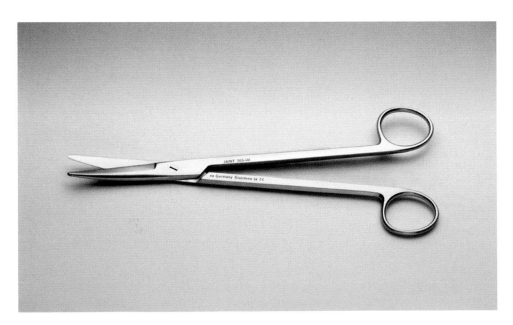

Instrument: MAYO UTERINE SCISSORS
Other Names: Uterine scissors
Category: Cutting and Dissecting
Description: These are long heavy scissors with curved or straight blades. The straight blades are usually used for cutting suture and the curved blades for cutting tissue.
Use(s): These are used for cutting the heavy uterine ligaments and vessels during a total abdominal hysterectomy.

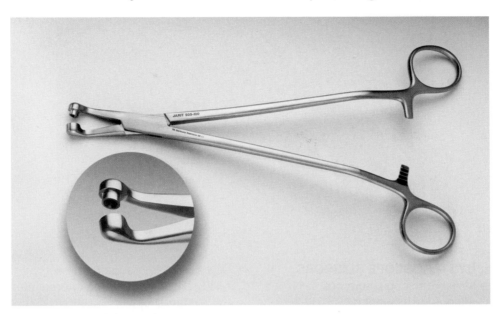

Instrument: THOMAS-GAYLOR UTERINE BIOPSY FORCEPS
Other Names: Gaylor punch
Category: Cutting and Dissecting
Description: It is a ringed instrument with a curved cup tip. The cup tips are sharp, and as they are closed, they bite into tissues.

Use(s): These are used for taking small bites of uterine tissue for examination.

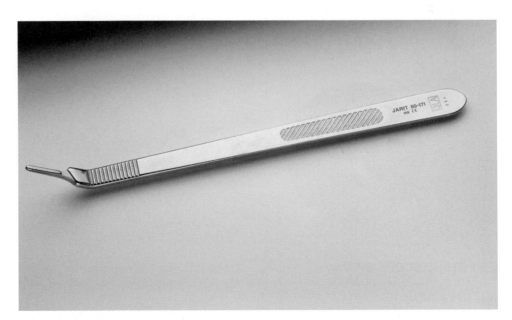

Instrument: LONG ANGLED NO. 3 KNIFE HANDLE
Other Names: Cold cone knife
Category: Cutting and Dissecting
Description: It is a long no. 3 handle that is angled at the blade end.

Use(s): It is used for removing abnormal cervical tissues during a cold conization of the cervix.
Instrument Insight: Generally, for a conization procedure, the handle is loaded with a no. 11 blade.

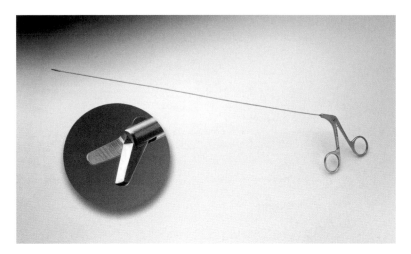

Instrument: HYSTEROSCOPE SCISSORS
Other Names: Hysteroscopic scissors
Category: Cutting and Dissecting
Description: These scissors have right-angled finger rings at the proximal end that lead to a long flexible wire that turns into straight scissor blades on the distal end. These are very small and will fit through the working channel on the hysteroscope.

Use(s): These are used for excising tissues and taking biopsies from the internal uterus through the hysteroscope.
Instrument Insight: These are delicate and should be handled with care; the wire portion should not be kinked, and heavy items should never be placed on top of them.

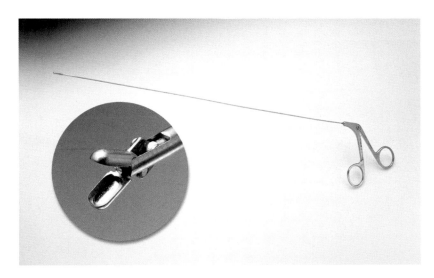

Instrument: HYSTEROSCOPE BIOPSY FORCEPS
Other Names: Biopsy forceps
Category: Cutting and Dissecting
Description: These forceps have right-angled finger rings at the proximal end that lead to a long flexible wire that turns into rounded sharp-cup forceps on the distal end. These are very small and will fit through the working channel on the hysteroscope.

Use(s): These are used for excising tissues and taking biopsies from the internal uterus through the hysteroscope.
Instrument Insight: These are delicate and should be handled with care; the wire portion should not be kinked, and heavy items should never be placed on top of them.

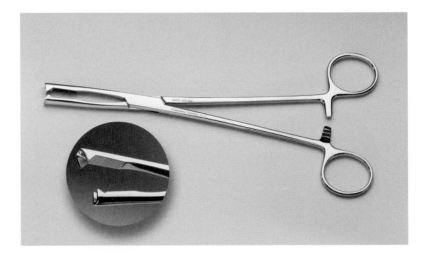

Instrument: JACOBS VULSELLUM
Other Names: Vulsellum, Jacobs uterine forceps, Jacobs tenaculum
Category: Grasping and Holding
Description: These are curved or straight heavy forceps with a flat, squared tip. Each inner jaw contains two heavy sharp teeth at the outer edge that interlock over each other when compressed. Horizontal serrations extend from the teeth to approximately one-fourth of the way down the inner jaw.
Use(s): It is used for grasping the anterior lip of the cervix for manipulation. The sharp teeth penetrate the fibrous tissue for greater control. Commonly used during vaginal procedures such as D&C or vaginal hysterectomy.
Instrument Insight: Because of penetration of the tissue, after removal of the forceps, the site should be assessed for bleeding. Hemostasis can be achieved with silver nitrate sticks, cautery, or Monsel's solution.

⚠ **CAUTION:** Care should be taken when handling this instrument because the sharp teeth can easily puncture gloves and/or skin.

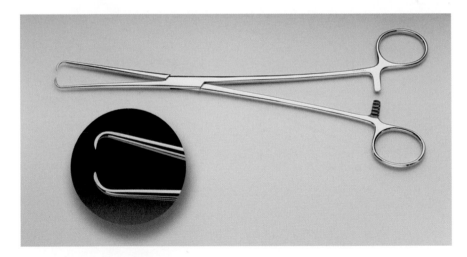

Instrument: SCHROEDER TENACULUM
Other Names: Single-tooth tenaculum, Braun tenaculum
Category: Grasping and Holding
Description: It has smooth round jaws that extend to sharp, inward-curved prongs.
Use(s): It is used for grasping the anterior lip of the cervix for manipulation. The sharp prongs on each jaw penetrate the fibrous tissue for greater control. It is commonly used during vaginal procedures such as D&C and vaginal hysterectomy.
Instrument Insight: Because of penetration of the tissue, after removal of the forceps, the site should be assessed for bleeding. Hemostasis can be achieved with silver nitrate sticks, cautery, or Monsel solution.

⚠ **CAUTION:** Care should be taken when handling this instrument because the sharp prongs can easily puncture gloves and/or skin.

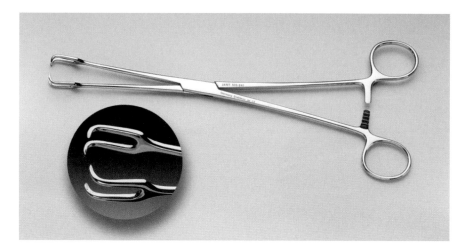

Instrument: SCHROEDER VULSELLUM
Other Names: Double-tooth tenaculum
Category: Grasping and Holding
Description: These are curved or straight forceps with smooth round jaws that bifurcate into two sharp, cupped prongs.
Use(s): It is used for grasping the anterior lip of the cervix for manipulation. The sharp prongs on each jaw penetrate the fibrous tissue for greater control. Commonly used during vaginal procedures such as D&C or vaginal hysterectomy.

Instrument Insight: Because of penetration of the tissue, after removal of the forceps, the site should be assessed for bleeding. Hemostasis can be achieved with silver nitrate sticks, cautery, or Monsel solution.

⚠ **CAUTION:** Care should be taken when handling this instrument because the sharp prongs can easily puncture gloves and/or skin.

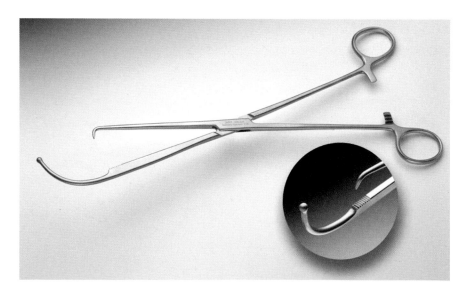

Instrument: HULKA TENACULUM
Other Names: Uterine manipulator
Category: Grasping and Holding
Description: One of the jaws has a long ball-tip probe extending to heavy horizontal serrations. The other side is shorter and has smooth round jaws that extend to a sharp, inward-curved prong. The heavy serrations and the curved prong interlock when compressed.
Use(s): It is used to manipulate the uterus and thereby facilitate visualization of and access to

pelvic structures during laparoscopic procedures. The probe tip is inserted into the cervical os, and the sharp prong penetrates the anterior cervical lip.

⚠ **CAUTION:** Care should be taken when handling this instrument because of the sharp prong that can easily puncture gloves and skin.

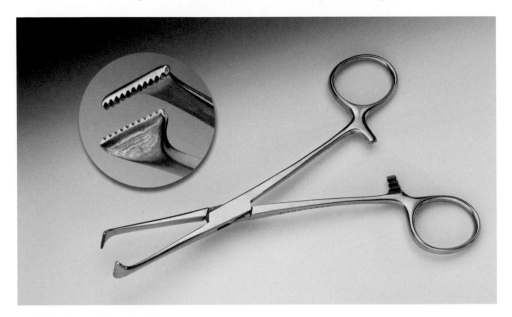

Instrument: ALLIS-ADAIR FORCEPS
Other Names: Big Allis forceps
Category: Grasping and Holding
Description: It has wide heavy tip with multiple interlocking fine teeth at the tip that reduce injury to the tissues. The jaws are much wider and heavier than regular Allis forceps.
Use(s): These are used for lifting, holding, and retracting slippery dense tissue that is being removed. In obstetric and gynecologic (OB/GYN) procedures, it is commonly used to grasp vaginal tissue during an anterior and posterior repair.
Instrument Insight: Will often need multiple Allis-Adair forceps to grasp the excess tissue in anterior and posterior (A&P) repair.

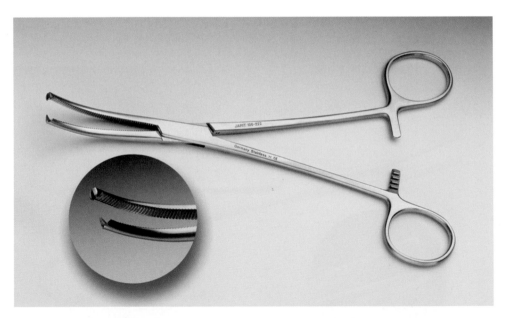

Instrument: CURVED OCHSNER FORCEPS
Other Names: Curved Kocher forceps
Category: Grasping and Holding
Description: The curved inner jaws have transverse serrations that run the length of the jaws. At the tip of the jaws are three large interlinking teeth. This instrument is available with both straight and curved jaws.
Use(s): These are used for grasping tough, fibrous, slippery tissues.

⚠ **CAUTION:** Care should be taken when handling this instrument because the sharp teeth can easily puncture gloves and skin.

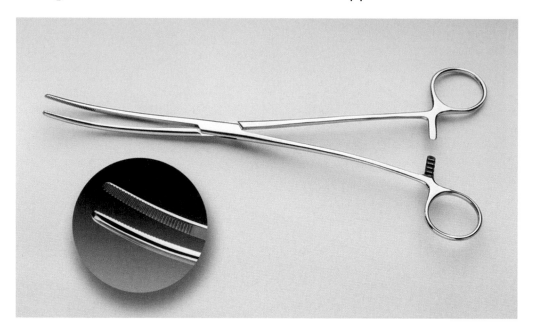

Instrument: BOZEMAN UTERINE DRESSING FORCEPS

Other Names: Dressing forceps, packing forceps

Category: Grasping and Holding

Description: These are long curved forceps with horizontal serrations running one-fourth of the way down the inner jaws.

Use(s): These are used for placing vaginal packing in the vagina after vaginal procedures.

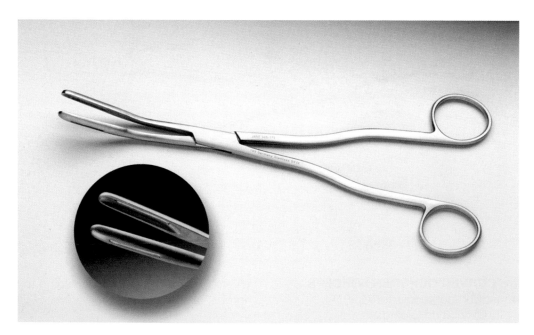

Instrument: OVERSTREET ENDOMETRIAL POLYP FORCEPS

Other Names: Polyp forceps

Category: Grasping and Holding

Description: These are curved or straight forceps with two fenestrated, oval-cupped tips.

Use(s): These are used for removal of endometrial polyps and other intrauterine tissue.

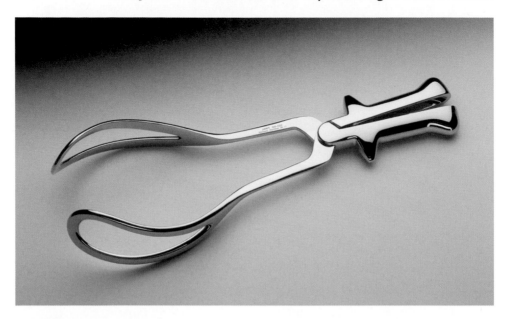

Instrument: SIMPSON OBSTETRICAL FORCEPS
Other Names: Tongs forceps
Category: Grasping and Holding
Description: It has two large, curved, teardrop-shaped blades that extend into two shafts that interlock at the handle. The interlocking handle is not fixed; therefore the two sides can be completely separated for ease in placement.
Use(s): These are used for facilitating fetal descent and delivery when the fetus is lodged in the birth canal. The blades are placed properly around the fetal head, and pulling the handle will aid in fetal descent.

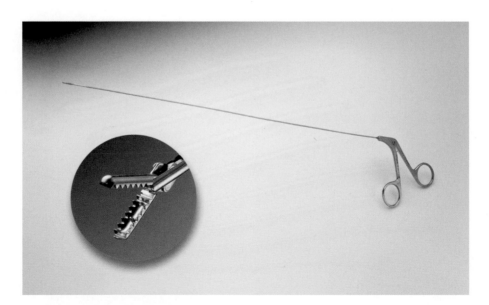

Instrument: HYSTEROSCOPE GRASPING FORCEPS
Other Names: Graspers
Category: Grasping and Holding
Description: These graspers have right-angled finger rings at the proximal end that lead to a long flexible wire that turns into rounded-tip forceps with multiple interlocking teeth on the distal end. These are very small and will fit through the working channel on the hysteroscope.
Use(s): These are used for grasping tissues in the internal uterus when excising or taking biopsies through the hysteroscope.
Instrument Insight: These are delicate and should be handled with care; the wire portion should not be kinked, and heavy items should never be placed on top of them.

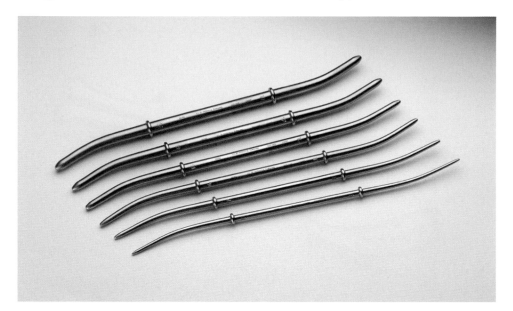

Instrument: HANK DILATORS
Other Names: Uterine dilators, cervical dilators
Category: Probing and Dilating
Description: It has double-ended probe with an elevated cuff designed to limit uterine penetration. Hank dilators are sized from 9–10F to 19–20F with one end of the dilator larger than the other.

Use(s): These are used for progressive dilation of the cervical os for intrauterine procedures such as D&C, suction and curettage (S&C), dilation and evacuation (D&E), or hysteroscopy.
Instrument Insight: Arrange dilators in a line from smallest to largest on the back table. Place the middle of the dilator in the surgeon's hand like a pencil, with the smaller end facing the field.

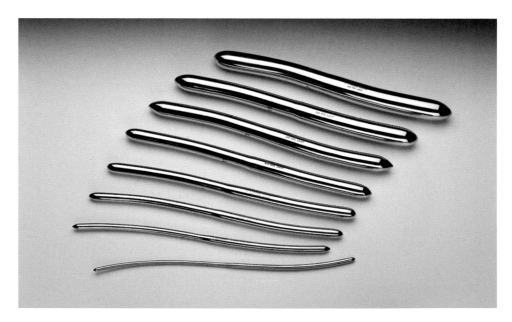

Instrument: HEGAR DILATORS
Other Names: Uterine dilators, cervical dilators
Category: Probing and Dilating
Description: It has double-ended heavy probe; range in size from 1–2 mm to 17–18 mm, with one end of the dilator larger than the other.
Use(s): These are used for progressive dilation of the cervical os for intrauterine procedures such as D&C, S&C, D&E, or hysteroscopy.
Instrument Insight: Arrange dilators in a line from smallest to largest on the back table. Place the middle of the dilator in the surgeon's hand like a pencil, with the smaller end facing the field.

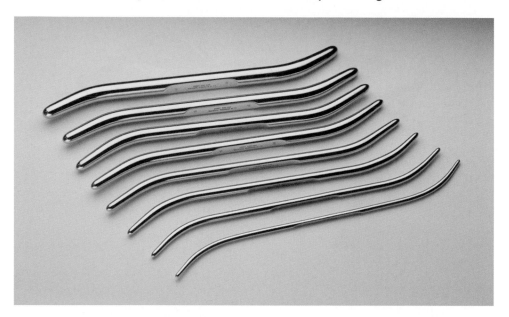

Instrument: PRATT UTERINE DILATORS
Other Names: Uterine dilators, cervical dilators
Category: Probing and Dilating
Description: It has double-ended probe that graduates up by 2F from 13–15F to 41–43F with one end of the dilator larger than the other.
Use(s): These are used for progressive dilation of the cervical os for intrauterine procedures such as D&C, S&C, or hysteroscopy.

Instrument Insight: Arrange dilators in a line from smallest to largest on the back table. Place the middle of the dilator in the surgeon's hand like a pencil, with the smaller end facing the field.

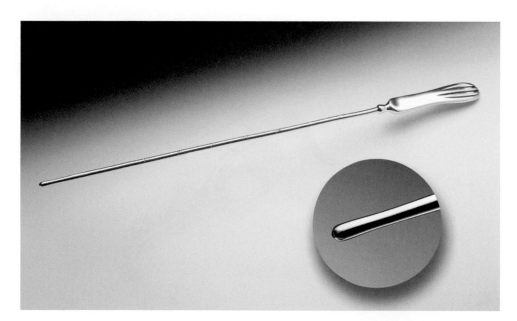

Instrument: SIMS UTERINE SOUND
Other Names: Sound, depth gauge
Category: Probing and Dilating
Description: It has a long narrow probe that is malleable and is calibrated in inches or centimeters.
Use(s): This instrument is inserted into the cervical os to measure the depth of the uterus from the cervix to the back of the uterus or the fundus. The purpose for measuring the uterus is to prevent perforation of the uterus while curetting of the endometrial lining during a D&C.

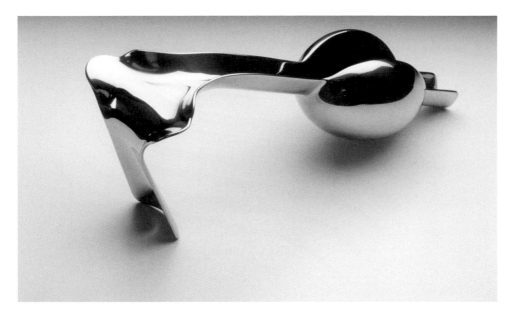

Instrument: AUVARD WEIGHTED VAGINAL SPECULUM
Other Names: Weighted speculum
Category: Retracting and Exposing
Description: It is a self-retaining retractor with angled concave blades that extend to a widened oblong lip. From this lip, there is a concave channel that leads to the bottom. At approximately two-thirds of the way down the channel is the round weighted ball.

Use(s): It is used for retraction of the posterior vaginal wall. The blade is placed into the vaginal vault, and the weight of the speculum allows it to hang in place.
Instrument Insight: The average weight of this retractor is 2.5 pounds. A sterile glove may be placed over the bottom of the retractor to catch any fluid.

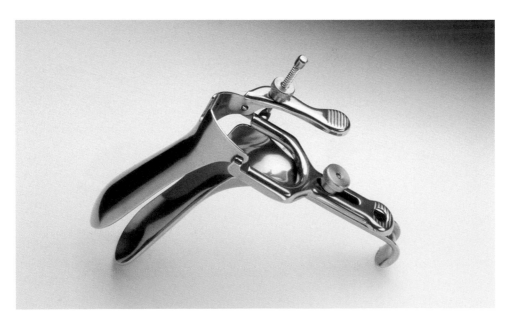

Instrument: GRAVES VAGINAL SPECULUM
Other Names: Duckbill speculum, bivalve speculum
Category: Retracting and Exposing
Description: It is a self-retaining retractor with inner upper and lower concave blades that are held open by a nut and screw mechanism.

Use(s): It is used for retraction of the anterior and posterior vaginal walls.
Instrument Insight: This speculum is available in different sizes; the size to be used is determined by the size of the patient.

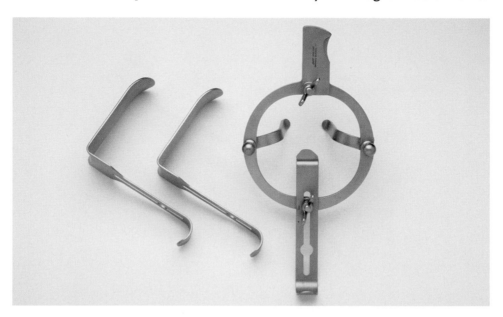

Instrument: O'SULLIVAN-O'CONNOR RETRACTOR
Other Names: Irish retractor, O'Sullivan retractor, O'Connor retractor
Category: Retracting and Exposing
Description: It is a ring frame self-retaining retractor with attached lateral blades and interchangeable upper and lower blades.

Use(s): It is used for retraction of the abdominal wall during open abdominal and pelvic procedures.
Instrument Insight: Each individual piece of the retractor is included separately as part of the count.

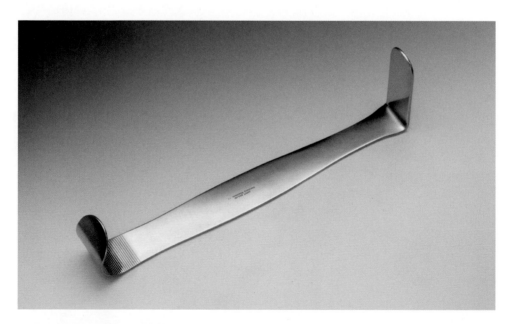

Instrument: HEANEY RETRACTOR
Other Names: Lateral retractor, right angle retractor
Category: Retracting and Exposing
Description: It is a 90-degree-angle flat blade that extends to a curved hook on the handle end.

Use(s): It is used for retraction of the anterior vaginal wall.
Instrument Insight: The retractor is placed in the palm of the hand with the hook up and over the top of the hand for easier holding.

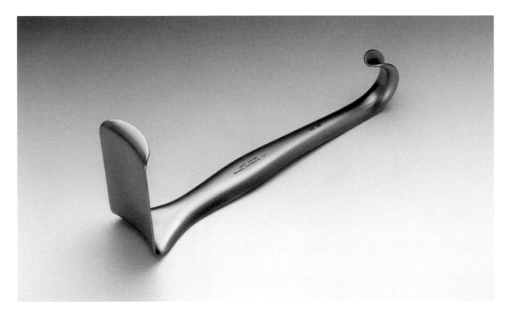

Instrument: EASTMAN RETRACTOR
Other Names: Lateral retractor
Category: Retracting and Exposing
Description: It has a hook-end handle that extends to a widened, lateral, right-angled blade that is slightly concave with a downward-bent, crescent-shaped lip.

Use(s): It is used for retracting the anterior vaginal wall.
Instrument Insight: The retractor is placed in the palm of the hand with the hook up and over the top of the hand for easier holding.

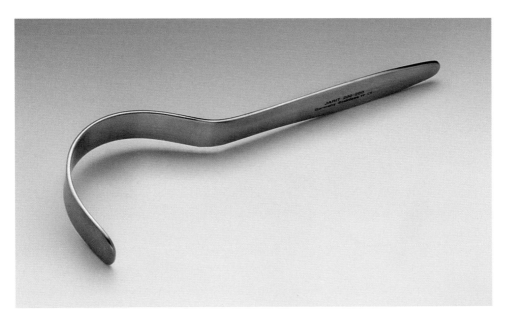

Instrument: BABY DEAVER RETRACTOR
Other Names: Small Deaver retractor
Category: Retracting and Exposing
Description: It is a flat, narrow, stainless steel strip that resembles a question mark.

Use(s): It is used for retraction of the anterior vaginal wall. It is also used for pediatric abdominal procedures.

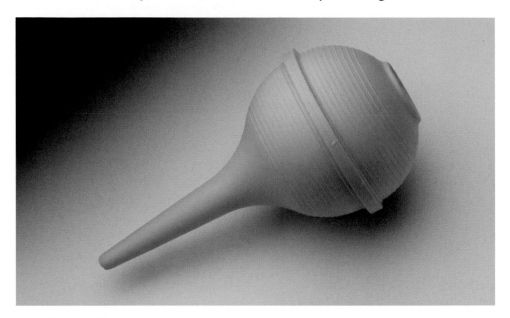

Instrument: BULB SYRINGE
Other Names: Baby sucker, ear syringe
Category: Suctioning and Aspirating
Description: It is a disposable, pliable hollow bulb that extends to a soft pliable tube.

Use(s): It is used for aspiration of mucus and fluid from the mouth and nose of a neonate.
Instrument Insight: Have readily available upon birth of a neonate.

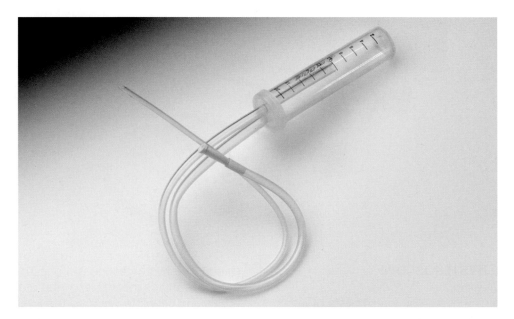

Instrument: DELEE SUCTION
Other Names: Mucus trap, baby sucker
Category: Suctioning and Aspirating
Description: It is an oral or mechanical suction device with a 20-mL canister that has a mucus trap and filter. This prevents the mucus or fluid from entering the baby's mouth. On the canister lid is a 10F flexible suction catheter and a suction tube.

Use(s): It is used for aspiration of mucus and fluid from the mouth, nose, and throat of a neonate during a cesarean delivery.
Instrument Insight: This should be immediately available upon delivery of the fetal head.

⚠ **CAUTION: This suction device should be hooked to regulated suction.** Do not hook the Delee to a regulator on full suction because this would be too strong.

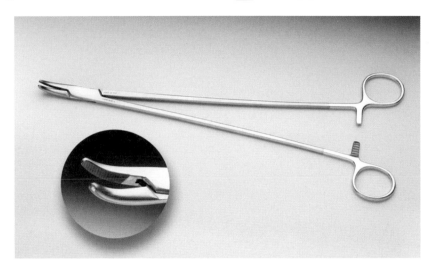

Instrument: HEANEY NEEDLE HOLDER
Other Names: Curved needle holder, Heaney needle driver, curved needle driver
Category: Suturing and Stapling
Description: It is a curved heavy needle holder with a carbide cross-hatch pattern of serrations on the inner jaws.

Use(s): It is used for proper placement of a suture needle when suturing around curved structures and in confined spaces, such as during a vaginal hysterectomy.
Instrument Insight: The needle should be positioned on the jaws of the needle holder with its curve toward the swaged end of the suture.

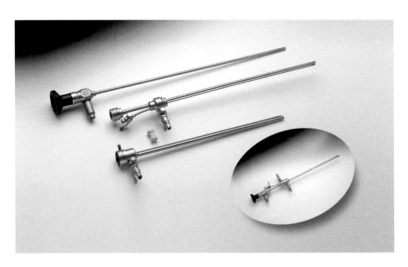

Instrument: HYSTEROSCOPE
Category: Viewing
Description: The hysteroscope consists of a telescope lens, outer sheath, and inner sheath. The outer sheath is a hollow metal tube with a stopcock on the side for the inflow of irrigation at the proximal end and a rounded angled tip at the distal end. The inner sheath is a smaller hollow tube that at the proximal end accepts the telescope lens. It also has a stopcock on the side for the inflow of irrigation and a working channel on the other side in which instruments are inserted. The working channel is fitted with a reducer cap to prevent fluid from leaking out during insertion and removal of instruments.

Use(s): The hysteroscope is a sheath and telescope that is inserted into the uterus via the vagina and cervix to visualize the internal structures of the uterus and the tubal orifices, endocervical canal, cervix, and vagina. Hysteroscopy can be performed for diagnostic or therapeutic indications.
Instrument Insight: The stopcocks should be closed before irrigation is opened. If the handle of the stopcock is aligned with the port, the stopcock is open. If the handle is up or down, the stopcock is closed. The port on the working channel should have a reducer cap and the stopcock closed to control the leakage of irrigation.

8 Genitourinary Instruments

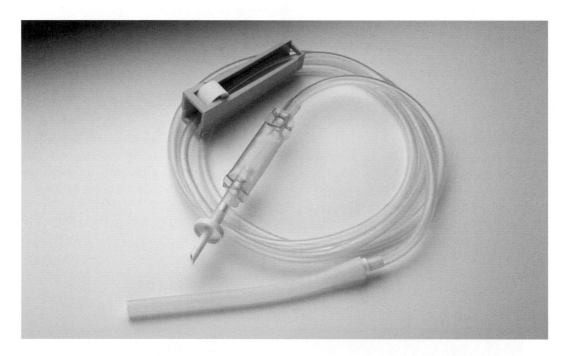

Instrument: IRRIGATION TUBING
Other Names: Water tubing, Cysto tubing ·
Category: Accessory
Description: It is a clear synthetic tubing with a spike, a drip chamber, and a roller clamp at the distal end and flexible rubber tubing on the working end.
Use(s): It is used for instillation of irrigation fluids into the urinary bladder, causing distention.

It is also used for visualizing the interior. This is done during endoscopic urologic procedures.
Instrument Insight: The spike end of the tubing is handed off the sterile field. A Luer-Lok adaptor is often attached to the rubber end of the tubing for connection to the scopes.

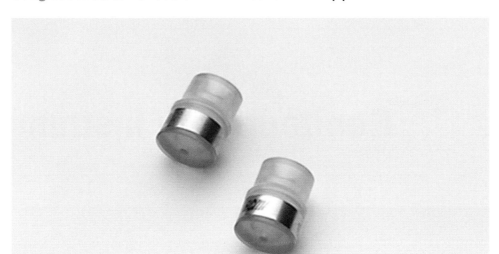

Instrument: REDUCER CAPS

Other Names: Seals

Category: Accessory

Description: These are reusable flexible caps with a small hole on the working end. Reducers are available in different sizes depending on the size of the device to be used.

Use(s): These are used to reduce leakage of irrigation when inserting a device into the working channels of bridges, the catheter-deflecting element, and flexible scopes.

Instrument Insight: The seals are stretched over the opening of the working channels.

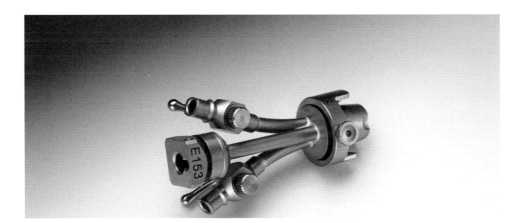

Instrument: TELESCOPE BRIDGE

Other Names: Lens Bridge

Category: Accessory

Description: The proximal end of the telescope bridge accepts the telescope and has a working channel on each side. The distal end is the connection to the cystoscope sheath. Bridges are available in several styles. They can be an adaptor only or be manufactured with one or two working ports.

Use(s): It is used to adapt the telescope lens to fit into the cystoscope sheath and may allow

insertion of one or two accessories. These would include guidewires, ureteral catheters, stents, and other flexible devices.

Instrument Insight: The lens will not fit into the cystoscope sheath without a bridge. The ports on bridges are covered with a reducer cap and have stopcocks to control the leakage of irrigation. If the handle of the stopcock is aligned with the port, the stopcock is open. If the handle is up or down, the stopcock is closed.

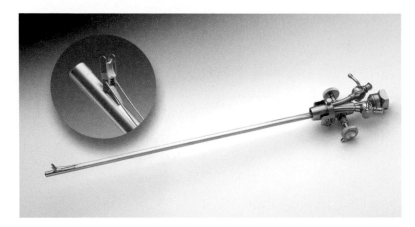

Instrument: CATHETER DEFLECTING ELEMENT
Other Names: Cath element, deflecting bridge, deflector, deflecting mechanism
Category: Accessory
Description: The proximal end of the catheter deflecting element accepts the telescope lens, which is slid through the hollow tube to the end for viewing. There are working channels on each side in which the ureteral catheter is inserted. Below the channels are thumb wheels to manipulate the lid or tip up and down. The deflecting element fits into the cystoscope sheath for use.
Use(s): This device allows the surgeon to aim the tip of the accessory at a specific area or anatomic structure. A deflecting element is commonly used during a cystoscopy for retrograde pyelograms to direct the catheter into the ureteral orifice.
Instrument Insight: To prevent damage to the urethra and the lid apparatus, it is important to remember to return the lid to the neutral position before handing the catheter-deflecting element to the surgeon. The ureteral catheter is inserted into the side port and pulled down to the lid at the tip of the sheath. The lid is lowered and the element is inserted into a cystoscope for use. Once inside the bladder, the lid is manipulated to guide the catheter into the ureteral orifice.

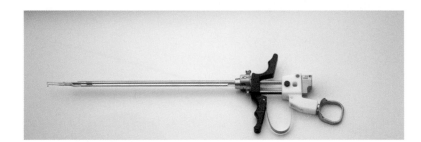

Instrument: WORKING ELEMENT
Other Names: Iglesias
Category: Accessory
Description: The proximal end of the working element accepts the telescope, which is slid through the sheath to the working end for viewing. The handle has a spring mechanism that draws the electrode back into the resectoscope sheath. Attaching the electrode is accomplished by sliding the wire end through the guide below the telescope sheath and into the handle where it is seated. The small black button on the side releases the electrode. It is not necessary to depress the button to seat the electrode. The small hole next to the black button is for active cord connection. The small silver button at the top of the sheath will release the working element from the resectoscope sheath.
Use(s): It is used with a resectoscope, telescope, and electrode to resect tissue and coagulate bleeders during a transurethral resection of the prostate or a bladder tumor.
Instrument Insight: A 30-degree telescope is loaded into the working element, and this enables the electrode to be seen during the procedure. Activation of the working element is accomplished when the surgeon steps on the foot pedal and compresses the handle, which draws the electrode through the tissue and back into the resectoscope sheath.

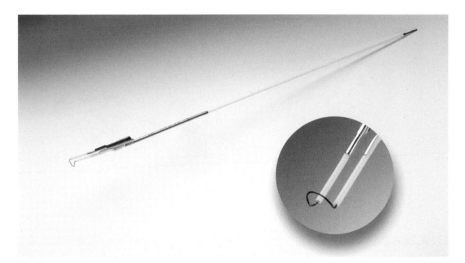

Instrument: LOOP ELECTRODE
Other Names: Loop
Category: Accessory
Description: It is an insulated wire that bifurcates at the working end and leads to a metal crescent-shaped wire between the two prongs.
Use(s): It is commonly used for resection and coagulation of prostatic and bladder tissues during transurethral procedures. A loop electrode vaporizes the tissue in its immediate area as it resects a piece of tissue. Bleeders may also be coagulated simultaneously or individually.
Instrument Insight: The electrode is seated into the working element by sliding the proximal end through the small hollow tube under the telescope sheath and into the handle. The small trough lies on top of the electrode and slides over the sheath, securing it to the working element. The electrodes are color coded to fit the proper size resectoscope.

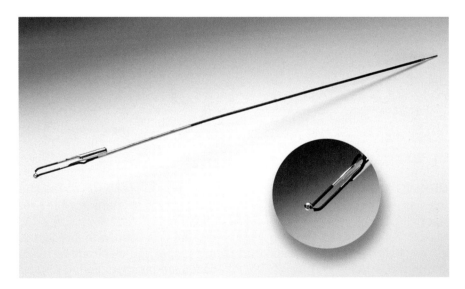

Instrument: BALL LOOP ELECTRODE
Category: Accessory
Description: It is an insulated wire that bifurcates at the working end and leads to a metal roller ball at the working end.
Use(s): It is used for coagulation of a larger surface area of the bladder.
Instrument Insight: The electrode is seated into the working element by sliding the proximal end through the small hollow tube under the telescope sheath and into the handle. The small trough lies on top of the electrode and slides over the sheath, securing it to the working element. The electrodes are color coded to fit the proper size resectoscope.

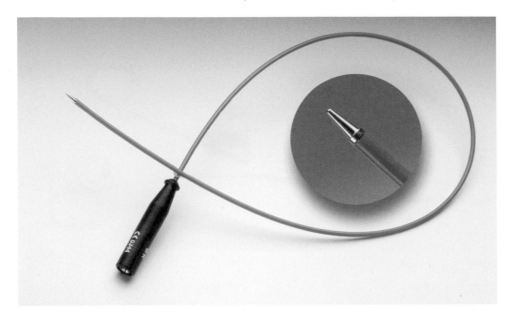

Instrument: BUGBEE ELECTRODE
Category: Accessory
Description: The Bugbee electrode is a flexible monopolar cautery electrode available in various diameters and lengths.

Use(s): It is used for coagulating small areas, usually after a bladder biopsy.
Instrument Insight: The Bugbee electrode is a reusable electrode that is generally packaged with the cord that attaches to the generator.

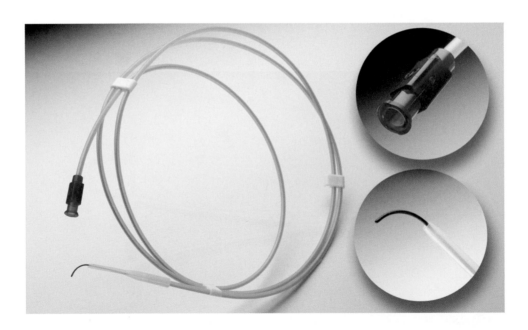

Instrument: GUIDEWIRE
Other Names: Glidewire
Category: Accessory
Description: It is a long, thin wire with a curved or straight flexible tip. Depending on the manufacturer, the wire will be constructed of a metal or synthetic material, which may be covered with a lubricious coating to ease insertion. The wire is a single-use item that comes packaged inside a hard plastic coil that

has an irrigation port at the proximal end and an insertion guide at the working end.
Use(s): It is used for guiding stents, dilatators, baskets, and other devices into the ureters.
Instrument Insight: Moistening the guidewire will ease the insertion through the working channel of the scope. This can be accomplished by injecting water through the irrigation port on the plastic coil or by dipping the wire itself in a basin of water.

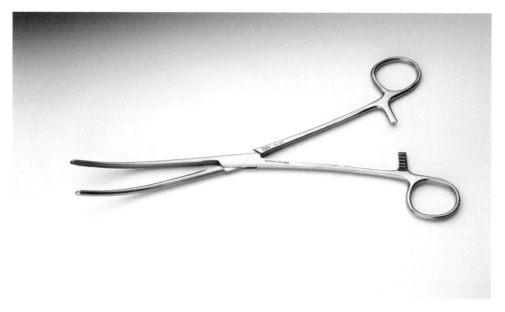

Instrument: YOUNG RENAL CLAMP
Category: Clamping and Occluding
Description: It is a long, heavy, curved clamp with longitudinal serrations and with cross-serrations at the tip.

Use(s): It is used for clamping heavy tissues and the pedicles during open kidney procedures.

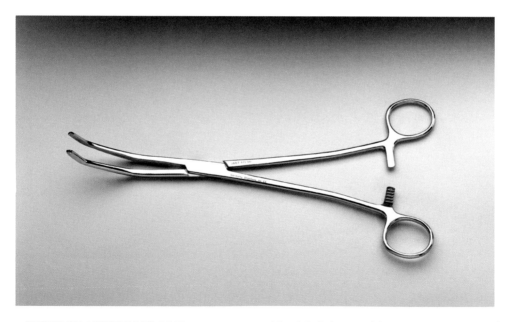

Instrument: HERRICK KIDNEY CLAMP
Other Names: Pedicle clamp
Category: Clamping and Occluding
Description: It is a long, heavy, double-angle clamp with longitudinal serrations.

Use(s): It is used for clamping heavy tissues and the pedicles during open kidney procedures.

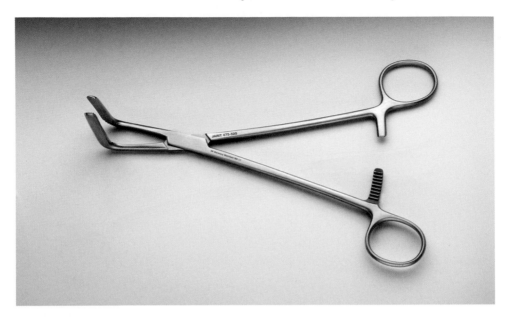

Instrument: WERTHEIM-CULLEN PEDICLE CLAMP
Other Names: Pedicle clamp
Category: Clamping and Occluding
Description: It is a broad right-angle clamp with longitudinal serrations that run from the tip to the curvature.

Use(s): It is used for clamping heavy tissues and the pedicles during open kidney procedures.

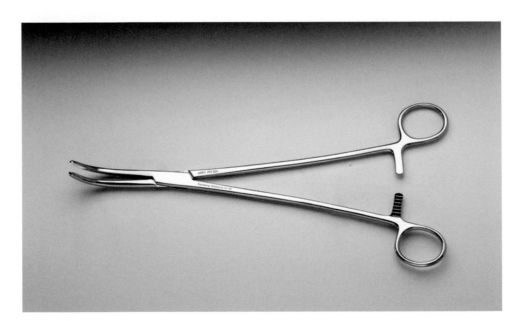

Instrument: WERTHEIM CLAMP
Category: Clamping and Occluding
Description: It is a long, heavy, curved clamp with horizontal serrations running the length of the jaws.

Use(s): It is used for clamping heavy tissue and vessels during open urological procedures.

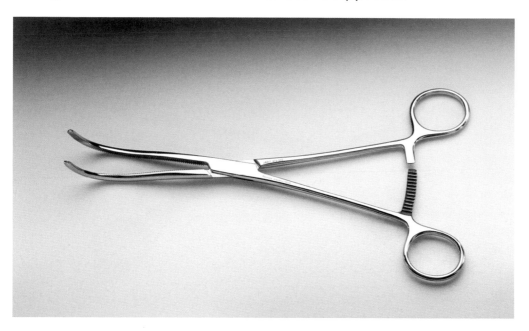

Instrument: MAYO-GUYON VESSEL CLAMP
Category: Clamping and Occluding
Description: It is a heavy clamp with long, curved jaws and horizontal serrations running the length of the jaws.

Use(s): It is used for clamping heavy tissue and vessels during open urologic procedures.

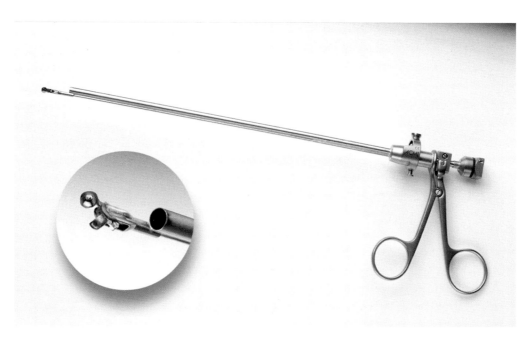

Instrument: BIOPSY FORCEPS
Category: Cutting and Dissecting
Description: The proximal end of the biopsy forceps accepts the telescope lens, and the finger rings open and close the cup-shaped jaws at the working end. The biopsy forceps are attached to the cystoscope sheath.

Use(s): These are used to remove small bites of tissue in the bladder for examination.
Instrument Insight: To prevent crushing or damaging the biopsy tissue, it can be swished in saline or pushed out of the jaws with a fine needle.

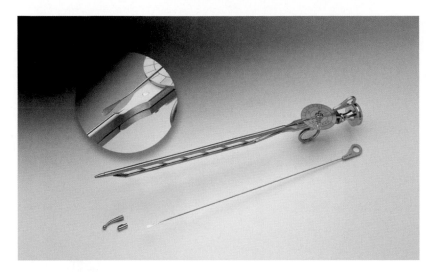

Instrument: OTIS URETHROTOME
Category: Cutting and Dissecting
Description: This has two pieces, a urethrotome and a blade. The urethrotome is a straight dilator that is expanded open when the round knob on the distal end is turned. The dial below the knob allows the surgeon to determine the amount of dilation that is occurring when the knob is turned. The blade fits down into the dilating rod and is pushed upward as the dilator is opened. When the dilator is expanded to the appropriate diameter, the surgeon will pull the blade out, cutting the stricture.

Use(s): It is used to perform a blind urethrotomy for strictures.
Instrument Insight: The Otis urethrotome is inserted into the urethra and is dilated to the desired width. The blade is pulled out and cuts the stretched urethra, releasing the strictures.

⚠ **CAUTION:** When loading the blade onto urethrotome, always use the handle on the blade to do so. The blade is very sharp and can cut through your gloves and skin.

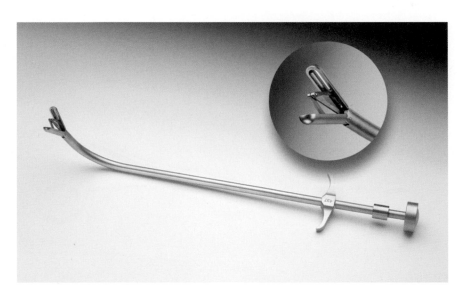

Instrument: LOWSLEY PROSTATIC TRACTOR
Category: Grasping and Holding
Description: It is a slender curved instrument with cupped blades at the tip that open and close by rotation of the handle at the proximal end.
Use(s): It is used for manipulating the prostate downward in the direction of the perineum during a perineal prostatectomy.

Instrument Insight: The Lowsley prostatic tractor is passed through the urethra into the bladder and then opened; therefore, it should be handed to the surgeon with the blades closed.

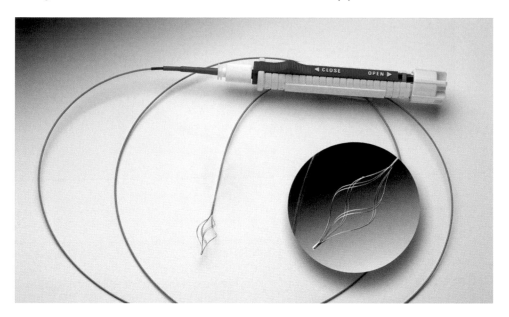

Instrument: STONE BASKET
Category: Grasping and Holding
Description: It is a single-use device that consists of a plastic handle with a thumb-slide mechanism for opening and closing the basket, a catheter sheath, and a wire catheter with expandable wire basket. These devices are available in a variety of lengths, tip designs, and basket configurations, depending on the manufacturer.
Use(s): It is used for entrapping and removing renal calculi via a ureteroscope or a cystoscope.
Instrument Insight: When the thumb slide on the handle is slid forward, the basket collapses into the outer sheath, and when pulled backward, the basket is expanded.

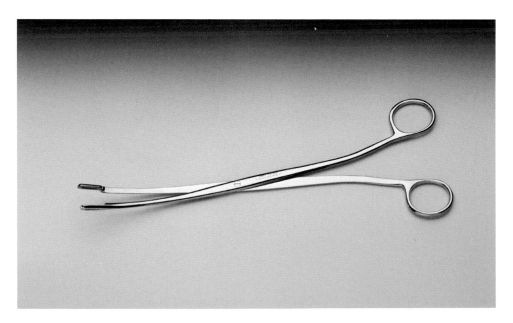

Instrument: RANDALL STONE FORCEPS
Category: Grasping and Holding
Description: These are curved, nonratcheted grasping forceps with fenestrated, oval-cup jaws with horizontal serrations. The Randall stone forceps are available in different degrees of curvature, ranging from one-fourth, one-half, and three-fourths of a curve to a full curve.
Use(s): These are used for grasping renal stones.

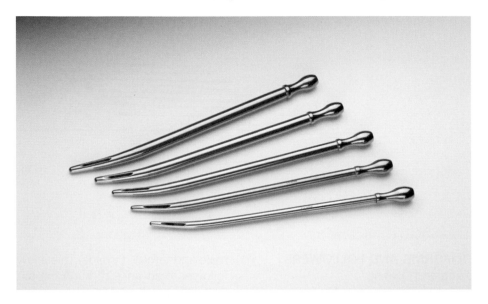

Instrument: WALTHER FEMALE URETHRAL SOUNDS

Other Names: Female sounds, female dilators, urethral dilators

Category: Probing and Dilating

Description: It is a stainless steel tube with a narrowed curved tip and oval drainage lumen. The sound size is measured on the French (F) scale with even numbers only that range from 12F to 38F.

Use(s): These are used to provide gradual dilation of the female urethra. Often used before placement of the cystoscope or resectoscope to ease insertion. The female sounds can also be used to obtain a urine specimen or drain the bladder.

Instrument Insight: The sounds should be arranged on the back table from smallest to largest.

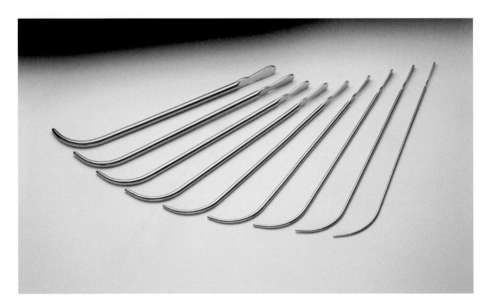

Instrument: VAN BUREN URETHRAL SOUNDS

Other Names: Male sounds, Van Buren sounds, urethral dilators

Category: Probing and Dilating

Description: It is a long stainless steel rod with a narrowed curved tip. The sound size is measured on the French scale with even numbers only that range from 8F to 40F.

Use(s): These are used to provide gradual dilation of the male urethra. Often used before placement of the cystoscope or resectoscope to ease insertion.

Instrument Insight: The sounds should be arranged on the back table from smallest to largest.

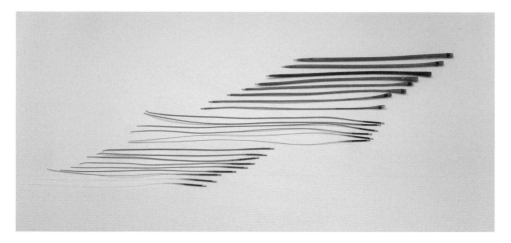

Instrument: FILIFORMS AND FOLLOWERS
Category: Probing and Dilating
Description: Filiforms are a made of a woven material and range in size from 2F to 6F. The tip may be straight, spiral, or Coude, and has a female thread at the distal end. The followers are hollow tubes made of the same woven material. The tip has a male thread and a hole for drainage, and ranges in size from 10F to 24F. Followers screw into the filiforms by way of male and female threads. This allows for the follower to advance through the stricture and dilate the urethra open.
Use(s): Filiforms are used to get past difficult urethral strictures, whereas followers are used for dilation and drainage.
Instrument Insight: Woven material softens in the body, allowing filiform tips to curl in the bladder while the urethra is being dilated.

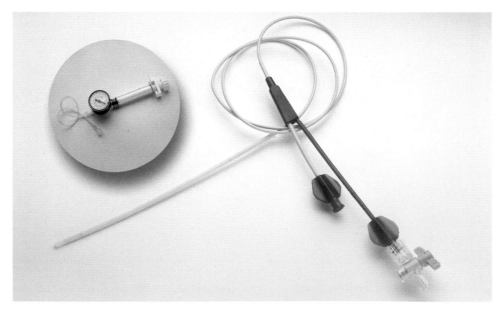

Instrument: BALLOON DILATOR
Category: Probing and Dilating
Description: It is a long plastic ureteral catheter with a high-pressure balloon tip on the distal end. At the proximal end is a balloon inflation port with a stopcock and a guidewire insertion port.
Use(s): It is used for dilation of ureteral strictures.
Instrument Insight: The balloon is inflated with a contrast medium solution for visualization by fluoroscopy.

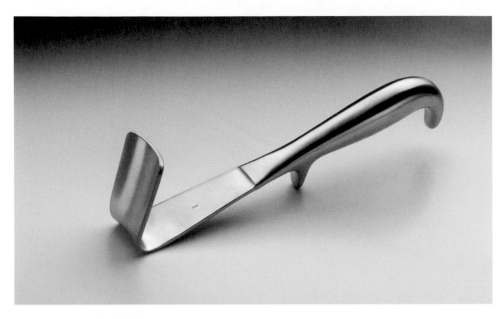

Instrument: YOUNG ANTERIOR RETRACTOR
Other Names: Anterior prostate retractor
Category: Retracting and Exposing
Description: It is a smooth, concave, anterior-bent blade with a solid grip handle.

Use(s): It is used for retracting muscles and tissues during a radical perineal prostatectomy.

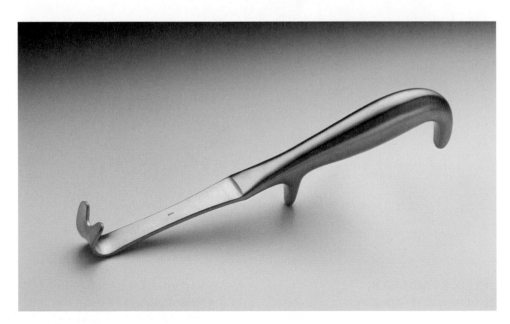

Instrument: YOUNG BULB RETRACTOR
Other Names: Notched retractor, bulb retractor
Category: Retracting and Exposing
Description: It is a short bent blade with a U-shaped notch at the end and a solid grip handle.

Use(s): It is used for retracting muscles and tissues during a radical perineal prostatectomy.
Instrument Insight: The U shape allows the catheter to be placed at the notch to prevent bending or crushing of the catheter.

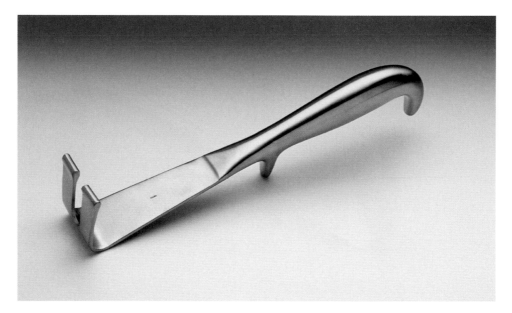

Instrument: YOUNG BIFURCATED RETRACTOR

Other Names: Bifurcated prostate retractor
Category: Retracting and Exposing
Description: It is a smooth, lateral-bent retractor with a U-shaped bifurcation in the blade and a solid grip handle.

Use(s): It is used for retracting muscles and tissues during a radical perineal prostatectomy.
Instrument Insight: The U shape allows the catheter to be placed at the notch to prevent bending or crushing of the catheter.

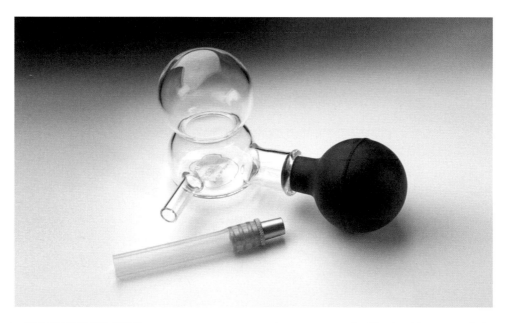

Instrument: ELLIK EVACUATOR

Category: Suctioning and Aspirating
Description: It is a glass double bowl and bulb with adaptor tip. The silicone tubing slides over the glass arm of the bowl. The adaptor is required to connect the evacuator to the inner sheath of the resectoscope.
Use(s): It is used for removing prostatic tissue segments and/or blood clots from the bladder.
Instrument Insight: All air must be eliminated from the bulb and glass bowl before use. After

the evacuator is filled with water, it is attached to the resectoscope sheath. The bulb is squeezed and released, causing whirling action of the water in and out of the bladder. The tissue pieces are trapped in the bottom portion of the glass bowl. To avoid reintroduction of the tissue back into the bladder, the tissue should be removed between uses.

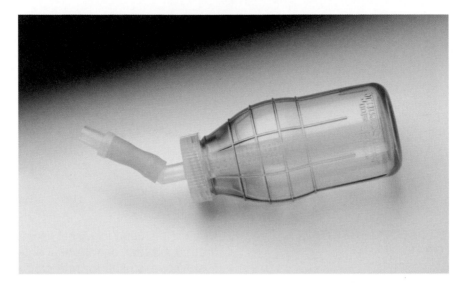

Instrument: MICROVASIVE EVACUATOR
Other Names: Disposable evacuator
Category: Suctioning and Aspirating
Description: It is a pliable plastic container with a screw on the lid that has a filter mechanism attached to the inside and an adaptor arm on the exterior. The adaptor fits inside the inner sheath of the resectoscope.
Use(s): It is used for removing tissue segments and/or blood clots from the bladder.

Instrument Insight: All air must be removed from the container before use. After the evacuator is filled with water, it is attached to the resectoscope sheath. The container is squeezed and released, causing a whirling action of the water in and out of the bladder. The filter mechanism inside the container traps the specimen, which allows for reuse without removing the tissue.

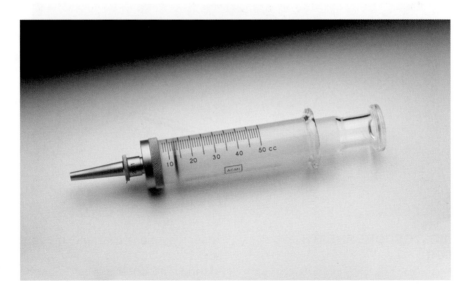

Instrument: TOOMEY SYRINGE
Category: Suctioning and Aspirating
Description: It is a glass syringe calibrated in milliliters with a stainless steel catheter adaptor tip.
Use(s): It is used for aspirating specimens and blood clots from the bladder. Often used to check for bleeding after a transurethral resection; this is done by injecting irrigation through the

urethral catheter and aspirating it back out, checking the color of the return.
Instrument Insight: When assembling the Toomey syringe, wetting the plunger portion will ease insertion into the barrel. A Toomey syringe may also be a single-patient use that is entirely made of plastic.

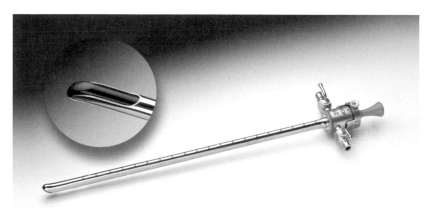

Instrument: **CYSTOSCOPE SHEATH AND OBTURATOR**

Category: Viewing

Description: The cystoscope sheath is a hollow tube with a rounded tip and mouth at the distal end. The proximal end is the insertion port for the obturator, bridge, telescope, deflecting mechanism, biopsy forceps, and other devices. It also has a stopcock on each side for the inflow of irrigation. The size of the cystoscope is measured according to the French (F) scale. A 21F cystoscope is the most widely used. The obturator is a removable core that has a rounded end that protrudes to the far opening of the sheath.

Use(s): It is used for visual examination of the urethra, bladder, and ureteral orifices. The cystoscope is used for retrograde pyelograms, bladder biopsies, ureteral stone manipulation, stent placement, and other endoscopic urologic procedures. The obturator is used to ease initial insertion of the cystoscope into the bladder.

Instrument Insight: Cystoscope sheaths and obturators are color coded to assist with proper assembly. Each manufacturer has its own color code, but if you spend time working with these instruments, it is beneficial to commit the colors to memory.

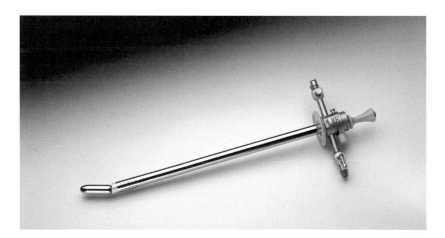

Instrument: **RESECTOSCOPE SHEATH AND OBTURATOR**

Category: Viewing

Description: The resectoscope sheath is a hollow stainless steel tube with a beveled ceramic tip at the distal end. The proximal end is an insertion port for the obturator, working element, telescope, and electrode; the proximal end also has a stopcock on each side for the inflow of irrigation. The obturator is a removable core that has a bullet-shaped end that protrudes through and beyond the far opening. The

resectoscope is available in two sizes: 25F and 27F.

Use(s): The outer sheath is used with the working element, telescope, and electrode to resect tissues and coagulate bleeders during a transurethral resection of the prostate or bladder tumor. The obturator is used to ease initial insertion of the resectoscope into the bladder.

Instrument Insight: Resectoscope sheaths and obturators are color coded to assist with proper assembly.

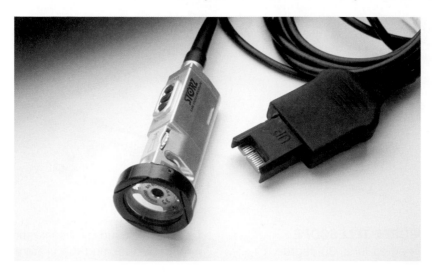

Instrument: ENDOSCOPIC CAMERA
Category: Viewing
Description: At the distal end of the camera is the coupler that attaches the camera to the eyepiece of the rigid scope. The coupler is attached to the camera head, which provides the image quality. Attached to the camera head is the cord, which relays images back to the video system.

Use(s): It is used for transmission images from the rigid telescope to the video monitor.
Instrument Insight: Most camera failures are related to a damaged cord. Care should be exercised when handling the camera and cord. They should never be placed under a heavy object, dropped, twisted, kinked, or immersed in water or any liquid.

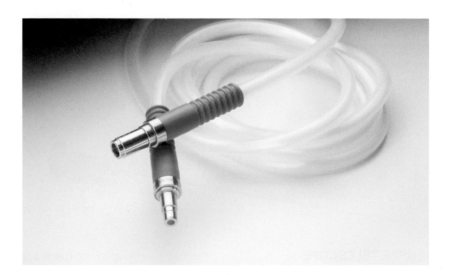

Instrument: FIBEROPTIC LIGHT CORD
Other Names: Light cord
Category: Viewing
Description: It is a 10-foot fiber-optic cable with an endoscope adaptor at the proximal end and a light source adaptor at the distal end.
Use(s): It is used for delivering high-intensity light to the endoscope for illumination of the interior bladder.
Instrument Insight: Care must be exercised when handling a fiberoptic cord. It should never

be placed under a heavy object, dropped, twisted, or kinked; the tiny glass fibers inside can be easily damaged.

⚠ **CAUTION:** When not in use, the light source should be turned off. The intense beam can ignite the drapes or any flammable vapors; it can also burn through the drapes and injure the patient.

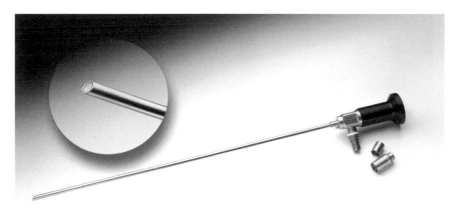

Instrument: 30-DEGREE TELESCOPE
Other Names: 30-degree lens, 30-degree endoscope
Category: Viewing
Description: It is a rigid stainless steel tube containing an optical chain of precisely aligned glass lenses and spacers. The objective lens is located at the distal tip of the scope. This determines the viewing angle. The stainless steel cylinder rod is called the optical element of the telescope, providing both images and light. The light connector allows attachment of the light cord to the telescope. At the proximal end is the eyepiece or ocular lens; this attaches to the camera coupler, or the surgeon may view the field directly.

Use(s): It is used for visualization of the urethra, interior bladder, and the ureteral orifices.
Instrument Insight: The 30 degrees is the angle in which the objective lens views. The 30-degree lens is the lens most often used in urology because it delivers the best panoramic view and allows for visualization of the urethra and the trigone area in the bladder.

⚠ **CAUTION:** Endoscopes are expensive and fragile. Care should be exercised when handling an endoscope; it should never be picked up by the distal telescope end, placed under heavy objects, or dropped.

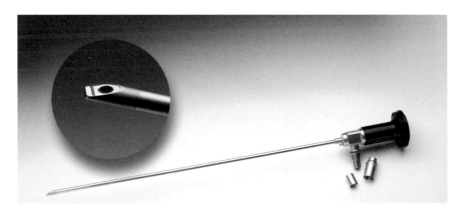

Instrument: 70-DEGREE TELESCOPE
Other Names: 70-degree lens, 70-degree endoscope
Category: Viewing
Description: It is a rigid stainless steel tube containing an optical chain of precisely aligned glass lenses and spacers. The objective lens is located at the distal tip of the scope. This determines the viewing angle. The stainless steel rod cyinder is called the optical element of the telescope, providing both images and light. The light connector allows attachment of the light cord to the telescope. At the proximal end is the eyepiece or ocular lens; this attaches to

the camera coupler, or the surgeon may view the field directly.
Use(s): It is used for visualization of the urethra, interior bladder, and the ureteral orifices.
Instrument Insight: The 70 degrees is the angle in which the objective lens views. The 70-degree lens is often used to inspect the bladder walls.

⚠ **CAUTION:** Endoscopes are expensive and fragile. Care should be exercised when handling an endoscope; it should never be picked up by the distal telescope end, placed under heavy objects, or dropped.

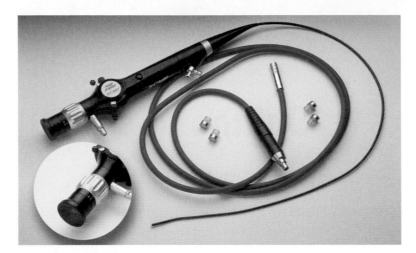

Instrument: FLEXIBLE URETEROSCOPE
Category: Viewing
Description: The proximal end of the flexible ureteroscope is comprised of the eyepiece; the light connection post; a deflecting control knob that operates the bending section, suction, and air and water valves; and the biopsy port. The central body is attached to an insertion tube, which is a flexible tube that contains channels for suction, biopsy, irrigation, and fiber-optic light and image bundles. At the distal end is a bending section that contains the objective lens and light lens, and can be manipulated in various directions within the internal structures.

Use(s): It is used for visual examination of the urinary tract, including the ureters and the renal pelvis. Ureteroscopy is commonly performed for removal of ureteral or renal calculi. It also can be used for other urologic procedures such as diagnosis, fulguration of bleeders, removal of neoplasm, and retrieval of migrated stents.
Instrument Insight: When using a flexible ureteroscope, it should never be placed under a heavy object, dropped, twisted, or kinked because the tiny glass lens and fibers inside can be easily damaged.

9

Ophthalmic Instruments

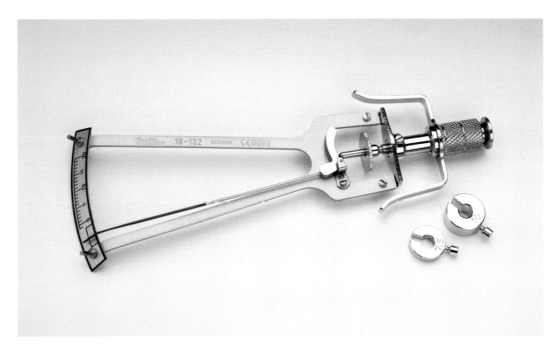

Instrument: TONOMETER
Other Names: Schiotz tonometer
Category: Accessory
Description: The distal working end of the tonometer is a concave plunger, which is gently placed onto the cornea. A small round weight is slid into the center section of the tonometer, which pushes down on the plunger and flattens the cornea. The needle on the proximal end moves to register the pressure. Weights of 5.5, 7.5, and 10 g are used.
Use(s): It is used for measuring intraocular pressure of the eye by recording the resistance of the cornea to weight.

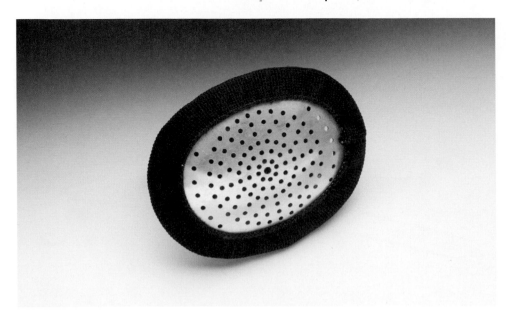

Instrument: FOX EYE SHIELD
Category: Accessory
Description: It is a lightweight, malleable, metal eye shield that is oval and convex to fit over the eye.

Use(s): It is used for protection of the eye after ophthalmic surgery.
Instrument Insight: It is generally placed over the dressing and taped in place.

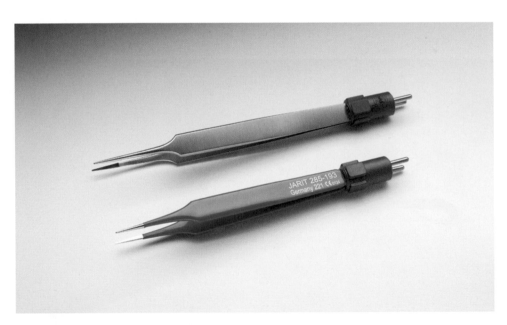

Instrument: JEWELER'S BIPOLAR FORCEPS
Other Names: Eye bipolar forceps, eye cautery forceps
Category: Accessory
Description: It resembles tissue forceps, is either insulated or noninsulated, and has straight forceps with fine tips.

Use(s): These are used for coagulating small blood vessels of the eye and the eyelids.
Instrument Insight: There are many different types of bipolar forceps that can be used in eye procedures.

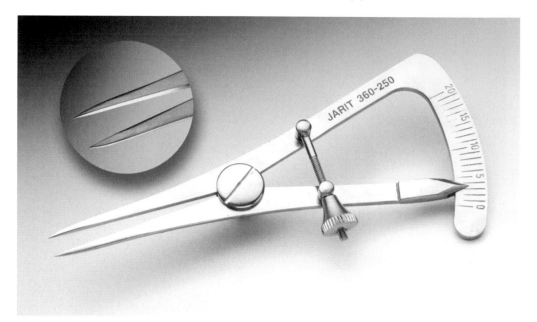

Instrument: CASTROVIEJO CALIPER
Other Names: Caliper
Category: Accessory
Description: The proximal end of the Castroviejo caliper measures from 0 to 20 mm in 1-mm increments. When the screw device is tightened or loosened, the smooth narrowed tips open or close.
Use(s): It is used for precise measuring of eye structures such as the cornea, lens, pupils, or lids.

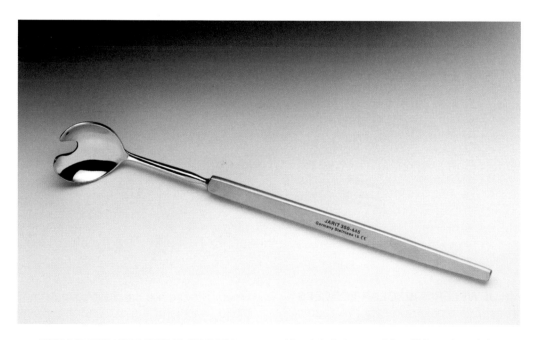

Instrument: WELLS ENUCLEATION SPOON
Category: Accessory
Description: It is an angled spoon-shaped instrument with a rounded notch at the distal end.
Use(s): It is used for lifting the globe upward to dissect the optic nerve during enucleation.

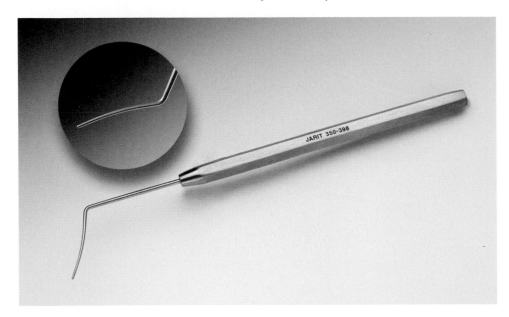

Instrument: BARRAQUER IRIS SPATULA
Other Names: Iris spatula
Category: Accessory

Description: It has a blunt angled tip with a gently curved flat blade and a short hexagonal handle.
Use(s): It is used for repositioning the iris.

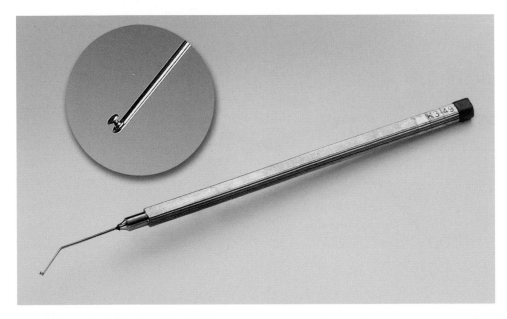

Instrument: GRAETHER COLLAR BUTTON
Other Names: Greather button, button
Category: Accessory
Use(s): It is used for iris retraction and polishing the capsule.

Description: It has a 45-degree-angled shaft that is 10 mm from bend to tip with a button on the end.

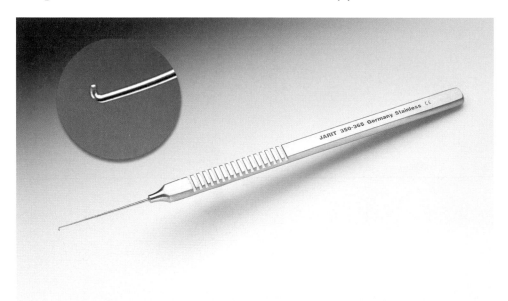

Instrument: SINSKEY HOOK
Category: Accessory
Description: It is a blunt right-angle hook with a flattened handle.
Use(s): It is used for manipulating the lens.

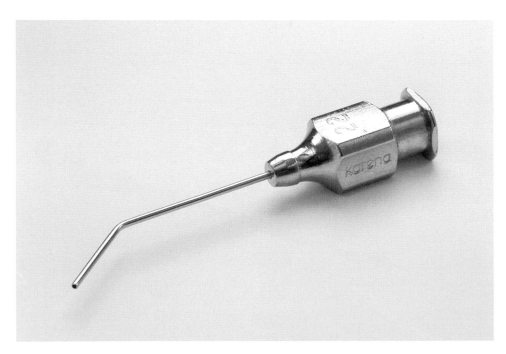

Instrument: IRRIGATING NEEDLE
Other Names: Irrigating Cannula
Category: Accessory
Description: It is an angled, blunt all-metal needle.

Use(s): It attaches to the balanced salt solution (BSS) bottle or a syringe to irrigate the cornea.
Instrument Insight: These can be either reusable or disposable.

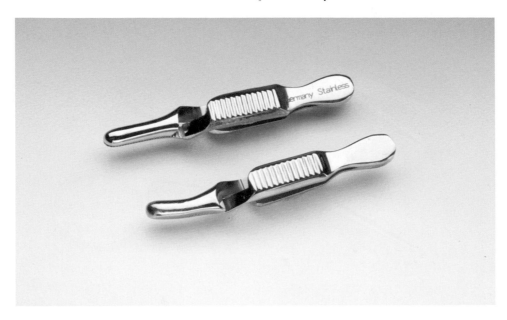

Instrument: SERREFINE CLAMPS
Category: Clamping and Occluding
Description: It is a spring-action clamp with curved or straight jaws with horizontal serrations and a blunt tip.

Use(s): These are used to tag and hold bridle or fine sutures.
Instrument Insight: These are also used in vascular surgery to occlude small vessels.

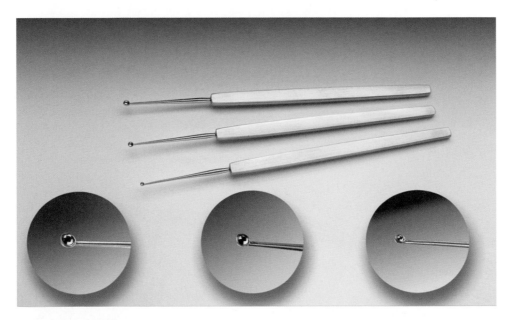

Instrument: MEYHOEFFER CHALAZION CURETTES
Category: Cutting and Dissecting
Description: These have small, sharp, scoop-shaped tips with a flattened handle.

Use(s): These are used for removing chalazion contents by scraping.
Instrument Insight: Tips range from 1 to 3.5 mm in diameter.

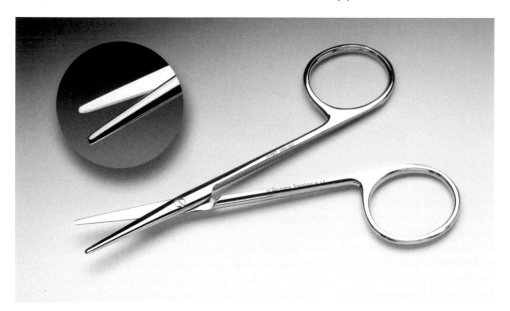

Instrument: KNAPP STRABISMUS SCISSORS
Category: Cutting and Dissecting
Description: These are straight or curved fine, blunt-tip scissors.

Use(s): These are used for dissecting the lateral and medial muscles during recession and resection.

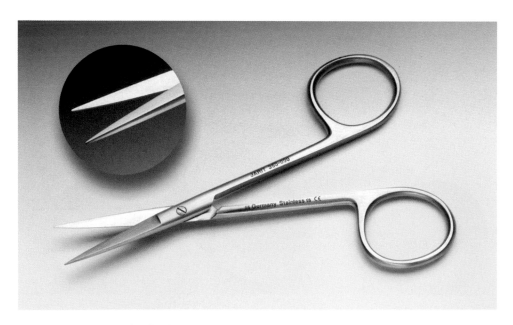

Instrument: KNAPP IRIS SCISSORS
Category: Cutting and Dissecting
Description: These are straight or curved sharp, fine-tip scissors.

Use(s): These are used for incising and dissecting the iris.

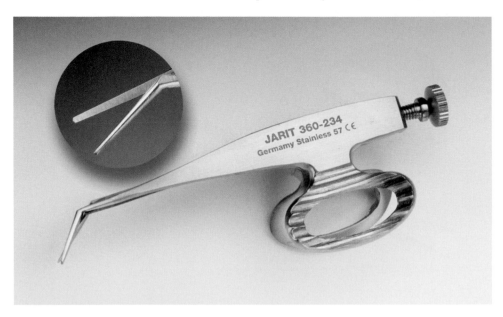

Instrument: BARRAQUER IRIS SCISSORS
Category: Cutting and Dissecting
Description: These are micro scissors with oval fingertip pads and angled, blunt-tip ped blades.
Use(s): These are used for incising and dissecting the iris.

Instrument Insight: Squeezing the finger pads between the thumb and forefinger will close these scissors.

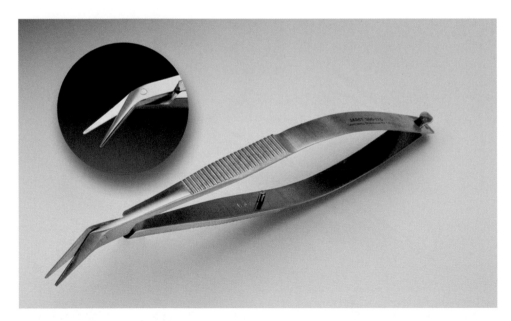

Instrument: CASTROVIEJO CORNEAL SCISSORS
Other Names: Castro scissors
Category: Cutting and Dissecting
Description: These are microsurgical spring-action scissors with angled blades. The blades may be straight or curved. The curved blades will have a right and a left scissors.
Use(s): These are used for incising and dissecting the cornea. During a corneal implant procedure, these scissors are commonly used to complete the trephination.

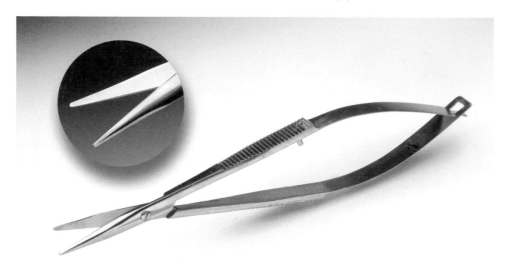

Instrument: WESTCOTT TENOTOMY SCISSORS
Category: Cutting and Dissecting
Description: These are spring-action scissors with fine, narrowed, blunt tips that can be curved or straight.

Use(s): These are used for incising the cornea, sclera, and iris and for dividing eye muscles.

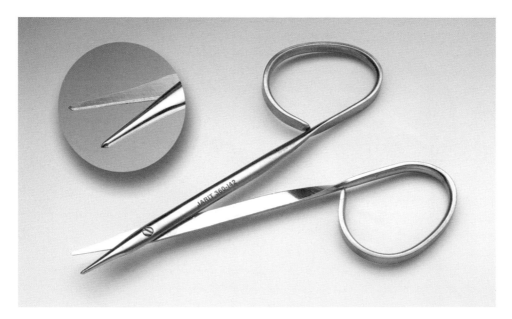

Instrument: STEVENS TENOTOMY SCISSORS
Other Names: Stevens scissors
Category: Cutting and Dissecting
Description: These are small fine scissors that can have curved or straight blades that narrow to blunt tips.

Use(s): These are used for dividing and dissecting the muscles and tendons of the eye. These are commonly used for dividing the lateral and medial tendons and muscles of the eye during recession and resection for strabismus.

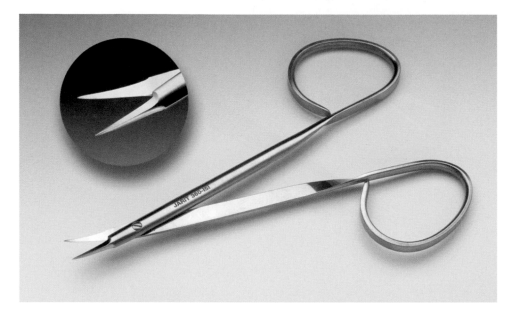

Instrument: EYE SUTURE SCISSORS
Category: Cutting and Dissecting
Description: These are small fine scissors with straight beveled blades that taper to sharp tips.

Use(s): They are used to cut fine eye sutures.
Instrument Insight: These scissors should be used to cut sutures only.

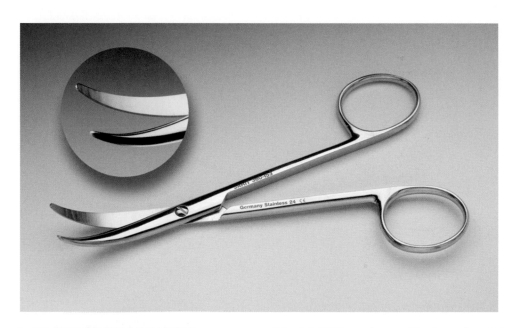

Instrument: ENUCLEATION SCISSORS
Category: Cutting and Dissecting
Description: These are extremely curved scissors that narrow to a blunt tip.

Use(s): These are used to free the globe from the orbit and transect the optic nerve.

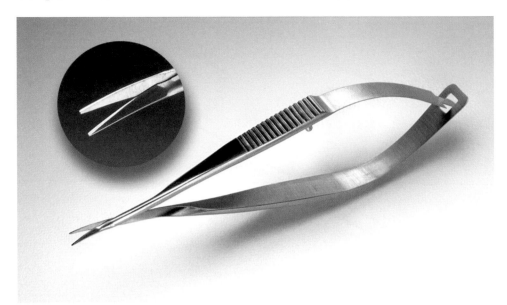

Instrument: VANNAS CAPSULOTOMY SCISSORS
Other Names: Vannas scissors
Category: Cutting and Dissecting
Description: These are micro spring-action scissors with fine, curved, or straight blunt-tipped blades.

Use(s): These are used to incise into the capsule tissue.

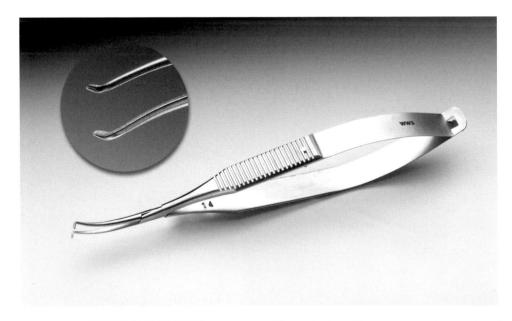

Instrument: LENS INSERTION FORCEPS
Other Names: Clayman lens forceps, lens inserter
Category: Grasping and Holding

Description: These are spring-action forceps with smooth curved jaws and angled tips.
Use(s): These are used for grasping, inserting, and positioning an intraocular lens implant.

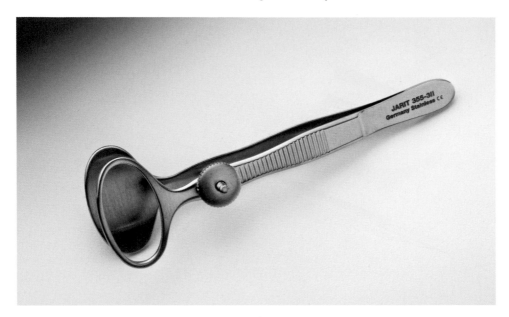

Instrument: **DESMARRES CHALAZION CLAMP**
Other Names: Oval chalazion clamp
Category: Grasping and Holding
Description: These are forceps with a flattened oval plate at the end of one arm and a matching open oval ring on the other arm with a screw-locking device that holds the clamp in place.

Use(s): These are used to stabilize and evert the eyelid to expose the chalazion.
Instrument Insight: This clamp provides hemostasis and a rigid surface against which the cyst can be incised.

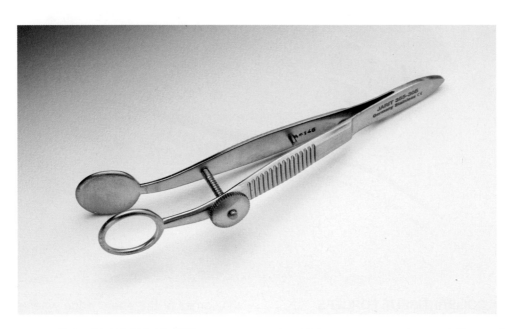

Instrument: **HUNT CHALAZION CLAMP**
Other Names: Round chalazion clamp
Category: Grasping and Holding
Description: These are forceps with a flattened round plate at the end of one arm and a matching open ring on the other arm with a screw-locking device that holds the clamp in place.

Use(s): These are used to stabilize and evert the eyelid to expose the chalazion.
Instrument Insight: This clamp provides hemostasis and a rigid surface against which the cyst can be incised.

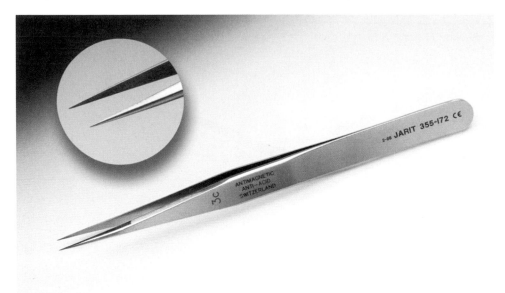

Instrument: JEWELER'S FORCEPS
Category: Grasping and Holding
Description: These are smooth forceps with narrowed, pointed tips.
Use(s): These are used for grasping the intraocular lens.

Instrument Insight: The tips are very sharp and can easily puncture gloves or drapes.

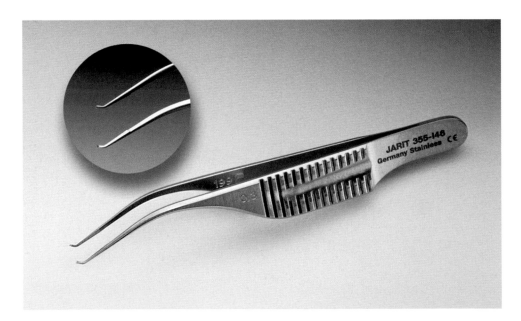

Instrument: COLIBRI TISSUE FORCEPS
Category: Grasping and Holding
Description: It has long, thin, downward-curving jaws with angled toothed tips and a smooth platform behind the tips.
Use(s): These forceps are designed for several functions. The tooth at the tip is used for holding the cornea or the scleral edge when suturing. The platform behind the tip allows for tying sutures. It can also be used to grasp the iris.
Instrument Insight: *Colibri* means bird in Italian and refers to the design of the forceps. The long, thin body ensures optimal viewing during surgical procedures.

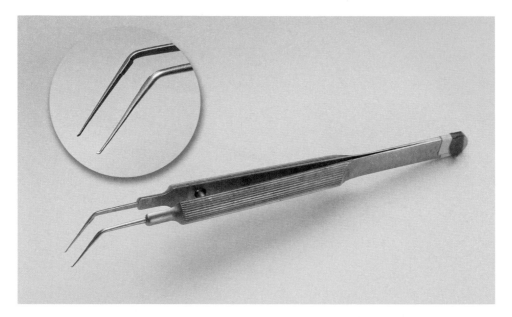

Instrument: CAPSULORHEXIS FORCEPS
Category: Grasping and Holding
Description: These forceps have angled shaft with a length of 12 mm from the bend to tip. Also these have fine, serrated sharp tips.
Use(s): These are used for grasping the capsule, and the sharp point enables the surgeon to initiate the capsule tear during cataract extraction.
Instrument Insight: It is important to check the fine tips of the forceps to make sure they are aligned and in proper working order.

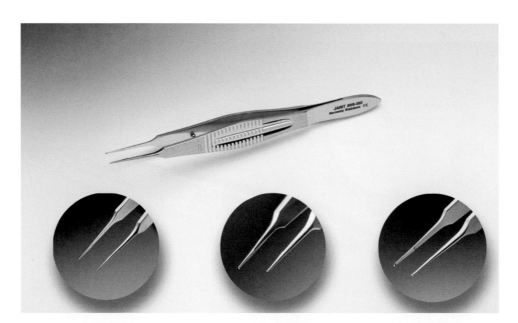

Instrument: CASTROVIEJO SUTURING TISSUE FORCEPS
Other names: .12 mm, .3 mm, .5 mm, point one twos, point threes, point fives
Category: Grasping and Holding
Description: These are small, fine tissue forceps with long, thin jaws that have smooth tying platforms and three interlocking teeth at the tips. Tip sizes are 0.12, 0.3, and 0.5 mm.
Use(s): These are used to grasp and manipulate tissues and tie fine sutures.
Instrument Insight: The area of the eye on which surgery is performed determines the size of the tissue forceps that will be used.

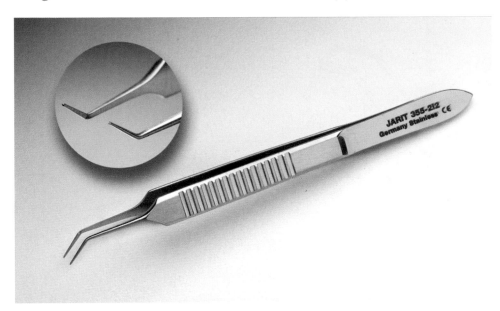

Instrument: McPHERSON TYING FORCEPS
Category: Grasping and Holding
Description: These are small, fine tissue forceps that can have angled or straight jaws with smooth tying platforms.

Use(s): These are designed for tying fine sutures; commonly used in corneal grafting and cataract surgery.
Instrument Insight: This should not be used for grasping tissues because it will crush them.

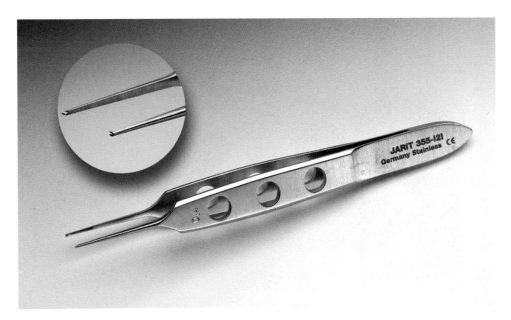

Instrument: BISHOP-HARMON IRIS TISSUE FORCEPS
Category: Grasping and Holding
Description: These are small, fine tissue forceps with long, thin jaws and three interlocking teeth at the tips.

Use(s): These are used for grasping tissue in and around the eye.

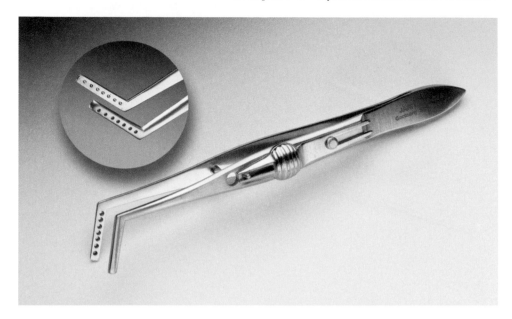

Instrument: JAMESON FORCEPS
Other Names: Muscle clamp
Category: Grasping and Holding
Description: It is a flat, serrated handle with a side lock and a right-angle shaft with six 1-mm teeth on one jaw that fit into the holes on the other jaw.
Use(s): These are used to clamp and hold the extrinsic muscles and provide hemostasis during strabismus procedures.

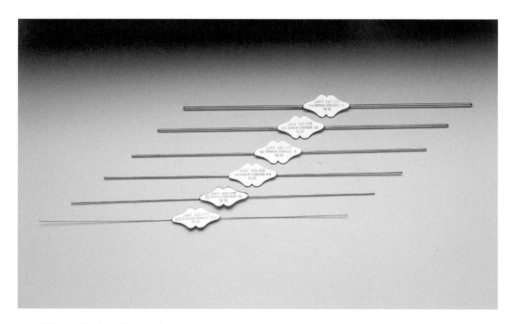

Instrument: BOWMAN LACRIMAL PROBE
Other Names: Lacrimal dilators, duct probes
Category: Probing and Dilating
Description: It is a thin wire on each side of a diamond-shaped plate, with the wire on one side larger than that on the other. The plate is designed to grasp and steady the probe.
Use(s): It is used for probing and gradually dilating the lacrimal duct. This instrument is also used to dilate the salivary duct opening under the tongue.
Instrument Insight: Manufactured in sets of six.

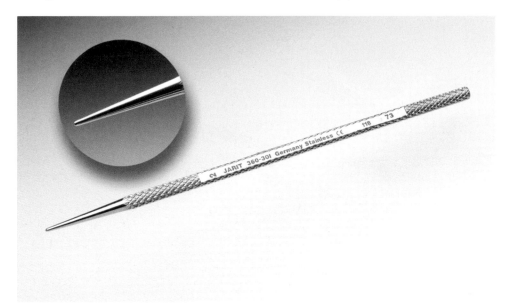

Instrument: WILDER LACRIMAL DILATOR
Other Names: Punctal lacrimal dilator
Category: Probing and Dilating
Description: It has a tapered blunt tip with a round, rough handle.

Use(s): It is used for dilating the lacrimal punctum.

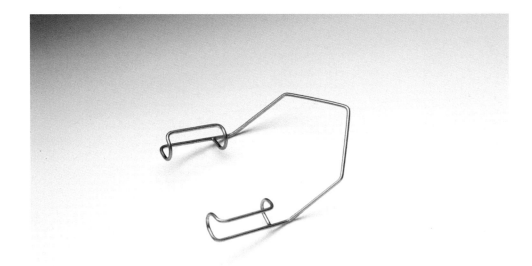

Instrument: BARRAQUER EYE SPECULUM
Other Names: Paper clip, wire speculum
Category: Retracting and Exposing
Description: It has a rigid wire frame with open, curved blades.

Use(s): It holds open the upper and lower eyelids. It is commonly used for cataract extraction.

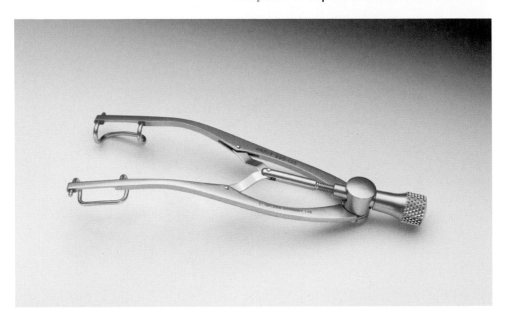

Instrument: CASTROVIEJO EYE SPECULUM
Category: Retracting and Exposing
Description: It is an adjustable self-retaining retractor with curved, open blades.
Use(s): It is used for wide retraction of the upper and lower eyelids. It is often used in strabismus and enucleation procedures in which wide retraction of the lids is needed.

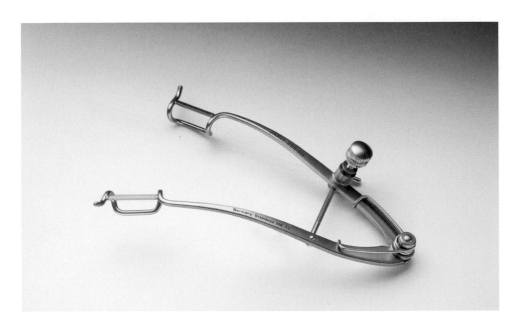

Instrument: WILLIAMS EYE SPECULUM
Category: Retracting and Exposing
Description: It is an adjustable self-retaining retractor with curved, open blades.
Use(s): It is used for wide retraction of the upper and lower eyelids. It is often used in strabismus and enucleation procedures in which wide retraction of the lids is needed.

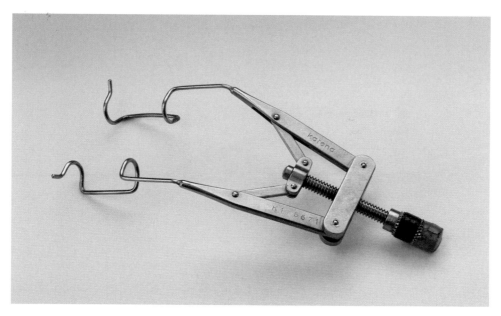

Instrument: LEIBERMAN EYE SPECULUM
Category: Retracting and Exposing
Description: It is an adjustable self-retaining retractor with open, curved, wire-like blades.

Use(s): It is used for wide retraction of the upper and lower eyelids. It is often used in strabismus and enucleation procedures in which wide retraction of the lids is needed.

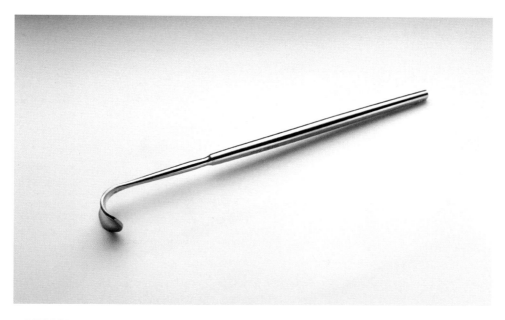

Instrument: DESMARRES LID RETRACTOR
Category: Retracting and Exposing
Description: It is a handheld retractor with a concave curved blade and a round smooth handle.

Use(s): It is used for retraction of the eyelids.

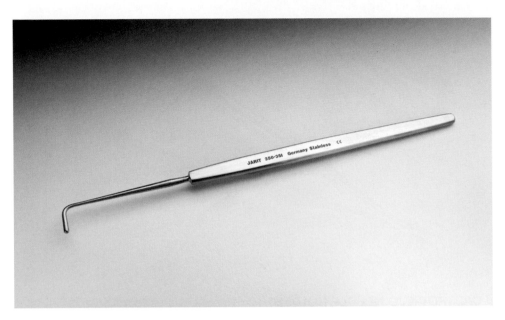

Instrument: VON GRAEFE STRABISMUS HOOK
Other Names: Muscle hook
Category: Retracting and Exposing
Description: It is a blunt right-angled hook with a flattened smooth handle.

Use(s): It is used for lifting and freeing the extrinsic eye muscles from the sclera during strabismus procedures.

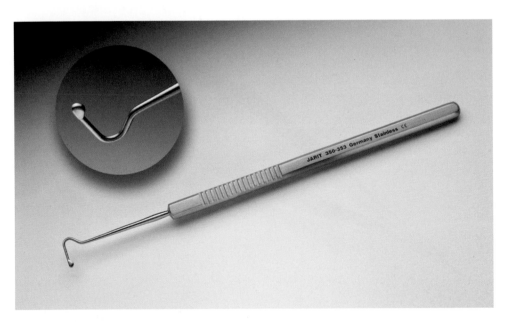

Instrument: JAMESON MUSCLE HOOK
Category: Retracting and Exposing
Description: It is an acute-angle hook with a round tip and a flattened handle.

Use(s): It is used for lifting and retracting the extrinsic eye muscles during strabismus procedures.

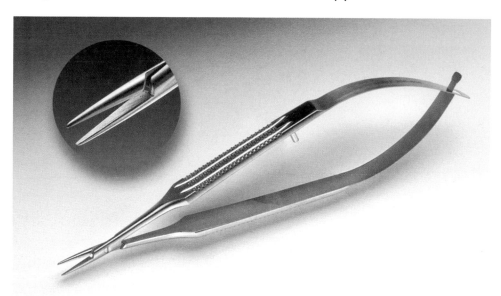

Instrument: CASTROVIEJO NEEDLE HOLDER
Category: Suturing and Stapling
Description: This can be a locking or nonlocking needle holder with narrowed blunt jaws.

Use(s): It is used for holding fine suture needles in eye procedures.

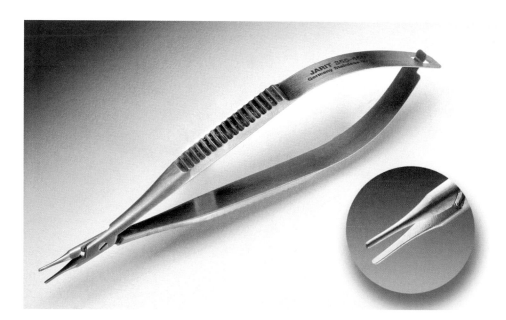

Instrument: McPHERSON NEEDLE HOLDER
Category: Suturing and Stapling
Description: It is a nonlocking needle holder with tapered blunt jaws.

Use(s): It is used for holding fine suture needles in eye procedures.

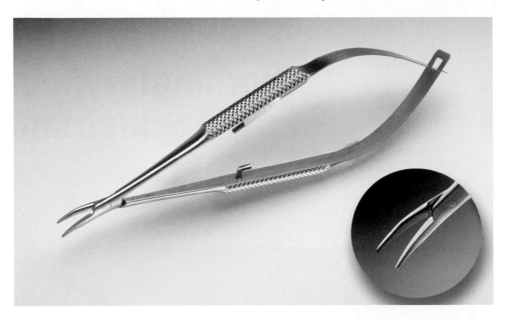

Instrument: BARRAQUER NEEDLE HOLDER
Category: Suturing and Stapling
Description: It is a locking needle holder with curved, narrowed, blunt jaws.

Use(s): It is used for holding fine suture needles in eye procedures.

10 Otorhinolaryngology Instruments

EARS

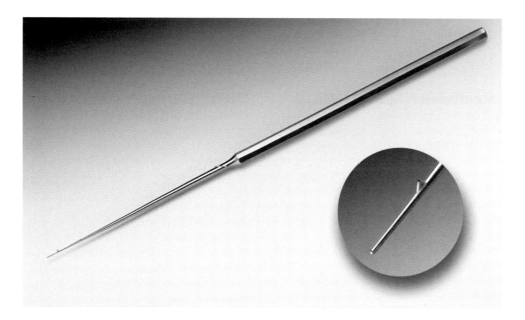

Instrument: HOUSE STRUT CALIPER
Other Names: Measuring tool, strut
Category: Accessory
Description: It is a sharp instrument with a barb toward the tip for measuring.

Use(s): It is used for measuring the ossicles and distances in the middle ear for repair or replacement, especially the stapes.

162

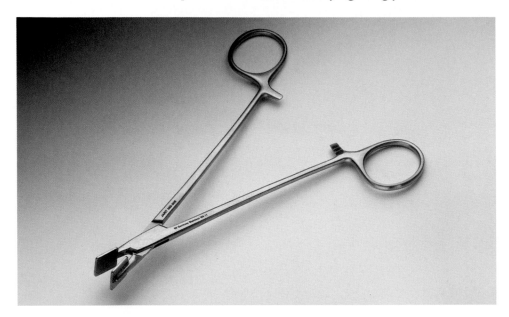

Instrument: HOUSE GELFOAM PRESS
Other Names: Gelfoam masher
Category: Accessory
Description: It has long shanks with finger rings and flat plates at its working tip.

Use(s): The press is used to compress Gelfoam into thin sheets that are cut into tiny squares and used for packing after middle ear procedures. This is done to support and position a graft or to stabilize the prosthesis.

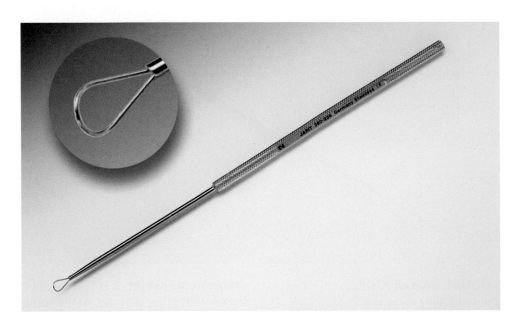

Instrument: BILLEAU EAR LOOP
Other Names: Ear curette
Category: Accessory
Description: It is a long handle with a loop of wire at its working end.

Use(s): It is used for removing cerumen from the ear canal.
Instrument Insight: Have a sponge ready to clean the tip of the instrument as the surgeon removes debris from the ear canal.

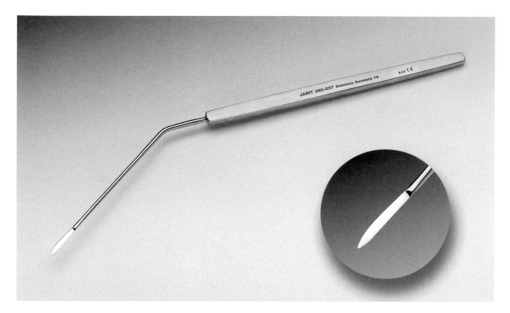

Instrument: MYRINGOTOMY KNIFE
Other Names: Tympanostomy knife, ear knife
Category: Cutting and Dissecting
Description: It is a long, narrow, angled knife with a lancet blade tip.

Use(s): It is used for incising the tympanic membrane for removal of fluid and insertion of aeration tubes.
Instrument Insight: May also use a Beaver knife handle with no. 377110 blades.

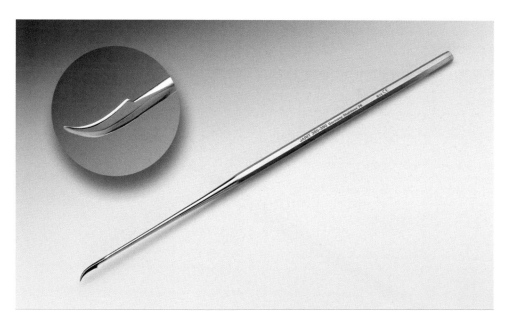

Instrument: HOUSE SICKLE KNIFE
Other Names: Ear knife
Category: Cutting and Dissecting
Description: It is a long handle with a sickle-type cutting edge at its working tip.
Use(s): It is used to cut tissue in the ear canal and middle ear; often used to create a tympanic flap when performing middle ear surgery.

Instrument Insight: It is commonly included in a rack with other delicate instruments for their protection.

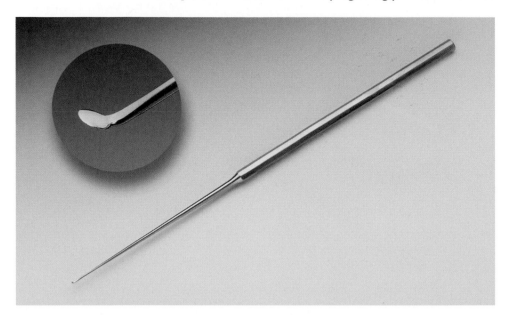

Instrument: HOUSE-SHEEHY KNIFE CURETTE
Other Names: Rosen knife, canal knife
Category: Cutting and Dissecting
Description: It is a long handle with a rounded, angled, sharp tip.
Use(s): It is used for removing tissue and bone from the ear canal and middle ear.
Instrument Insight: It is commonly included in a rack with other delicate instruments for their protection.

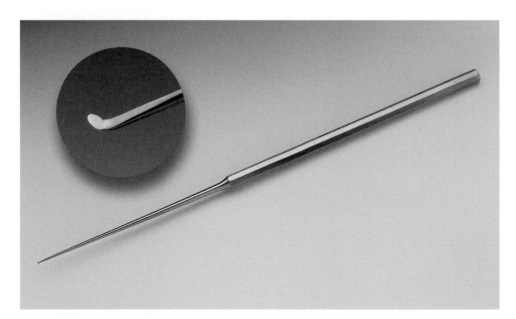

Instrument: HOUSE JOINT KNIFE
Other Names: Canal knife, flap knife
Category: Cutting and Dissecting
Description: It is a long handle with a rounded, angled, sharp tip.
Use(s): It is used for incising and dissecting tissue in the ear canal and middle ear, such as creating a tympanic flap, incising the canal during a tympanoplasty, or separating the incus from the stapes during a stapedectomy.
Instrument Insight: It is commonly included in a rack with other delicate instruments for their protection.

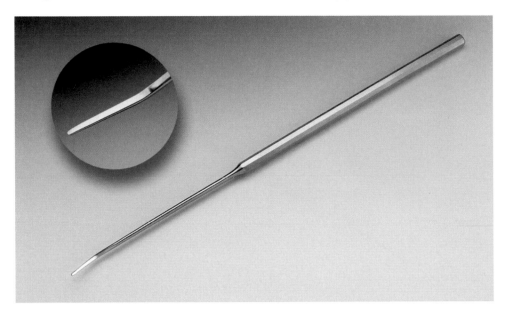

Instrument: HOUSE ELEVATOR
Other Names: Canal elevator, gimmick elevator
Category: Cutting and Dissecting
Description: It is a long handle with an angled, elongated, oval, blunt tip.
Use(s): It is used for manipulating and dissecting tissue in the middle ear and ear canal, such as elevating the annulus of the tympanic membrane.
Instrument Insight: It is commonly included in a rack with other delicate instruments for protection.

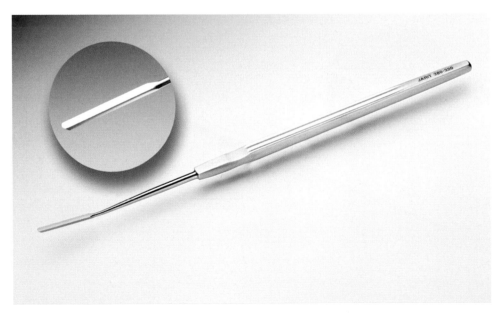

Instrument: LEMPERT ELEVATOR
Category: Cutting and Dissecting
Description: It is a long handle with a slightly angled, elongated, oval, blunt tip.
Use(s): It is used to cut and dissect tissue in the middle ear and ear canal.
Instrument Insight: It is commonly included in a rack with other delicate instruments for protection.

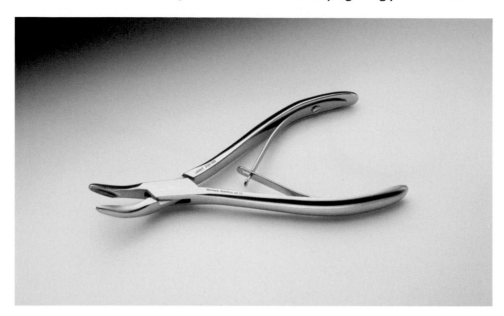

Instrument: CICHERELLI MASTOID RONGEUR
Other Names: Mastoid rongeur
Category: Cutting and Dissecting
Description: It is a small, single-action rongeur, which comes straight or angled.
Use(s): It is used to cut and remove bone and air cells from the mastoid area.
Instrument Insight: This rongeur is often used in other specialties involving bone or tough tissue removal. Always have a moistened sponge ready when handing the surgeon a rongeur. As the surgeon works to remove tissue and/or bone, the rongeur should be cleaned between uses. While focusing on the wound, the surgeon will point the tip of the rongeur toward the surgical technologist. Using a moistened sponge, the surgical technologist should remove the tissue from the jaws of the rongeur.

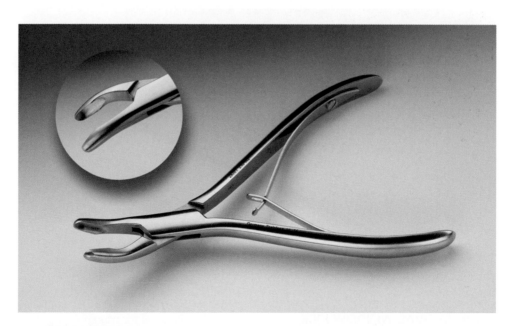

Instrument: DEAN RONGEUR
Category: Cutting and Dissecting
Description: It is a single-action instrument with a curved, sharp, cupped tip.
Use(s): It is used to remove bone.
Instrument Insight: Tissues should be removed between uses with a moistened sponge.

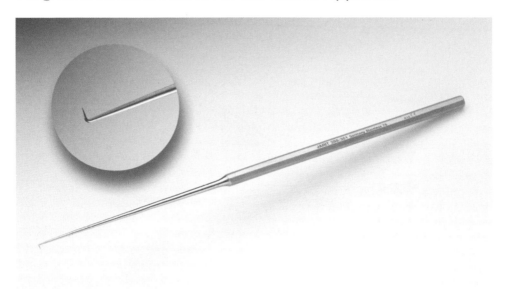

Instrument: HOUSE PICK
Category: Cutting and Dissecting
Description: It is a long handle with a 90-degree angle sharp tip.
Use(s): It is used to manipulate tissue in the middle ear.

Instrument Insight: It is commonly included in a rack with other delicate instruments for protection.

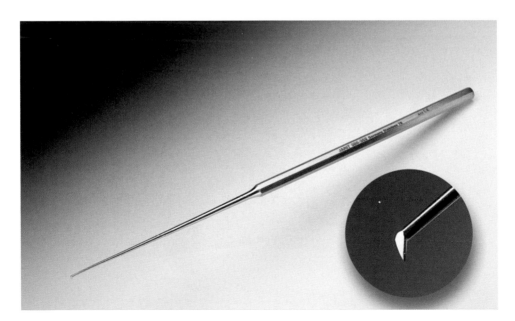

Instrument: HOUSE OVAL WINDOW PICK
Other Names: oval pick, window pick
Category: Cutting and Dissecting
Description: It is a long handle with an angled, sharp, triangular tip.

Use(s): It is used for manipulating the soft tissue graft over the oval window during a stapedectomy.
Instrument Insight: It is commonly included in a rack with other delicate instruments for protection.

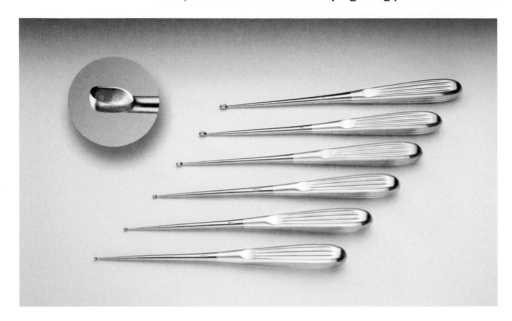

Instrument: SPRATT MASTOID CURETTES
Other Names: Ear curettes
Category: Cutting and Dissecting
Description: These are small, oval, cup-shaped curettes.

Use(s): These are used to remove diseased bone and tissue during a mastoidectomy.

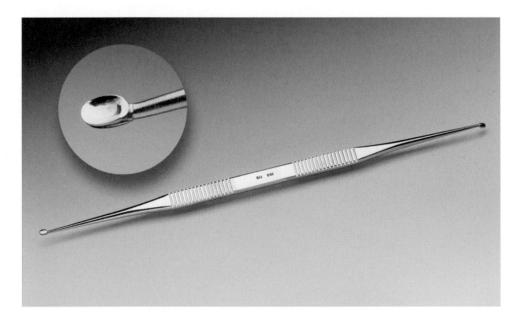

Instrument: HOUSE DOUBLE-ENDED CURETTE
Other Names: Ear curette, small bone curette
Category: Cutting and Dissecting
Description: It is a double-ended curette with cutting cups of different sizes at the ends.

Use(s): It is used to remove bone from the ear canal and middle ear.
Instrument Insight: It is commonly included in a rack with other delicate instruments for protection.

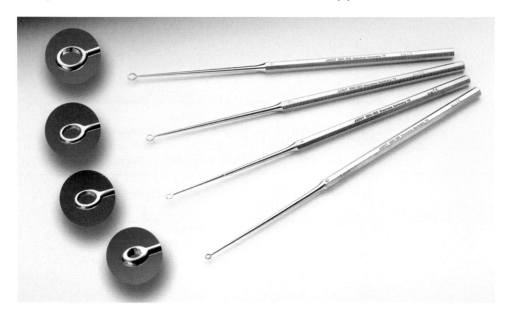

Instrument: BUCK EAR CURETTE
Other Names: Ring curette
Category: Cutting and Dissecting
Description: It is a long handle with a blunt or sharp open ringed tip.

Use(s): It is used to remove bone and tissue from the ear canal and middle ear.

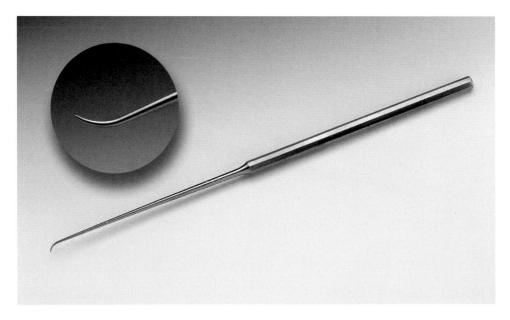

Instrument: ROSEN NEEDLE
Category: Cutting and Dissecting
Description: It is a long handle with a curved tip that tapers to a blunt point.

Use(s): It is used for manipulating tissue and ossicles in the middle ear.
Instrument Insight: It is commonly included in a rack with other delicate instruments for protection.

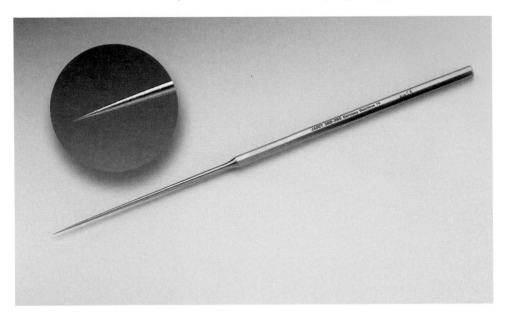

Instrument: HOUSE-BARBARA SHATTERING NEEDLE
Other Names: Barbara needle, shattering needle
Category: Cutting and Dissecting
Description: It is a long handle with a straight tip that tapers to a sharp point.

Use(s): It is used for manipulating tissue and ossicles in the middle ear. It also is used to fracture the superior portion of the stapes from the footplate during a stapedectomy.
Instrument Insight: It is commonly included in a rack with other delicate instruments for protection.

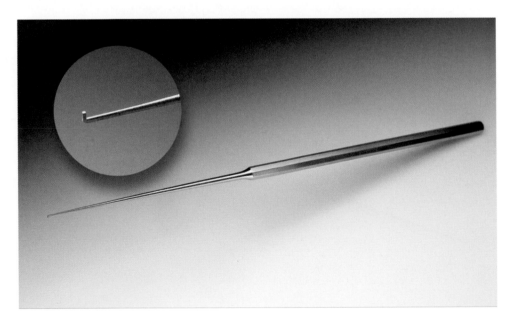

Instrument: HOUSE HOUGH
Category: Cutting and Dissecting
Description: It is a long handle with a 90-degree blunt hooked tip.
Use(s): It is used for manipulating the ossicles and tissues in the middle ear.

Instrument Insight: It is commonly included in a rack with other delicate instruments for protection.

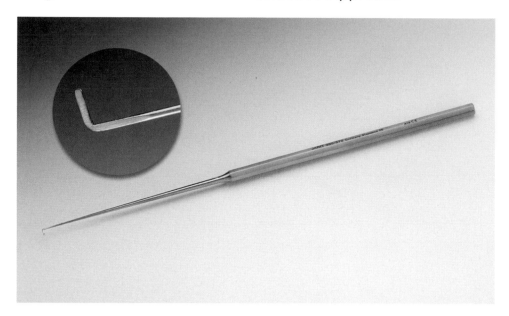

Instrument: CRABTREE DISSECTOR
Other Names: Jimmy dissector
Category: Cutting and Dissecting
Description: It is a long handle with a 90-degree blunt working tip.
Use(s): It is used for manipulating ossicles and tissue in the middle ear.
Instrument Insight: It is commonly included in a rack with other delicate instruments for protection.

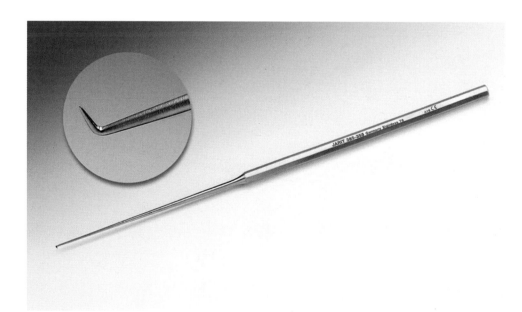

Instrument: HOUSE STRUT HOOK
Other Names: Ditto
Category: Cutting and Dissecting
Description: It is a long handle with a 90-degree sharp tip.
Use(s): It is used for dissecting and removing ossicles from the middle ear.
Instrument Insight: It is commonly included in a rack with other delicate instruments for protection.

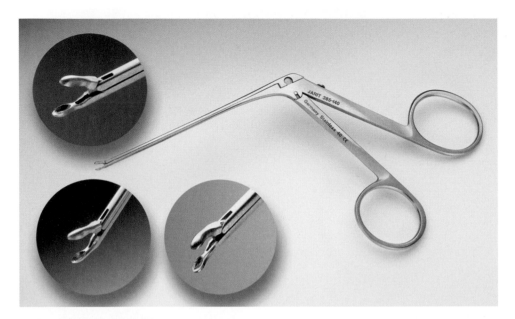

Instrument: OVAL CUP FORCEPS, STRAIGHT CUP FORCEPS, RIGHT CUP FORCEPS, LEFT CUP FORCEPS
Other Names: Micro cups, ear cup forceps
Category: Cutting and Dissecting
Description: These are small instruments with finger rings and an oval cupped working tip. The cup tips can be straight, left, right, up, or down biting for accessing the middle ear.
Use(s): These are used for removing tissue and ossicles from the middle ear.
Instrument Insight: These instruments should be cleaned with an instrument wipe between uses.

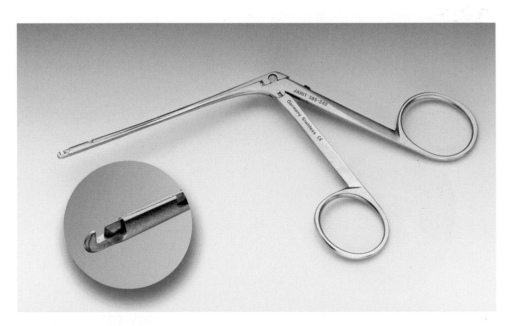

Instrument: HOUSE-DIETER MALLEUS NIPPER
Other Names: Nipper
Category: Cutting and Dissecting
Description: It is a small instrument with finger rings and a guillotine-type cutting tip.
Use(s): It is used for reshaping of the ossicles, especially the malleus, for ossicular reconstruction.

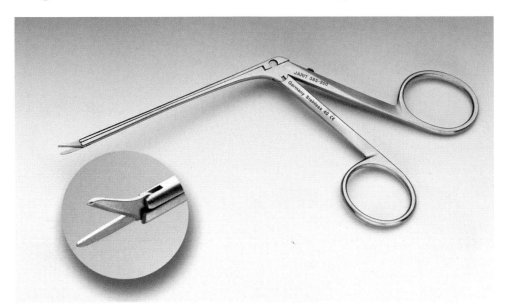

Instrument: BELLUCCI SCISSORS
Other Names: Middle ear scissors
Category: Cutting and Dissecting
Description: It is a small instrument with finger rings and delicate scissors on the working tip.

Use(s): It is used for cutting tissue in the middle ear.
Instrument Insight: These are very delicate instruments; do not use them to cut packing or sutures of any kind, as this will dull the blades.

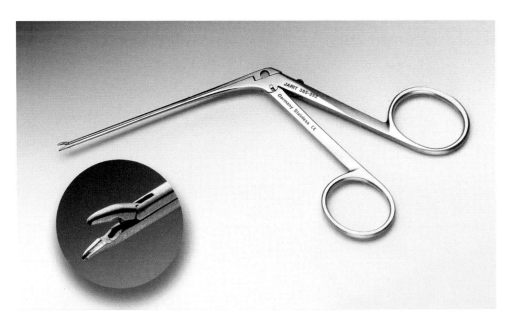

Instrument: McGEE WIRE CRIMPING FORCEPS
Other Names: Crimper forceps
Category: Grasping and Holding
Description: These are small instruments with finger rings and delicate working tip for use through the ear canal and into the middle ear.

Use(s): These are used for ossicular reconstruction to clip or bend the wire on the stapes prosthesis.
Instrument Insight: Instrument is delicate; do not drop or place heavier instruments on top of it. Keep its tip clean with an instrument wipe or dampened sponge.

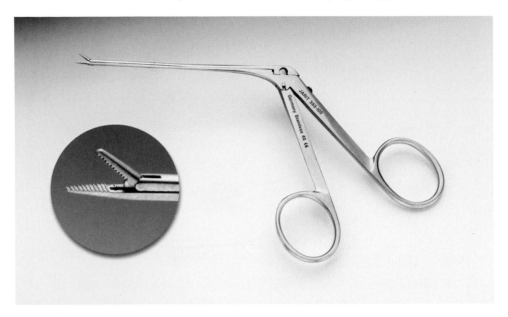

Instrument: WULLSTEIN EAR FORCEPS
Other Names: Alligator forceps
Category: Grasping and Holding
Description: These are small instruments with finger rings with tapered, serrated jaws.

Use(s): These are used for manipulating and removing tissue from the ear canal and middle ear, inserting aeration tubes, and placing Gelfoam packing when grafting.

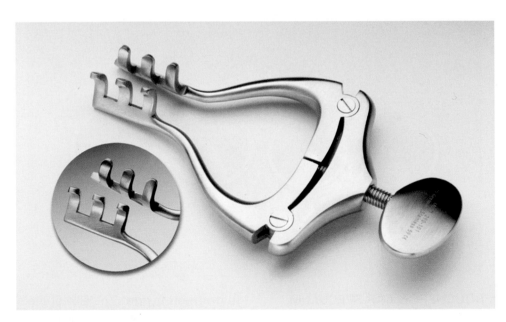

Instrument: JANSEN MASTOID RETRACTOR
Category: Retracting and Exposing
Description: It is a small self-retaining retractor with a screw-locking device at the proximal end that holds it open and two small arms that have three sharp or blunt outward-curving prongs on the working end.

Use(s): It is used for retracting a postauricular incision.

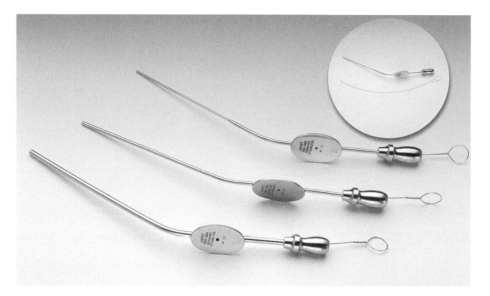

Instrument: BARON SUCTION TIPS
Other Names: Ear suction, finger control suction
Category: Suctioning and Aspirating
Description: It is a small, angled, cylindric tube with a relief opening/hole on the handgrip. The diameters are 3F, 5F, and 7F, and they are usually packaged with a metal stylet that fits inside the cylinder.
Use(s): These are used to remove excess fluid and blood from the operative site.
Instrument Insight: Suction can be increased by covering the relief opening. When the suction tip becomes clogged with tissue and debris, the stylet is used to remove it, or a syringe with sterile water can be used to flush it. Be sure to place a finger over the opening when irrigating the tip. If the stylet is inadvertently left in the suction tip during the sterilization process, do not just remove the stylet and hand it off the field. The inside of the Baron tip and the stylet is considered unsterile, and both should be removed from the field.

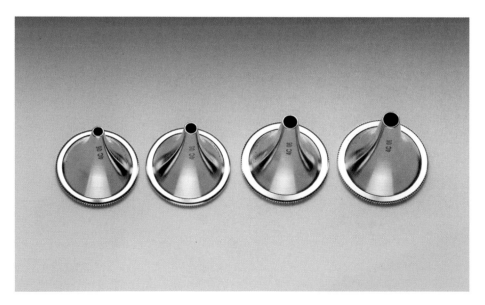

Instrument: BOUCHERON EAR SPECULUM
Category: Viewing
Description: It is a bell-shaped speculum with a round opening; available in a set of varying sizes.
Use(s): It is used for opening the ear canal for exposure of the tympanic membrane and portions of the middle ear.

Instrument Insight: The size of the speculum is determined by the size of the patient's ear canal.

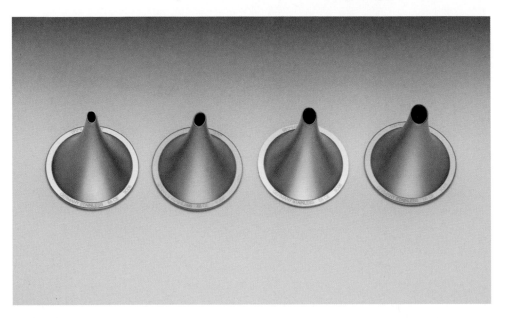

Instrument: FARRIOR EAR SPECULUM
Category: Viewing
Description: It is a bell-shaped speculum with an oval opening; available in a set of varying sizes.

Use(s): It is used for opening the ear canal for exposure of the tympanic membrane and portions of the middle ear.
Instrument Insight: The size of the speculum is determined by the size of the patient's ear canal.

NOSE

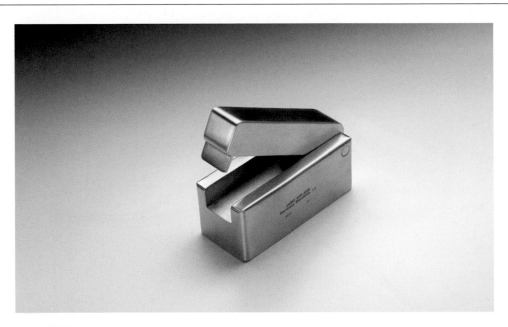

Instrument: COTTLE BONE CRUSHER
Category: Accessory
Description: A rectangular solid box with a channel in the middle and a solid lid that closes into the channel, compressing the object placed inside.

Use(s): It is used to flatten the septal cartilage before replacing it in the nose.
Instrument Insight: A mallet is used to impact the lid to prepare the cartilage.

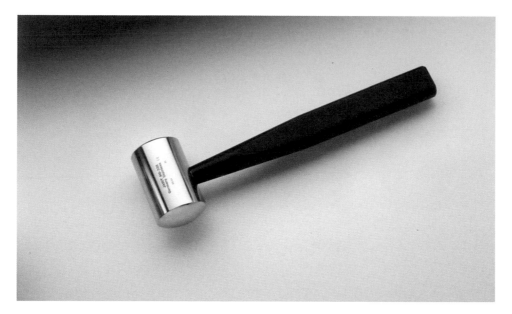

Instrument: COTTLE MALLET
Other Names: Mallet
Category: Accessory
Description: It is a solid stainless steel head with one flat face and one round face attached to a black aluminum handle. Mallets are hammering-type instruments that weigh between 5 ounces and 2 pounds.

Use(s): It is used to exert force on osteotomes, chisels, gouges, tamps, and other specially designed instruments.
Instrument Insight: The surgeon will use a "tap-tap" rhythm when hitting the osteotome. The second hit is usually slightly harder than the first.

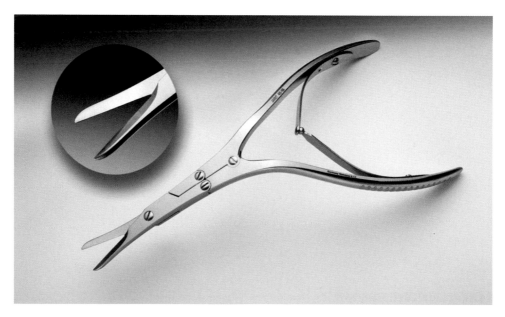

Instrument: CAPLAN SCISSORS
Category: Cutting and Dissecting
Description: These are double-action instruments with angled scissor blades and blunt tips.

Use(s): These are used for cutting tissue within the nasal cavity.

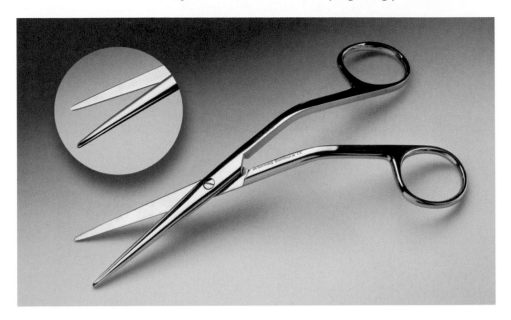

Instrument: COTTLE ANGULAR SCISSORS
Other Names: Turbinate scissors, posterior scissors
Category: Cutting and Dissecting
Description: These are angled scissors with long, narrow, blunt blades.

Use(s): These are used for trimming the turbinate (mucosal) tissue in the nose.
Instrument Insight: These scissors come in small and medium sizes.

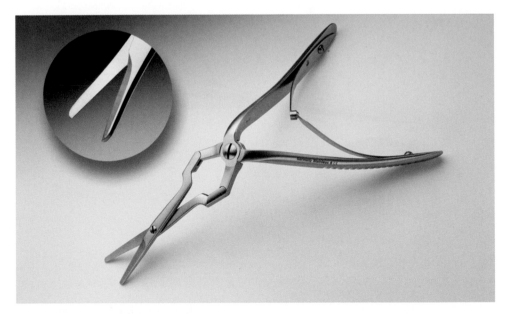

Instrument: BECKER SEPTUM SCISSORS
Category: Cutting and Dissecting
Description: These are angled double-action scissors with straight, blunt-tip ped blades.

Use(s): These are used for cutting tissue within the nasal cavity.

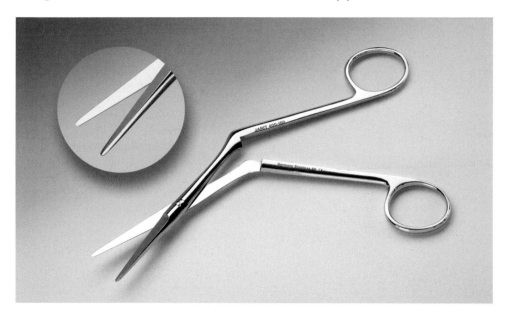

Instrument: KNIGHT ANGULAR SCISSORS
Other Names: Heymann-Knight angular scissors
Category: Cutting and Dissecting
Description: These are angled scissors with narrow, blunt blades.

Use(s): These are used for cutting tissue within the nasal cavity.

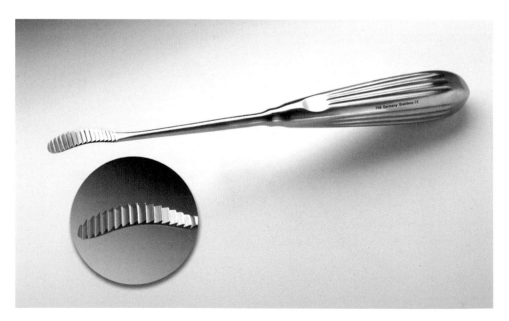

Instrument: AUFRICHT NASAL RASP
Category: Cutting and Dissecting
Description: This rasp is a round-handled instrument that has a rounded, slightly curved working end with sharp horizontal ridges.

Use(s): It is used for filing hard tissue and bone.
Instrument Insight: Bits of bone and tissue will accumulate in the ridges; clean the rasp by rinsing it in a small basin of water between uses.

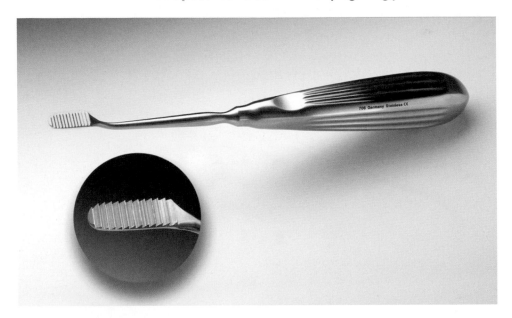

Instrument: LEWIS RASP
Category: Cutting and Dissecting
Description: This rasp is a round-handled instrument that has a rounded, straight working end with sharp horizontal ridges.

Use(s): It is used for filing hard tissue and bone.
Instrument Insight: Bits of bone and tissue will accumulate in the ridges; clean the rasp by rinsing it in a small basin of water between uses.

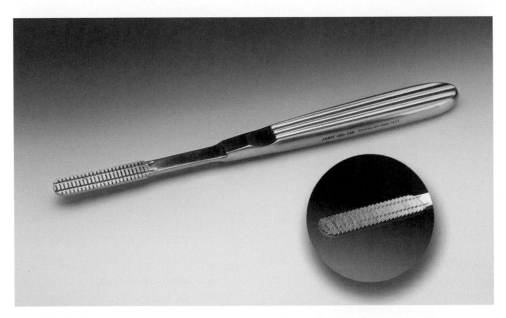

Instrument: MALTZ RASP
Other Names: Maltz-Lipsett rasp
Category: Cutting and Dissecting
Description: It has a rectangular sanding edge with horizontal and vertical ridges.

Use(s): It is used for filing hard tissue and bone.
Instrument Insight: Bits of bone and tissue will accumulate in the ridges; clean the rasp by rinsing it in a small basin of water between uses.

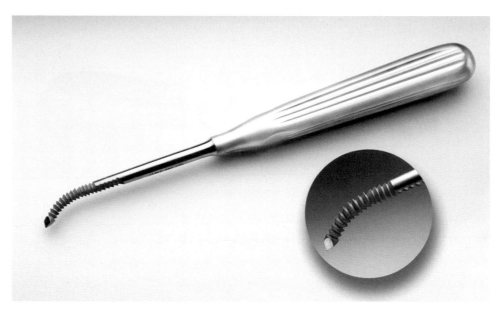

Instrument: WIENER ANTRUM RASP
Other Names: Antrum rasp
Category: Cutting and Dissecting
Description: It is a straight handle and shaft with a curved working end that has sharp, encircling, raised serrations and a trocar tip.

Use(s): It is used for creating an opening through the nasal wall to the maxillary sinus.

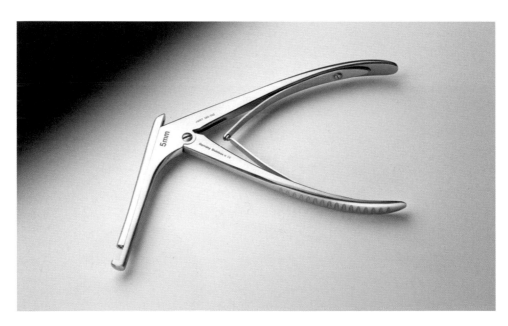

Instrument: KERRISON RONGEUR
Other Names: Up-biter
Category: Cutting and Dissecting
Description: It has gripped handles with a 4-inch shaft and chisel-edge punch at the working tip. The punch tip is available in 3-, 4-, 5-, and 6-mm bites.
Use(s): It is used for biting off bone.
Instrument Insight: This rongeur can also have the biting edge positioned downward, called a down-biter or back biter. Always have a moistened sponge ready when handing the surgeon a rongeur. As the surgeon works to remove tissue and/or bone, the rongeur has to be cleaned between uses. While focusing on the wound, the surgeon will point the tip of the rongeur toward the surgical technologist. Using a moistened sponge, the surgical technologist will clean the tissue and bone from the jaws.

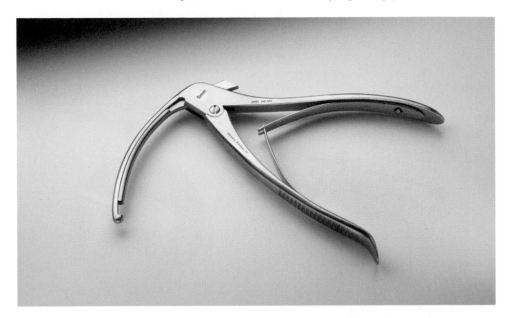

Instrument: KERRISON-COSTEN RONGEUR
Category: Cutting and Dissecting
Description: This instrument is a variation of the Kerrison rongeur, but this rongeur has an angled arm and the cutting end is facing downward.
Use(s): It is used for biting off bone.
Instrument Insight: Always have a moistened sponge ready when handing the surgeon a rongeur. As the surgeon works to remove tissue and/or bone, the rongeur has to be cleaned between uses. While focusing on the wound, the surgeon will point the tip of the rongeur toward the surgical technologist. Using a moistened sponge, the surgical technologist will clean the tissue from the jaws.

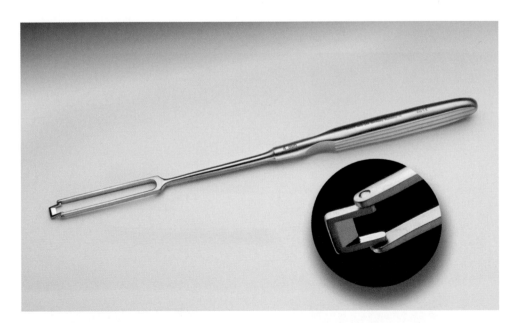

Instrument: BALLENGER SWIVEL KNIFE
Other Names: Swivel knife
Category: Cutting and Dissecting
Description: It is a handled instrument with a hinged cutting tip for ease of application through nasal tissue.

Use(s): It is used to cut and dissect nasal mucosa.

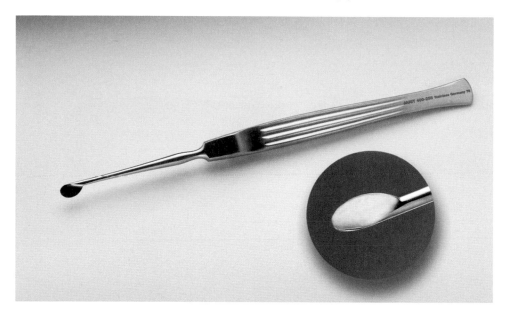

Instrument: FREER SEPTUM KNIFE
Other Names: Septal knife
Category: Cutting and Dissecting
Description: It is a flat-handled instrument with a rounded, sharp cutting end.
Use(s): It is used to cut and dissect septal mucosa.

Instrument Insight: It is commonly included in a tray or rack with other delicate instruments for protection.

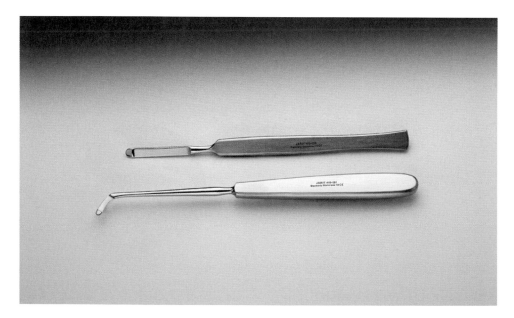

Instrument: JOSEPH BUTTON-END KNIFE
Category: Cutting and Dissecting
Description: It is a solid-handled instrument with either an angled or a straight blade.

Use(s): It is used for dissecting nasal mucosa from the septum.

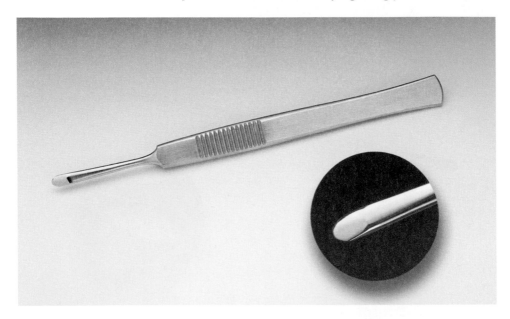

Instrument: COTTLE NASAL KNIFE
Category: Cutting and Dissecting
Description: It is a flat-handled instrument with a smaller, flattened, sharp tip.
Use(s): It is used for dissecting nasal mucosa from the septum.

Instrument Insight: It is commonly included in a tray or rack with other delicate instruments for protection.

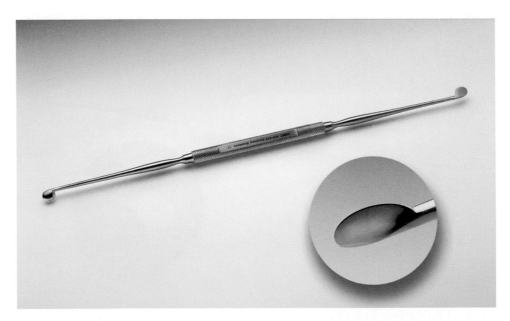

Instrument: PIERCE DOUBLE-ENDED ELEVATOR
Category: Cutting and Dissecting
Description: It is a double-ended elevator with two rounded sharp blades at each end, with one blade larger than the other.

Use(s): It is used to cut and dissect septal mucosa.
Instrument Insight: It is commonly included in a tray or rack with other delicate instruments for protection.

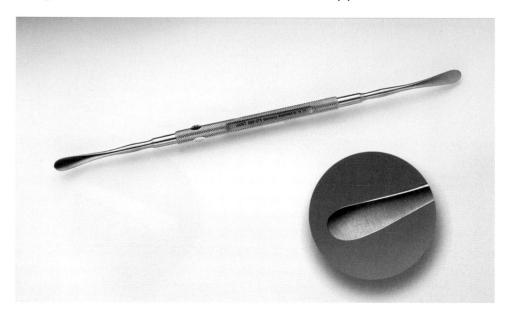

Instrument: FREER SEPTUM ELEVATOR
Other Names: Freer elevator
Category: Cutting and Dissecting
Description: It is a round handle with tear-shaped sharp tips at both ends.

Use(s): It is used to dissect nasal mucosa from the septum.

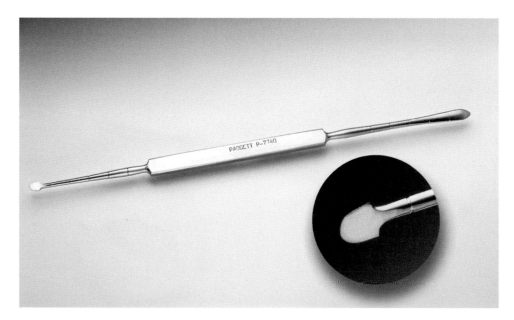

Instrument: COTTLE SEPTAL ELEVATOR
Category: Cutting and Dissecting
Description: It is a double-ended elevator with a flattened handle; one end is sharp and rounded and the other end is sharp, flattened, and tear-shaped. The instrument has calibrations on both arms.

Use(s): It is used for cutting and dissecting nasal mucosa.
Instrument Insight: It is commonly included in a tray or rack with other delicate instruments for protection.

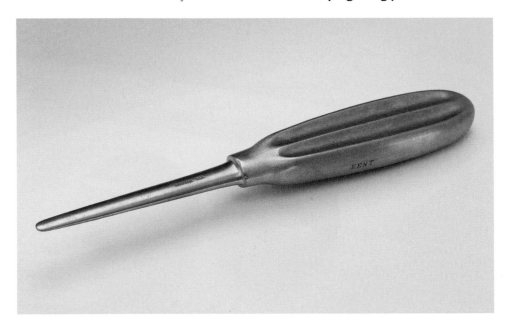

Instrument: **GOLDMAN SEPTUM ELEVATOR**
Other Names: Boies elevator, Butter knife
Category: Cutting and Dissecting
Description: It has a broad, smooth blade with a heavy, oval-shaped, grooved handle.

Use(s): The elevator is used to manipulate and realign cartilage and bone during a reduction nasal fracture. It can also be used to lift the mucoperichondrial flap in septoplasties.

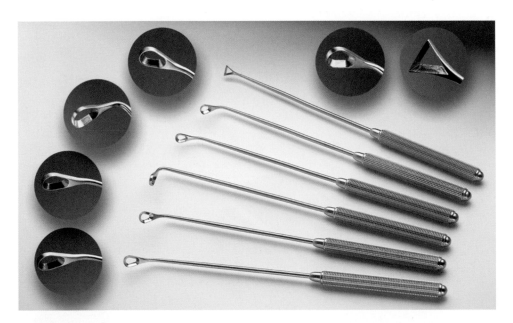

Instrument: **COAKLEY ANTRUM CURETTES**
Other Names: Nasal curettes
Category: Cutting and Dissecting
Description: It is a round-handled instrument with a circular cutting tip that is available in different sizes and different angles.

Use(s): It is used for removing polyps and diseased sinus tissue.

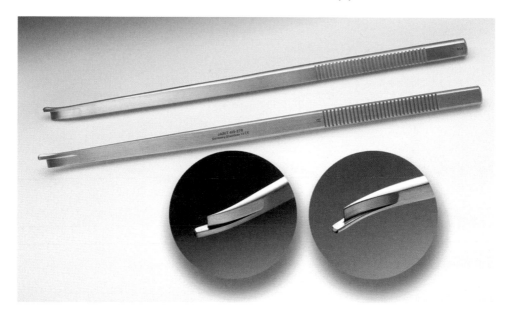

Instrument: ANDERSON-NEIVERT OSTEOTOME, GUARDED
Category: Cutting and Dissecting
Description: It is a flat-handled instrument with a tip beveled to a point for cutting. One side of the tip extends out and is blunt, which acts as a guard. These osteotomes vary in width.
Use(s): It is used for cutting bone.
Instrument Insight: Always hand it to the surgeon with a mallet.

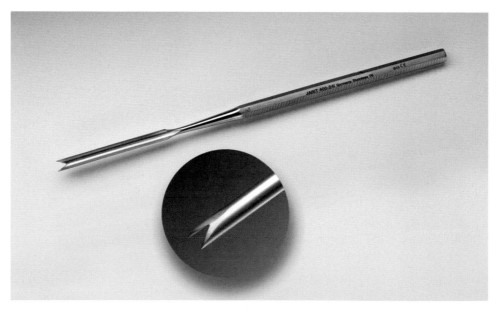

Instrument: BALLENGER V-SHAPED OSTEOTOME
Category: Cutting and Dissecting
Description: It is a rounded handle with a V-shaped cutting edge.
Use(s): It is used for removing bone.
Instrument Insight: This instrument is finer than other osteotomes but still requires a mallet for use.

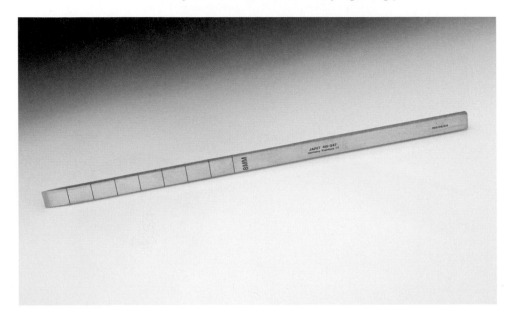

Instrument: COTTLE OSTEOTOME
Category: Cutting and Dissecting
Description: It is a solid stainless steel strip with a smooth, inclining, sharp-blade tip.

Use(s): It is used for dissecting and sculpting bone.
Instrument Insight: Always hand it to the surgeon with a mallet.

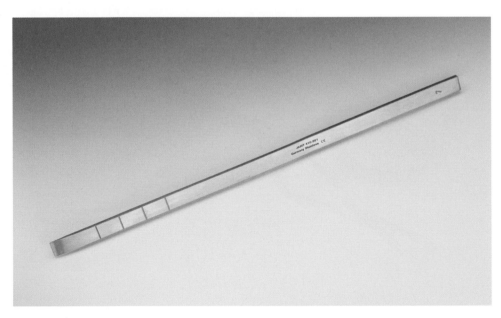

Instrument: COTTLE CHISEL
Other Names: Nasal chisels
Category: Cutting and Dissecting
Description: It is a solid stainless steel strip that ends in a beveled, sharp tip.

Use(s): It is used for cutting bone.
Instrument Insight: Always hand it to the surgeon with a mallet.

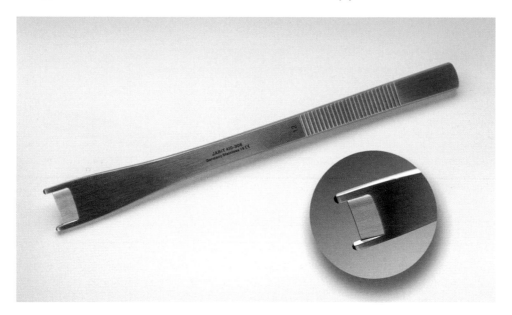

Instrument: CINELLI GUARDED OSTEOTOME
Category: Cutting and Dissecting
Description: It is a solid stainless steel strip with a widened blade that has a guard on each side.

Use(s): It is used to cut bone.
Instrument Insight: Always hand it to the surgeon with a mallet.

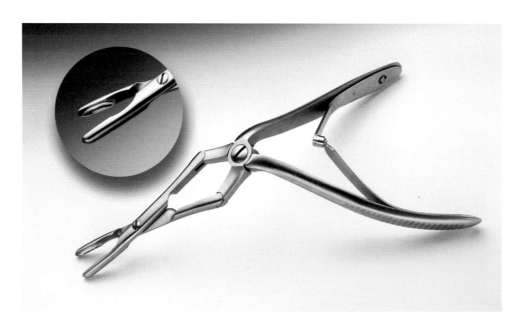

Instrument: JANSEN-MIDDLETON SEPTUM FORCEPS
Category: Cutting and Dissecting
Description: It is a double-action angled instrument with oval cup jaws.

Use(s): It dissects and removes nasal tissues.
Instrument Insight: Tissues should be removed between uses with a moistened sponge.

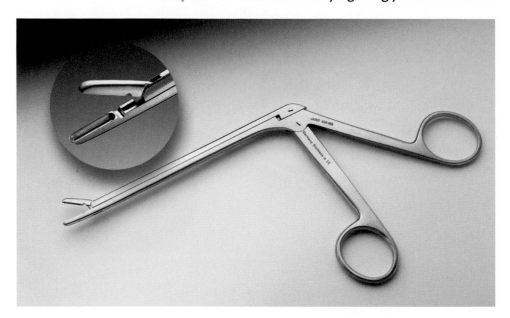

Instrument: TAKAHASHI NASAL FORCEPS
Category: Cutting and Dissecting
Description: It is a handle with finger rings and a long shaft, with an oval cup-shaped tip.

Use(s): It is used to grasp and remove nasal tissue and polyps.
Instrument Insight: Tissues should be removed between uses with a moistened sponge.

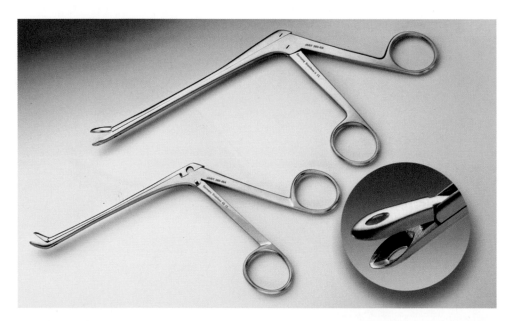

Instrument: WILDE ETHMOID FORCEPS
Category: Cutting and Dissecting
Description: It has a handle with finger rings, a long shaft, and an oval cup-shaped tip with fenestrations.
Use(s): It is used to remove infected or inflamed tissue that lines the nasal sinuses or to remove nasal polyps, especially in the ethmoid sinuses.
Instrument Insight: Instrument is available in straight and up-biting tips. Tissue should be removed between uses with a moistened sponge.

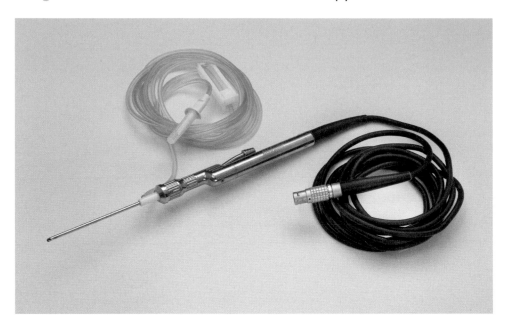

Instrument: STRAIGHTSHOT MICRODEBRIDER
Other Names: Sinus shaver, Straightshot shaver
Category: Cutting and Dissecting
Description: It is a headpiece with interchangeable blades and burrs that are determined by the procedure being performed.

The headpiece is hooked to suction, irrigation, and the console. The headpiece is activated by a foot pedal.
Use(s): It is used for incising or removing soft tissue, hard tissue, or bone. It is also used during endoscopic sinus, laryngeal, and tracheal procedures.

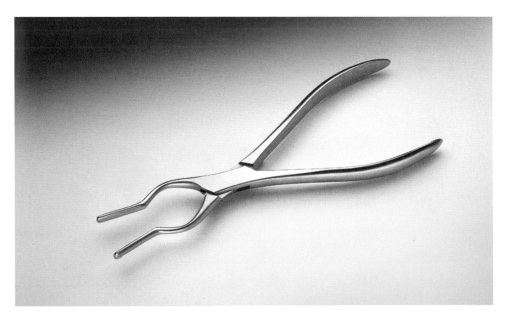

Instrument: WALSHAM SEPTUM STRAIGHTENER
Category: Grasping and Holding
Description: It is a single-action handle with a rounded jaw that extends to a flattened end approximately 1 inch on each side of the jaw.

Use(s): This instrument is placed inside the nose, on both sides of the septum, to straighten a displaced nasal fracture.
Instrument Insight: The ends are rounded at the tip to prevent injury to the septum during insertion.

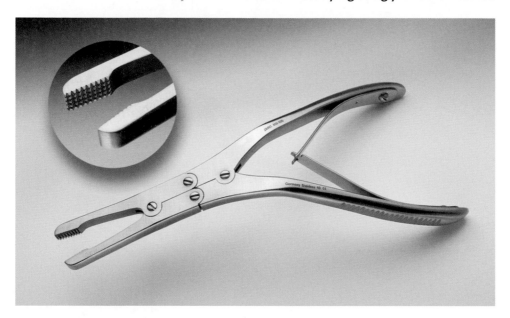

Instrument: RUBIN MORSELIZER
Category: Grasping and Holding
Description: It is a double-action instrument with a rectangular tip and cross-hatch serrations.

Use(s): It is used to grasp and soften nasal cartilage for reinsertion into the septum.

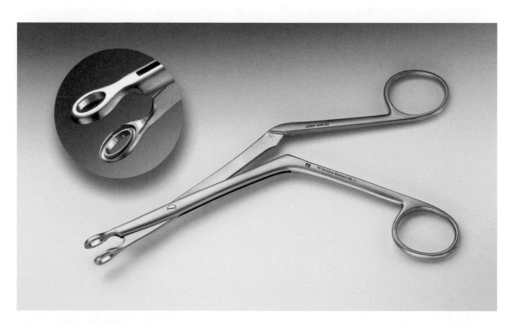

Instrument: BRUENING SEPTUM FORCEPS
Category: Grasping and Holding
Description: It is an instrument with finger rings and a cupped, perforated tip.

Use(s): It is used to grasp and hold nasal tissue.

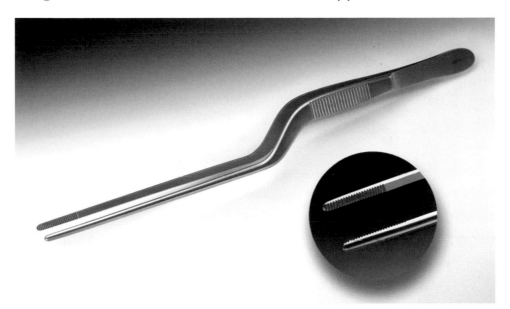

Instrument: JANSEN TISSUE FORCEPS
Other Names: Bayonet
Category: Grasping and Holding
Description: These are long bayonet-shaped tissue forceps with serrated, round tips.
Use(s): These are used for grasping and manipulating tissue and placing packing or nasal splints.

Instrument Insight: The bayonet has a curved shape to keep the instrument from obstructing the surgeon's view when in use.

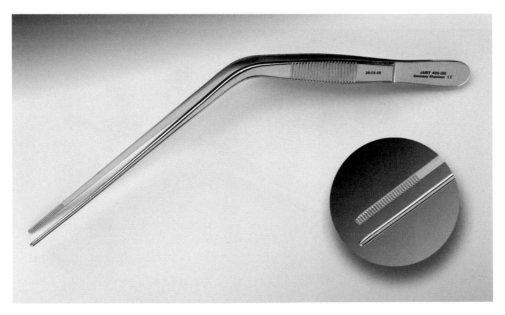

Instrument: WILDE TISSUE FORCEPS
Other Names: Wilde dressing forceps
Category: Grasping and Holding
Description: These are long, angled tissue forceps with serrated, round tips.

Use(s): These are used for grasping and manipulating tissue and placing packing or nasal splints.

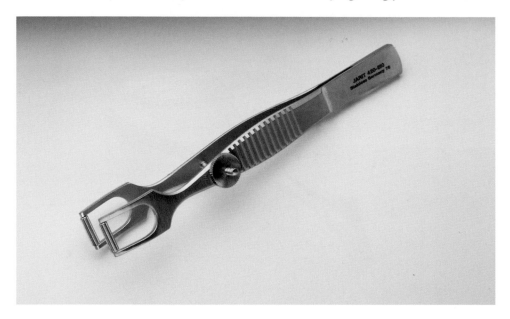

Instrument: COTTLE COLUMELLA FORCEPS
Other Names: Columella retractor
Category: Retracting and Exposing
Description: It is a two-bladed, self-retaining instrument with a screw-down mechanism to hold arms in place.

Use(s): It is used for manipulating and retracting the nasal columella.
Instrument Insight: This instrument fits onto the anterior part of the septum (columella) with one blade positioned on each side, and screws down to lock.

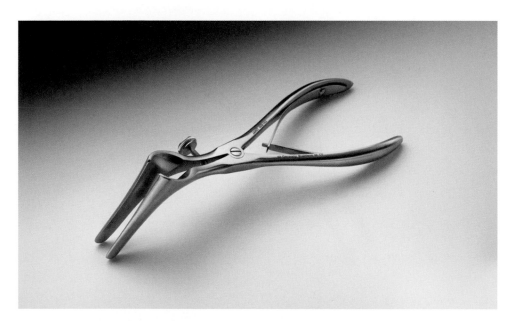

Instrument: COTTLE NASAL SPECULUM
Category: Retracting and Exposing
Description: It is a self-retaining instrument with double-bladed tips and a screw opening device. The speculum blades vary in length.

Use(s): It is used for retracting the nares for visualization.

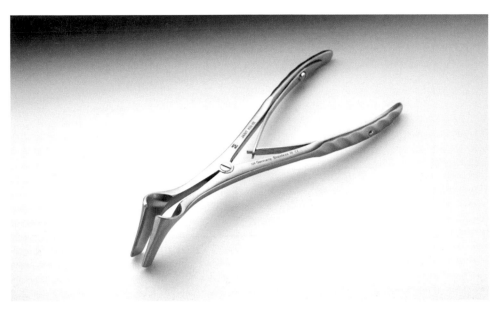

Instrument: VIENNA NASAL SPECULUM
Category: Retracting and Exposing
Description: It is a manually held double-bladed instrument with concave tips. The speculum blades vary in length.

Use(s): It is used for retracting the nares for visualization.

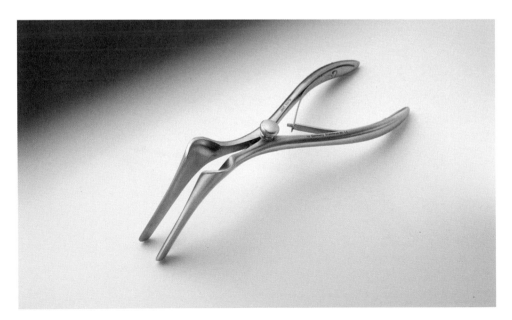

Instrument: KILLIAN NASAL SPECULUM
Category: Retracting and Exposing
Description: It is a self-retaining instrument with double-bladed tips and a screw opening device. The speculum blades vary in length.

Use(s): It is used for retracting the nares for visualization.

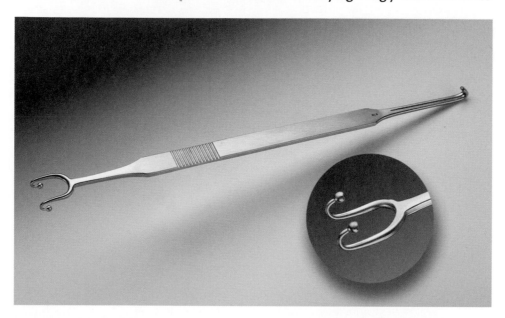

Instrument: COTTLE KNIFE GUIDE AND RETRACTOR
Category: Retracting and Exposing
Description: It is a double-ended retractor with a small blunt hook on one end and two curved ball-tip prongs on the other end.

Use(s): It is used for retracting the nares for visualization.

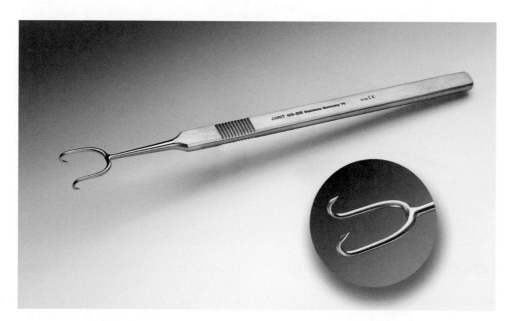

Instrument: COTTLE DOUBLE HOOK RETRACTOR
Category: Retracting and Exposing
Description: It is an instrument with a flat handle and two sharp hooks.

Use(s): It is used for retracting the nares for visualization.
Instrument Insight: Use caution not to perforate gloves or drapes with the sharp ends.

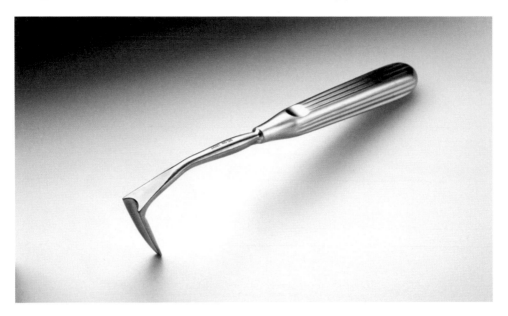

Instrument: AUFRICHT NASAL RETRACTOR
Category: Retracting and Exposing
Description: Round-handled instrument with a right-angled, slightly concave, blunt blade at its end.

Use(s): It is used for retracting the nares for visualization.

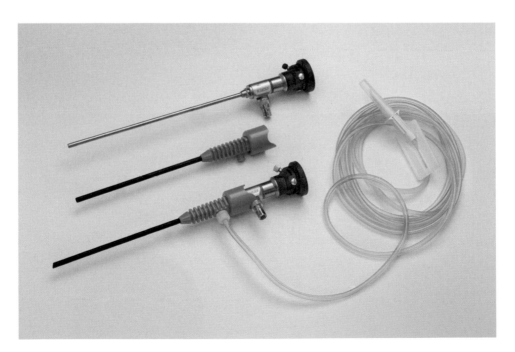

Instrument: ENDO-SCRUB LENS CLEANING SHEATH
Other Names: Endo-scrub sheath
Category: Viewing
Description: It is a plastic hollow sheath that fits over the lens which has a port on the side for water tubing attachment.
Use(s): It is used in maintaining visualization during endoscopic nasal and sinus surgery.

Irrigation prevents fogging and flushes debris from the tip of the lens.
Instrument Insight: The end scrub water tubing is attached to a fluid bag and the tubing is threaded through a pump that uses software settings to keep the lens clean and clear.

THROAT/NECK

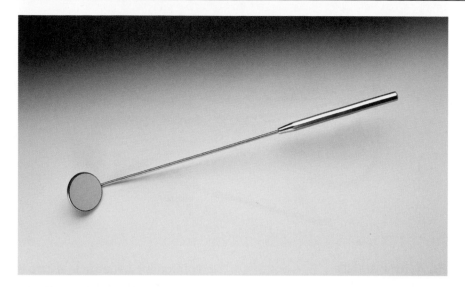

Instrument: LARYNGEAL MIRROR
Category: Accessory
Description: The laryngeal mirror is a round-handled instrument with a small rounded mirror on the end. Mirrors are available in different diameters.

Use(s): It is used for visualization of pharyngeal and laryngeal areas from the back of the throat.
Instrument Insight: Mirrors may fog when inserted into the oral cavity, so the mirrors are dipped into some type of antifog solution or possibly warm water.

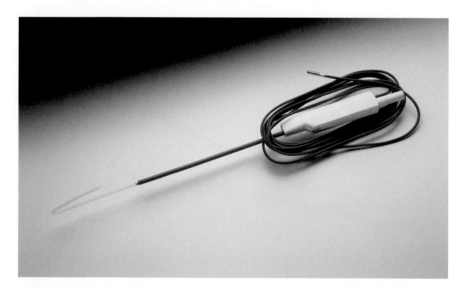

Instrument: SUCTION COAGULATOR TIP
Other Names: Neurocautery suction, suction coag
Category: Accessory
Description: It is a single-use insulated monopolar suction tip with a relief hole on the handgrip and with a monopolar cord and stylet.
Use(s): It is used for removing the tonsils and adenoids by cauterizing tissue and at the same time suctioning fluid, debris, and plume from the operative site.
Instrument Insight: During use, the tip may become plugged with charred debris. This can be remedied by inserting the stylet and wiping the tip with a moistened sponge. A dispersive pad must be placed on the patient before use.

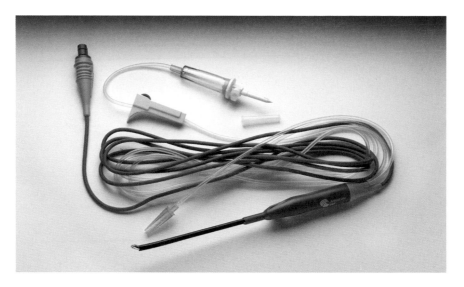

Instrument: COBLATION WAND

Category: Accessory

Description: It is a single-use wand with an attached Coblation cord, suction connector, and irrigation tubing.

Use(s): It is used for removing tonsils and adenoids.

Instrument Insight: Coblation technology is a controlled, non-heat-driven process that uses radiofrequency energy to excite the electrolytes in a conductive medium, such as saline solution, creating precisely focused plasma. The plasma's energized particles have sufficient energy to break molecular bonds within tissue, causing tissue to dissolve at relatively low temperatures. The result is removal of targeted tissue with minimal damage to surrounding tissue.

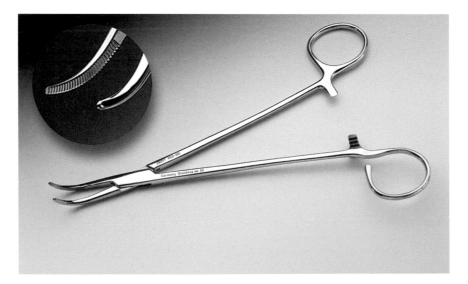

Instrument: ADSON TONSIL–SCHNIDT FORCEPS

Other Names: Adson forceps, Schnidt forceps, fancy clamp

Category: Clamping and Occluding

Description: The jaws of Adson Tonsil–Schnidt forceps may be curved or straight; they have horizontal serrations running half of their length, ending in fine blunt tips. The shanks are longer than those of a Crile or Kelly forceps.

Use(s): These are used for clamping small vessels in a deep wound and for holding tonsil sponges.

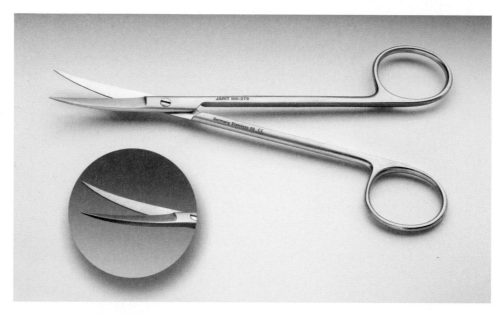

Instrument: JOSEPH SCISSORS
Category: Cutting and Dissecting
Description: These are small, delicate, curved scissors with very sharp points.

Use(s): These are used for cutting fine tissue.
Instrument Insight: Because of the sharp points, handle and pass with care.

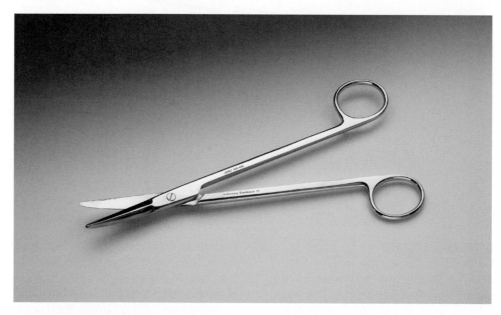

Instrument: BOETTCHER TONSIL SCISSORS
Other Names: Tonsil scissors
Category: Cutting and Dissecting
Description: These are long, narrow, curved scissors with beveled outer blades.

Use(s): These are used for cutting tissue, especially in the oral pharynx for a tonsillectomy.
Instrument Insight: These scissors are placed on the surgeon's fingers with the tips pointing downward.

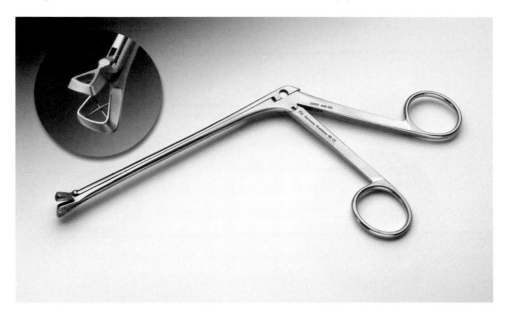

Instrument: MELTZER ADENOID PUNCH
Other Names: Punch
Category: Cutting and Dissecting
Description: It is a finger-ringed instrument with a long shaft and triangular sharp jaws that fit inside one another.

Use(s): It is used for dissecting adenoids.
Instrument Insight: Tissue is removed with a moistened sponge between uses.

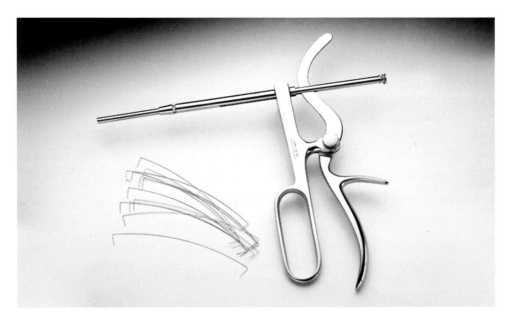

Instrument: TONSIL SNARE
Category: Cutting and Dissecting
Description: It is a handle grip that attaches to a metal cannula and an inner sliding rod. The inner rod has two small holes at the tip in which the snare wires are loaded.
Use(s): Snare wire is placed around the base of each tonsil, the handle is squeezed, and the wire is withdrawn into the cannula, severing the tonsil tissue through a guillotine action.

Instrument Insight: When loading the snare wires, expose the rod tip by opening the handles. The bent ends of the snare wire are then threaded into the holes. A slight compression of the handle then pulls the rough ends of the wire into the cannula, creating a loop. Wires become twisted and compressed after use; therefore, they should be discarded and replaced with new ones.

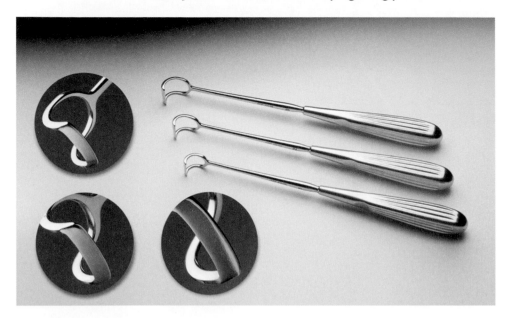

Instrument: BARNHILL ADENOID CURETTES
Category: Cutting and Dissecting
Description: These are rounded handles with a curved, open frame that contains a cutting edge.

Use(s): These are used for removing adenoid tissue via a scraping action.
Instrument Insight: Instruments come in sets with various sizes.

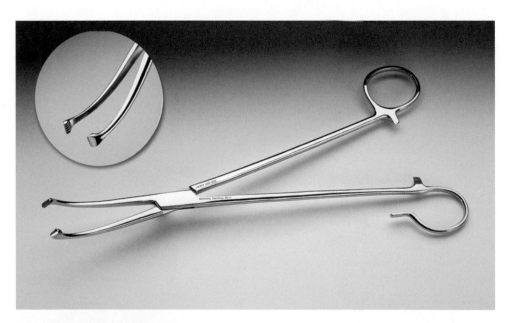

Instrument: CURVED ALLIS FORCEPS
Other Names: Tonsil grasper, tonsil forceps
Category: Grasping and Holding
Description: These are finger-ringed instruments with one open ring, long shanks with curved jaws, and intertwining fine teeth at the tip.

Use(s): These are used to grasp and hold tonsil tissue for removal.
Instrument Insight: The one ring is open so that after the tissue is grasped, a suture may slide down the instrument and secure the tissue.

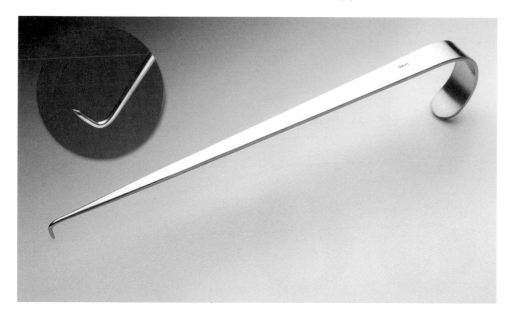

Instrument: HUPP TRACHEAL HOOK
Other Names: Trach hook
Category: Grasping and Holding
Description: It is a retracting instrument with a curved handle for easy holding and a hooked, sharp end.

Use(s): It is used to penetrate the trachea and pull it upward during a tracheotomy.
Instrument Insight: Use caution when handling to prevent puncture wounds on gloves or drapes.

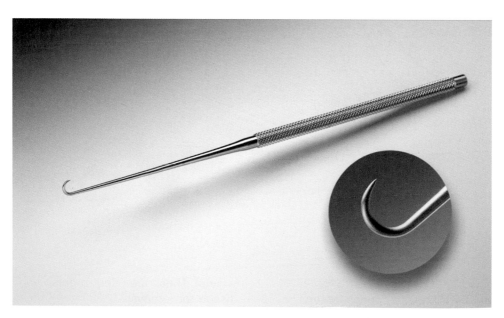

Instrument: JOSEPH SKIN HOOKS
Other Names: Single skin hook
Category: Retracting and Exposing

Description: It is a round-handled instrument with a single, sharp, hooked end.
Use(s): It is used for retracting tissues.

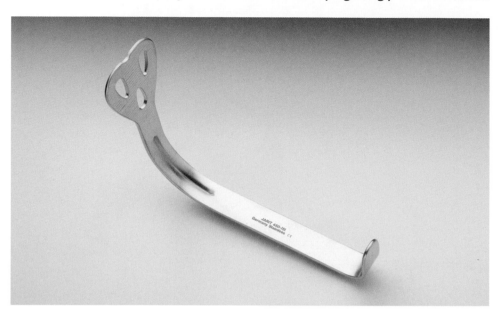

Instrument: WIEDER TONGUE BLADE
Other Names: Tongue depressor
Category: Retracting and Exposing
Description: It is a flat-handled instrument with a heart-shaped tip and three oval-shaped holes.

Use(s): It is used to depress and thus retract the tongue away from the operative site.

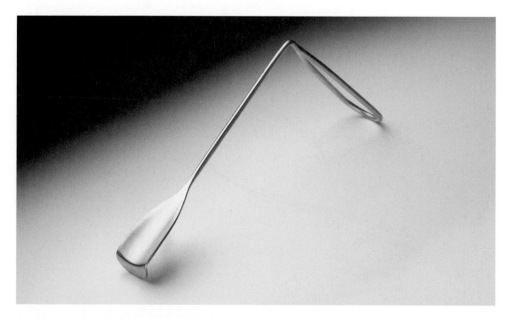

Instrument: LOTHROP UVULA RETRACTOR
Category: Retracting and Exposing
Description: It is an angled retractor with a looped handle and a flattened end with a lip at the distal end for retracting the soft palate.

Use(s): It is used for retracting the uvula and soft palate.

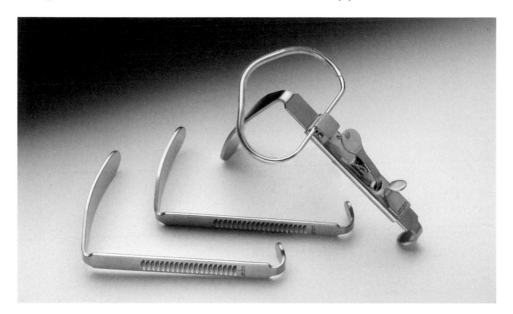

Instrument: McIVOR MOUTH GAG
Category: Retracting and Exposing
Description: It is a self-retaining loop-shaped frame retractor with an attachable tongue blade that slides onto the handle and has a ratchet for adjustment.
Use(s): It is used for retracting the mouth open and the tongue down for exposure of the oral cavity and the back of the throat.

Instrument Insight: The mouth gag is available with three different-sized tongue blades. The hook end of the tongue blade slips over the edge of the Mayo stand to hold the patient in proper alignment for maximum exposure.

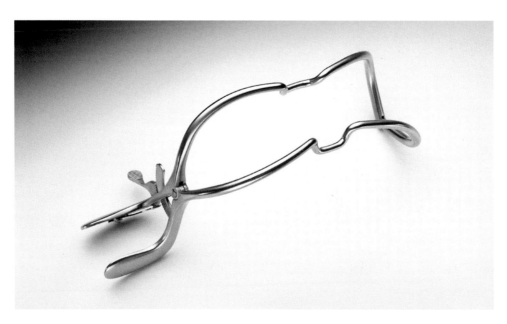

Instrument: JENNINGS MOUTH GAG
Category: Retracting and Exposing
Description: It is a self-retaining eye-shaped retractor with ratchets.

Use(s): It is used for retracting the mouth open for exposure of the oral cavity and the back of the throat.

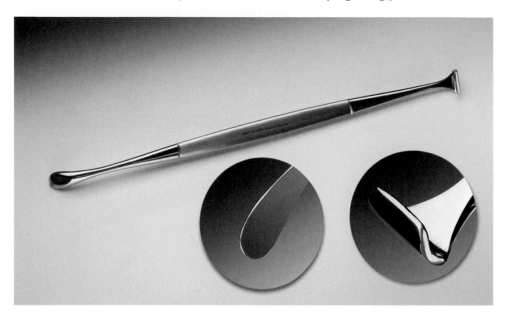

Instrument: HURD DISSECTOR
Other Names: Hurd elevator, pillar retractor
Category: Retracting and Exposing
Description: It is a flat-handled instrument with different ends: one is a rounded and slightly sharp end, the other curves into a lip.

Use(s): It retracts the soft palate for oral procedures and dissects tonsil tissue.

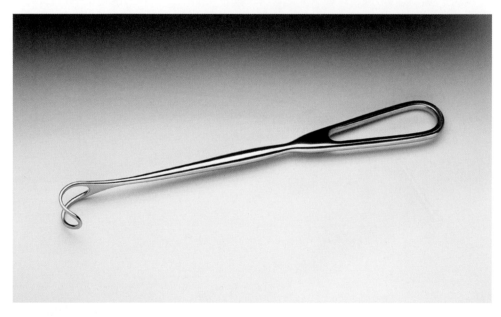

Instrument: GREEN RETRACTOR
Other Names: Thyroid retractor
Category: Retracting and Exposing
Description: It is a loop-handled retractor with a curved, oval, blunt-looped end.

Use(s): It is used for retracting tissue, particularly in the neck area.

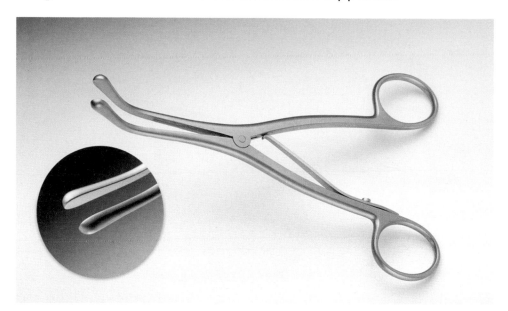

Instrument: TROUSSEAU TRACHEAL DILATOR
Other Names: Tracheal spreader
Category: Retracting and Exposing
Description: It is a finger-ringed handle with two blunt-angled ends that spread apart when the handle is compressed.

Use(s): It is used for retracting the tracheal edges. This allows for placement of a tracheotomy tube.

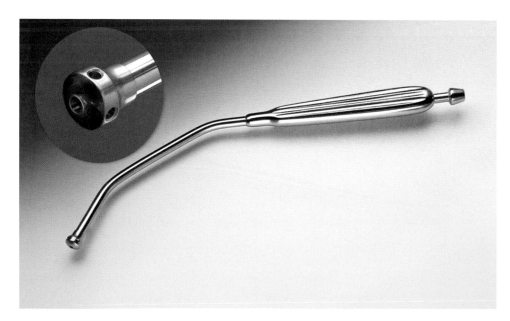

Instrument: NONDISPOSABLE YANKAUER SUCTION TIP
Other Names: Oral tip, oral suction tip
Category: Suctioning and Aspirating
Description: It is a hollow, curved, stainless steel tube with a ball tip and a grip handle.

Use(s): It is used for evacuating tissue, blood, and debris from the surgical site.
Instrument Insight: Note the tip of the suction tip is removable for cleaning. Make sure the tip is securely tightened before and after the procedure.

11

Oral Instruments

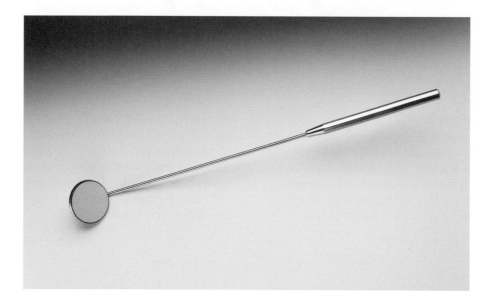

Instrument: MOUTH MIRROR
Other Names: Dental mirror, laryngeal mirror
Category: Accessory
Description: The mouth mirror is a round-handled instrument with a small rounded mirror on the end. Mirrors are available in different diameters.
Use(s): It is used for visualization of the mouth, including the teeth, gums, tongue, palate, and cheeks.

Instrument Insight: Mirror may fog when inserted into the oral cavity; the mirrors are dipped into some type of antifog solution or possibly warm water. Some oral surgeons will use the patient's saliva to prevent fogging of the mirrors.

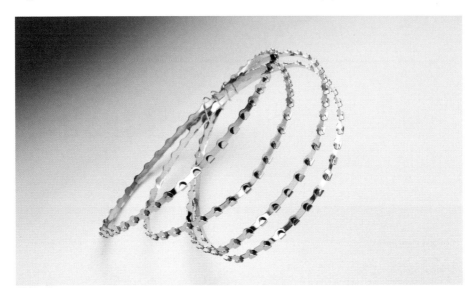

Instrument: ARCH BARS
Category: Accessory
Description: These appliances are rigid metal strips that have hooks to which wire is applied around both the top and bottom and twisted.
Use(s): Arch bars are used to manage a fracture of the mandible (jaw). A set of arch bars is placed with wires that will easily conform to the natural arch of the teeth. The arch bars are ideal to maintain a patient's natural bite in a stationary position until the patient's bone heals.
Instrument Insight: The hooks on the arch bars are placed downward on the lower teeth and upward on the upper teeth.

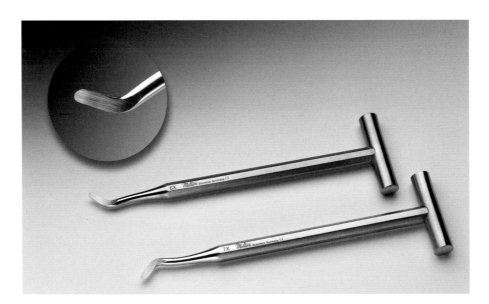

Instrument: POTTS ELEVATOR
Other Names: T-bar Potts elevator
Category: Cutting and Dissecting
Description: The working end of the Potts elevator is a right or left curve with a rounded tip in a range of sizes. Handles may be either T-bar style or designed with heavy tapering to the working end.
Use(s): It is used to loosen tooth or root from a bony socket before use of the extraction forceps.
Instrument Insight: These are in the set as right and left pairs.

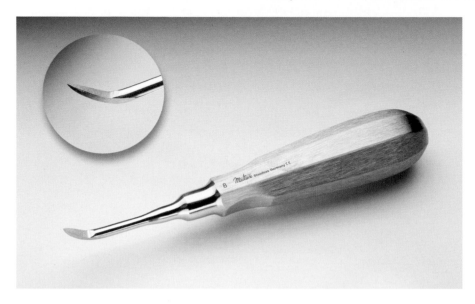

Instrument: CRANE ELEVATOR
Other Names: Crane pick, angular elevator, root tip pick
Category: Cutting and Dissecting
Description: The working end of the Crane elevator has an upward angle with a pointed tip.

Handles may be either T-bar style or designed with heavy tapering to the working end.
Use(s): It is used to loosen tooth or root from a bony socket before use of the extraction forceps.

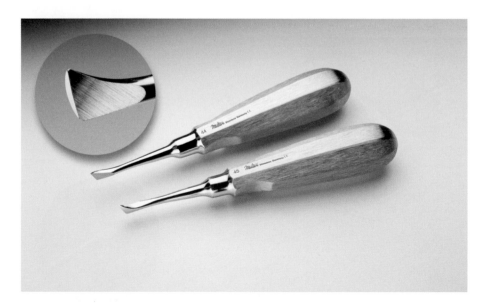

Instrument: CRYER ELEVATOR
Other Names: Flag elevator, root elevator
Category: Cutting and Dissecting
Description: The working end of the Cryer elevator is on the right or left with a triangular pointed tip in a range of sizes. Handles may be either T-bar style or designed with heavy tapering

to the working end.
Use(s): It is used to loosen tooth or root from a bony socket before use of the extraction forceps.
Instrument Insight: These are in the set as right and left pairs.

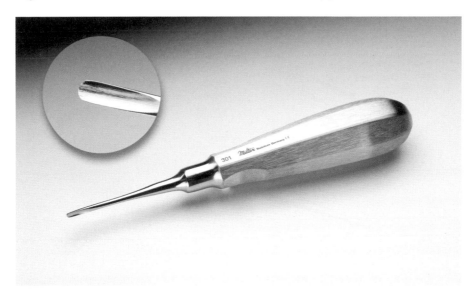

Instrument: APICAL ELEVATOR
Other Names: Straight elevator, luxating elevator
Category: Cutting and Dissecting
Description: It has a round trough-like tip in a range of sizes with a heavy rounded tapering handle.

Use(s): It is used to loosen tooth or root from a bony socket before use of the extraction forceps.
Instrument Insight: Common sizes are no. 1, 34, and 301; these are often referred to by number.

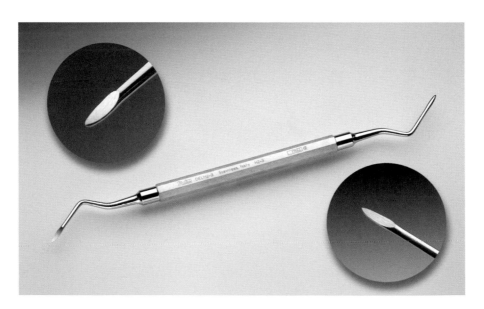

Instrument: ROOT TIP PICK
Other Names: Angle pick, dental pick
Category: Cutting and Dissecting
Description: It is a double-ended small elevator with a thin, angled pointed tip on one end and a blunt tip on the other.

Use(s): It is used to retrieve loose root fragments from the socket after an extraction.

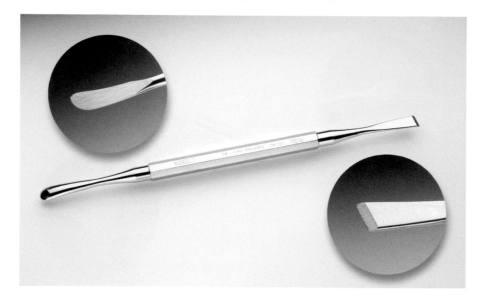

Instrument: WEST PERIOSTEAL
Other Names: Periosteal elevator
Category: Cutting and Dissecting
Description: It is a double-ended straight instrument with one curved, round end and one chisel-like end.

Use(s): It is primarily used to retract gingival tissue; also used during an incisional extraction to remove soft tissues from the tooth.

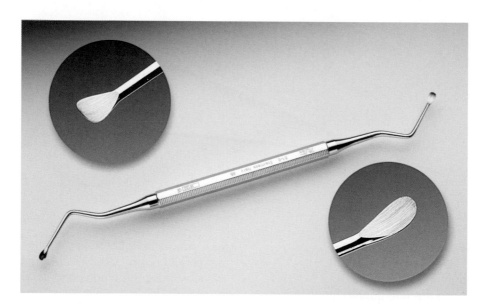

Instrument: LUCAS BONE CURETTE
Other Names: Angled curette
Category: Cutting and Dissecting
Description: It is an angular double-ended, angled, spoon-shaped scraping instrument in a range of sizes.

Use(s): It is often used after tooth extraction to make sure debris and tissue are removed from the socket.

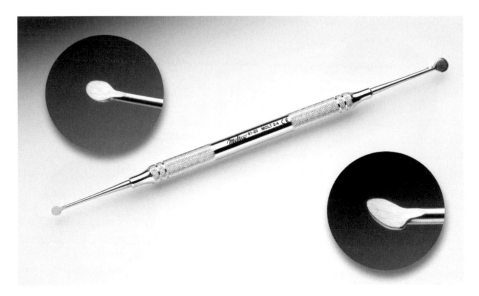

Instrument: MOLT BONE CURETTE
Other Names: Surgical curette, straight curette
Category: Cutting and Dissecting
Description: It is a double-ended, straight instrument with round working ends that are graduated in size. These come in a range of sizes.

Use(s): It is often used to remove tissue or debris from bony sockets.

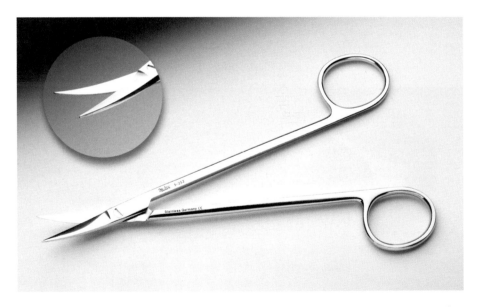

Instrument: KELLY SCISSORS
Other Names: Tissue scissors
Category: Cutting and Dissecting
Description: These are fine curved-tip blades.
Use(s): These are used for cutting and excising excess or diseased soft tissue.

Instrument Insight: These are tissue scissors and should not be used to cut other items, which will dull the blades and make them unsafe for patient use.

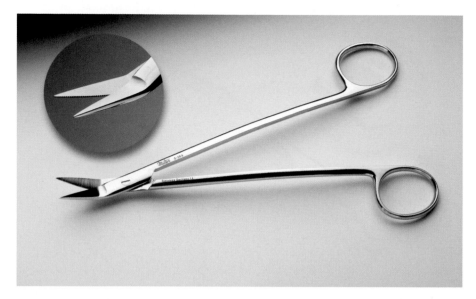

Instrument: DEAN SCISSORS
Other Names: Right-angle scissors
Category: Cutting and Dissecting
Description: These are scissors with fine blades that angle upward to a right angle. These have sharp tips, and the shaft is slightly curved.

Use(s): These are used for cutting and excising excess or diseased soft tissue.
Instrument Insight: These are tissue scissors and should not be used to cut other items, which will dull the blades and make them unsafe for patient use.

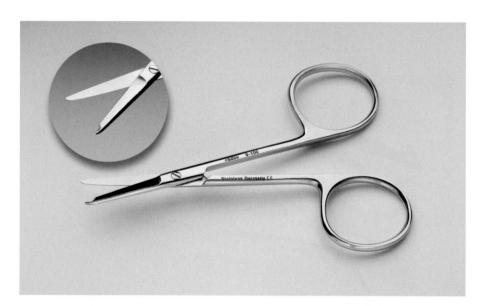

Instrument: SPENCER SUTURE SCISSORS
Other Names: Suture scissors
Category: Cutting and Dissecting
Description: These are fine scissors with straight blades.

Use(s): These scissors are used to cut sutures intraoperatively and to remove sutures postoperatively.
Instrument Insight: One blade has a hook-like tip to slip under a suture to hold the suture away from tissue while cutting.

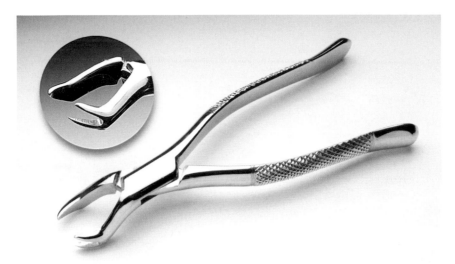

Instrument: LEFT UPPER MOLAR EXTRACTION FORCEPS (88L)

Other Names: Maxillary left forceps, no. 88L forceps

Category: Grasping and Holding

Description: The tip of the left upper molar extraction forceps (88L) has a bayonet design with one sharp projection on one jaw and two projections on the other. Each tip is designed to adjust to anatomic differences of the molar roots on the facial and lingual sides of the socket. The handles are straight and have nonslip diamond-cut grips.

Use(s): These are used for extracting the left first and second maxillary molars.

Instrument Insight: The two prongs are placed on the palate side of the tooth, and the single prong is placed on the cheek side. Extraction forceps are often asked for by number instead of by proper name.

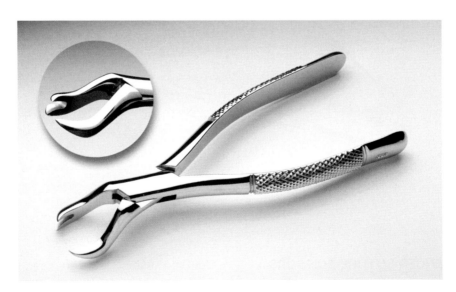

Instrument: RIGHT UPPER MOLAR EXTRACTION FORCEPS (88R)

Other Names: Maxillary right forceps, no. 88R forceps

Category: Grasping and Holding

Description: The tip of the right upper molar extraction forceps (88R) has a bayonet design with one sharp projection on one jaw and two projections on the other. Each tip is designed to adjust to anatomic differences of the molar roots on the facial and lingual sides of the socket. The handles are straight and have nonslip diamond-cut grips.

Use(s): These are used for extracting the right first and second maxillary molars.

Instrument Insight: The two prongs are placed on the palate side of the tooth, and the single prong is placed on the cheek side. Extraction forceps are often asked for by number instead of by proper name.

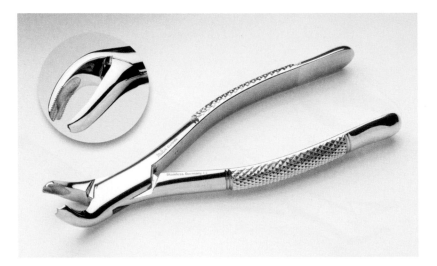

Instrument: LOWER MOLAR EXTRACTION FORCEPS (17)

Other Names: Mandibular forceps (17), no. 17 forceps

Category: Grasping and Holding

Description: The jaws of the lower molar extraction forceps (17) are curved with an oval cup-shaped trough on the inner aspect and one sharp projection in the middle of the tip. The tips are universal in design to conform to facial and lingual roots for both the right and left sides. The handles are straight and have nonslip diamond-cut grips.

Use(s): These are used for extracting the first and second maxillary molars of the right and left quadrants.

Instrument Insight: The no. 17 forceps are handed with the tip curved downward. Extraction forceps are often asked for by number instead of by proper name.

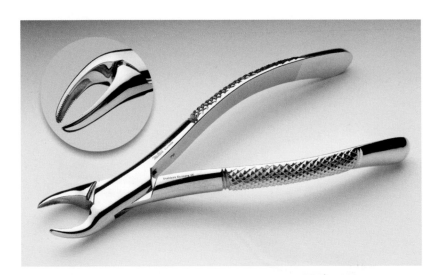

Instrument: UPPER ANTERIOR EXTRACTION FORCEPS (150)

Other Names: Maxillary universal forceps, Cryer forceps, no. 150 forceps

Category: Grasping and Holding

Description: The jaws of the upper anterior extraction forceps (150) are curved with an oval cup-shaped trough on the inner aspect. The tips are universal in design to conform to facial and lingual roots for both the right and left sides. The handles are curved and have nonslip diamond-cut grips.

Use(s): These are used for extracting the maxillary centrals, laterals, cuspids, premolars, and roots of the right and left quadrants.

Instrument Insight: These are maxillary counterpart to the no. 151 mandibular Cryer forceps; these should be placed on the Mayo stand together. Extraction forceps are often asked for by number instead of by proper name.

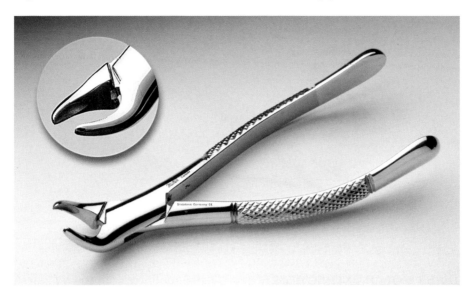

Instrument: LOWER ANTERIOR EXTRACTION FORCEPS (151)

Other Names: Mandibular universal forceps, Cryer forceps, no. 151 forceps

Category: Grasping and Holding

Description: The jaws of the lower anterior extraction forceps (151) are curved with an oval cup-shaped trough on the inner aspect. The tips are universal in design to conform to facial and lingual roots for both the right and left sides. The handles are curved and have nonslip diamond-cut grips.

Use(s): These are used for extracting the mandibular centrals, laterals, cuspids, premolars, and roots of the right and left quadrants.

Instrument Insight: Mandibular counterpart to the maxillary no. 150 Cryer forceps; these should be placed on the Mayo stand together. Extraction forceps are often asked for by number instead of by proper name.

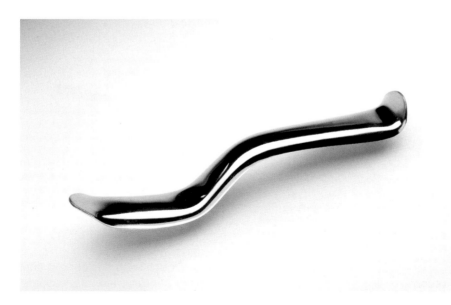

Instrument: MINNESOTA CHEEK RETRACTOR

Other Names: Cheek retractor, University of Minnesota retractor, Cawood retractor

Category: Retracting and Exposing

Description: It is a curved, bent, and angled ribbon of stainless steel.

Use(s): It is used to retract the tongue and cheek away from the surgical site.

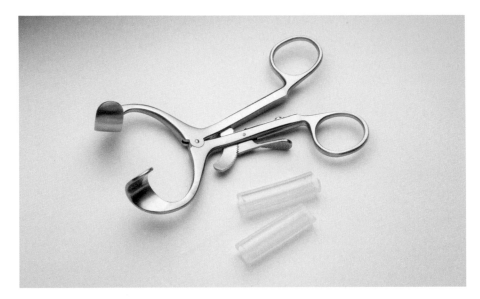

Instrument: MOLT MOUTH GAG
Other Names: Mouth gag, mouth prop
Category: Retracting and Exposing
Description: It is a self-retaining C-shaped retractor with blades that curve inward and ratcheted finger rings to hold it in place. The disposable rubber tubing slides onto the blades to protect the teeth and soft tissue.
Use(s): It is used to retract the mouth open during procedures.

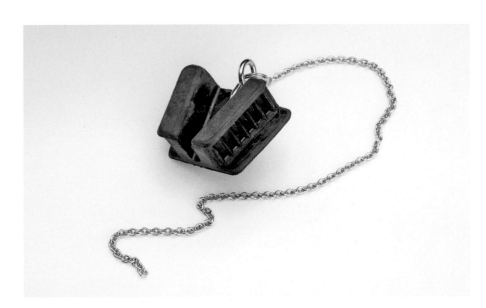

Instrument: MOUTH PROP
Other Names: Bite block, bite wedge
Category: Retracting and Exposing
Description: It is a rubber wedge that has a rim on both sides into which the upper and lower teeth fit. The mouth prop comes in four sizes for children and adults. The attached chain is for removal of the wedge.
Use(s): It is used to keep the mouth propped open during procedures.
Instrument Insight: The narrow end of the wedge is placed into the mouth first.

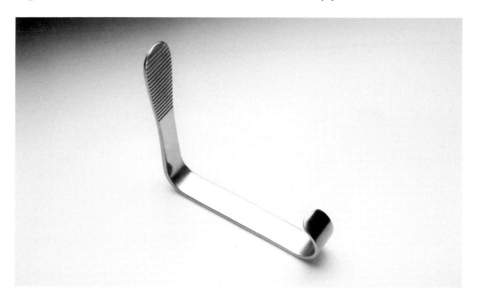

Instrument: ANDREWS TONGUE DEPRESSOR

Other Names: Tongue blade

Category: Retracting and Exposing

Description: It is a flat-handled right-angle retractor with a round, horizontal, serrated blade.

Use(s): It is used for retracting the mouth open and the tongue down for exposure of the oral cavity and the back of the throat.

12 Plastic and Reconstructive Instruments

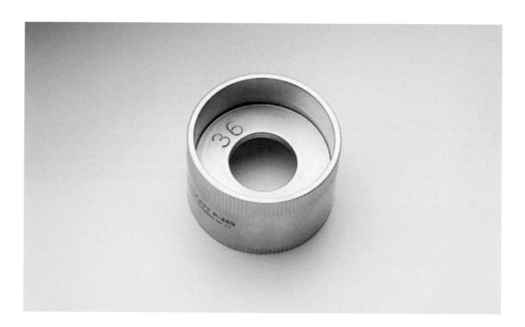

Instrument: FREEMAN AREOLA MARKER

Other Names: Areola marker, cookie cutter, nipple washer

Category: Accessory

Description: The areola marker is a circular tube with a flat metal ring in the center. These range in size from 24 to 50 mm in diameter.

Use(s): It is used for marking an incision line around the areola for a reduction mammoplasty and for marking tissue to become the new areola during reconstruction mammoplasty.

Instrument Insight: The breast incisions are commonly marked preoperatively with the patient standing. Always have sterile areola markers and a marking pen available for marking the new areola site during the procedure.

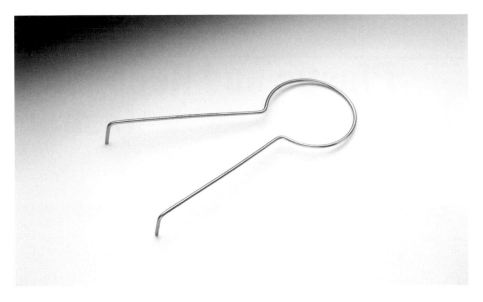

Instrument: McKISSOCK KEYHOLE
Other Names: Reduction marker
Category: Accessory
Description: It is a heavy stainless steel wire shaped like a keyhole.
Use(s): It is used for marking the incision outline for a reduction mammoplasty.

Instrument Insight: The breast incisions are commonly marked preoperatively with the patient standing. Always have a sterile keyhole and marking pen available during the procedure.

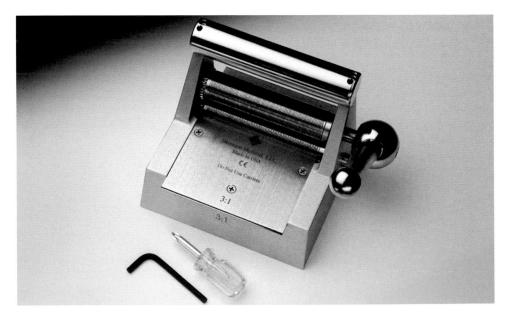

Instrument: DERMAMESHER
Other Names: Skin mesher
Category: Cutting and Dissecting
Description: It is a hand-cranked roller-cutting device that creates numerous identical perforations in the skin graft, giving it a mesh appearance. Meshing facilitates fluid drainage and allows the graft to be stretched over a larger surface area.
Use(s): It is used for expansion of a split-thickness skin graft.
Instrument Insight: Depending on the type and manufacturer, some meshers use a skin carrier and others take only skin.

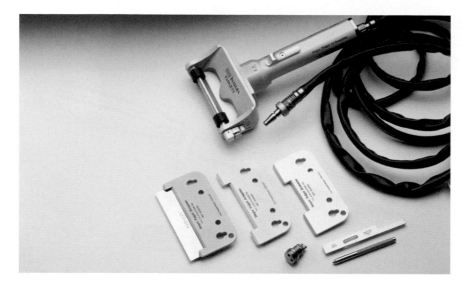

Instrument: DERMATOME
Other Names: Paget dermatome
Category: Cutting and Dissecting
Description: It is a power-driven dermatome that uses electricity or compressed gas to move the blade side to side to obtain a skin graft. This set includes the dermatome handpiece; power cord; 1-, 2-, and 3-inch width plates; calibration guide; and screwdriver. The dermatome blades are manufacturer packaged for one-time use. There are several manufacturers of mechanical dermatomes.
Use(s): Used for harvesting a split-thickness skin graft.
Instrument Insight: Attaching the blade onto the back of the handpiece assembles the dermatome. The width plate is then placed over the blade by lining up the outer holes with the screws on the handpiece. After this is completed, the plate is slid forward and locked in place by tightening the screws.

⚠ **CAUTION:** Before handing this instrument to the surgeon, the dermatome should always be connected to power and tested to ensure the blade is moving freely. Always have sterile mineral oil and tongue blades available for lubrication and tension at the donor site. The skin should be held taut while the dermatome is cutting.

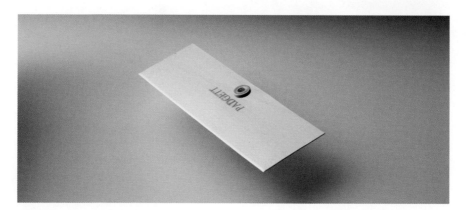

Instrument: DERMATOME BLADE
Other Names: Paget blade
Category: Cutting and Dissecting
Description: It is a disposable rectangular razor blade.
Use(s): It is used for harvesting a split-thickness skin graft.
Instrument Insight: The blade attaches onto the back of the handpiece with the bevel down. The dermatome blades are manufacturer packaged for one-time use.

⚠ **CAUTION:** The handpiece should always be tested after being assembled to verify that the blade is moving properly.

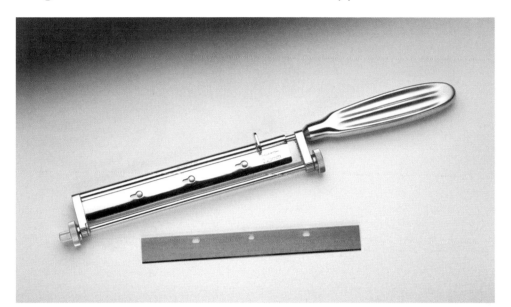

Instrument: WATSON SKIN GRAFT KNIFE
Other Names: Humby knife
Category: Cutting and Dissecting
Description: It is a handheld dermatome with an adjustable roller that determines the depth of the graft. The blade is manufacturer packaged for one-time use.

Use(s): It is used for harvesting a split-thickness skin graft or for wound debridement.
Instrument Insight: The blade is attached with the bevel up.

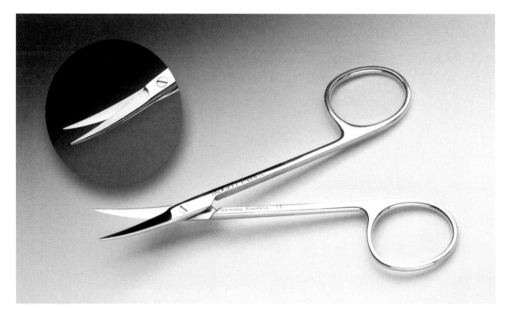

Instrument: IRIS SCISSORS
Category: Cutting and Dissecting
Description: These are small curved or straight scissors with fine blades and sharp tips.
Use(s): These are used to cut tissues during fine dissection.
Instrument Insight: Straight iris scissors are sometimes used to cut very delicate sutures. Curved scissors are for tissue dissection only.

⚠ **CAUTION:** Never place heavy instruments on top of delicate scissors. Never use curved delicate scissors for anything other than delicate tissue dissection because they will dull quickly.

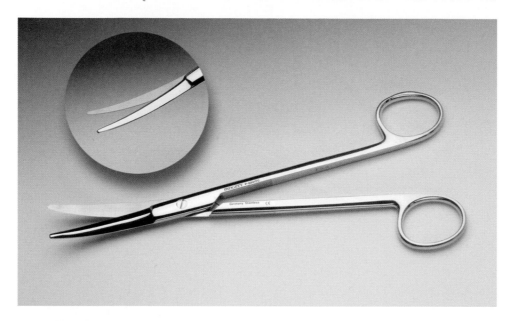

Instrument: KAYE FACELIFT SCISSORS
Other Names: Lift scissors
Category: Cutting and Dissecting
Description: These are fine scissors with curved, beveled blades and blunt tips.

Use(s): These are used for cutting and dissecting tissue during a rhytidectomy.

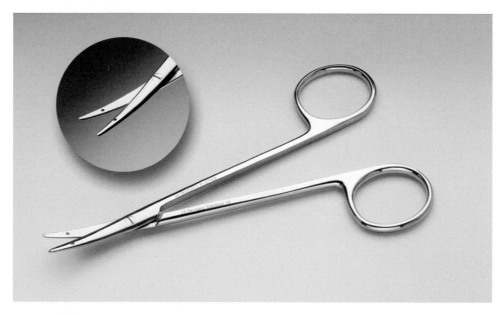

Instrument: LITTLER PLASTIC SURGERY SCISSORS
Other Names: Littler scissors
Category: Cutting and Dissecting
Description: These are fine scissors with curved, smooth blades and a single small hole close to the blunt tip.

Use(s): These are used to cut tissues during fine dissection.
Instrument Insight: Holes on blades serve as suture carriers.

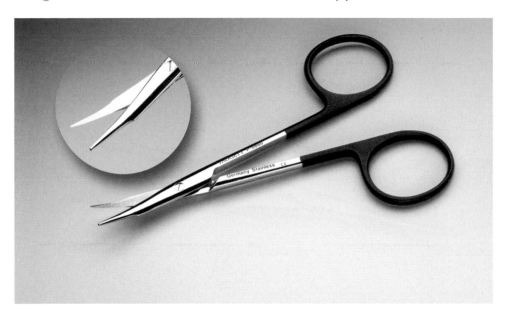

Instrument: STEVENS TENOTOMY SCISSORS
Category: Cutting and Dissecting
Description: These are small scissors with straight or slightly curved fine blades that narrow to blunt tips.

Use(s): These are used to cut tissues during fine dissection.

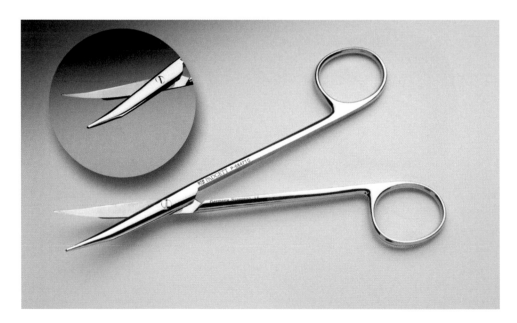

Instrument: JAMISON SCISSORS
Category: Cutting and Dissecting
Description: These are small scissors with curved elongated blades that narrow to blunt tips.

Use(s): These are used to cut tissues during fine dissection.

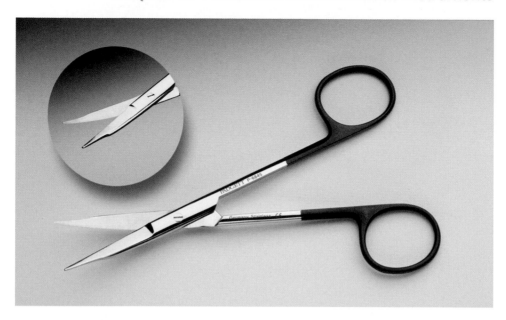

Instrument: REYNOLDS SCISSORS
Category: Cutting and Dissecting
Description: These are small scissors with curved, widened blades that narrow to blunt tips.

Use(s): These are used to cut tissues during fine dissection.

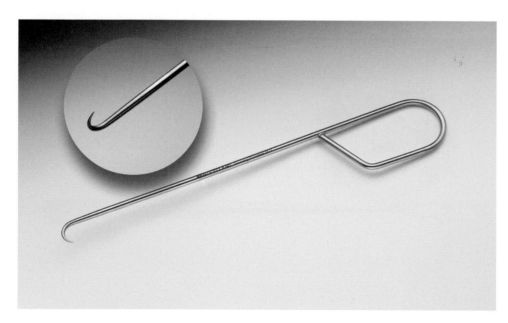

Instrument: MAMMOPLASTY HOOK
Other Names: Breast hook
Category: Retracting and Exposing
Description: It is a heavy, sharp hook retractor with a wire handle.
Use(s): It is used for retracting breast tissue during mastectomy or mammoplasty.

Instrument Insight: Always hand it to the surgeon with the hook pointed downward.

⚠ **CAUTION:** Care must be taken not to puncture gloves on the sharp point of the hook.

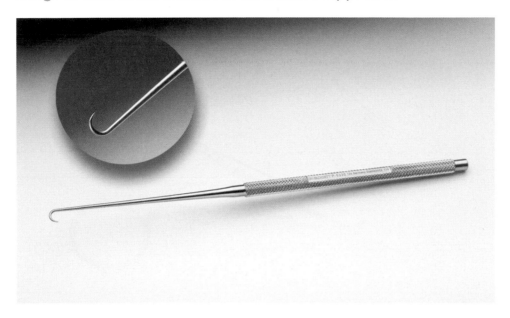

Instrument: JOSEPH SINGLE SKIN HOOK
Category: Retracting and Exposing
Description: It is a small, sharp hook retractor with a round grip handle.
Use(s): It is used for retracting skin edges of small wounds.

Instrument Insight: Hand to the surgeon with the hook pointing downward.

⚠ **CAUTION:** Care must be taken not to puncture gloves on the sharp point of the hook.

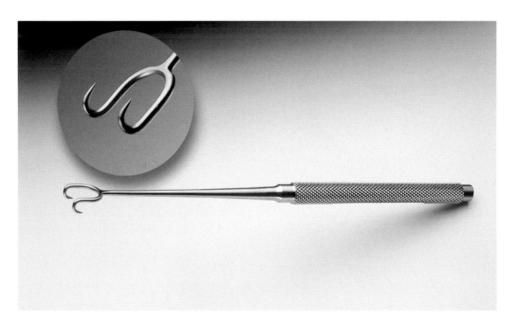

Instrument: JOSEPH DOUBLE SKIN HOOK
Category: Retracting and Exposing
Description: It is a small, sharp double-hook retractor with a round grip handle.
Use(s): It is used for retracting skin edges of small wounds.

Instrument Insight: Hand it to the surgeon with the hooks pointing downward.

⚠ **CAUTION:** Care must be taken not to puncture gloves on the sharp point of the hooks.

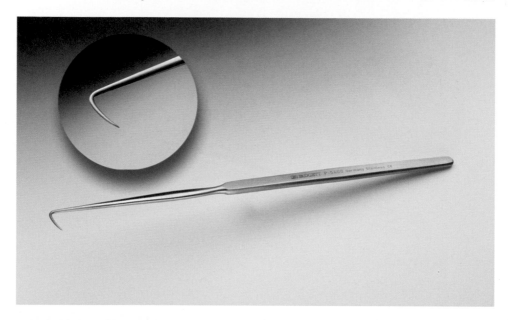

Instrument: SINGLE COTTLE TENACULUM
Category: Retracting and Exposing
Description: It is a small, sharp, L-shaped hook retractor with a flattened handle.
Use(s): It is used for retracting skin edges and deeper tissues of small incisions.

Instrument Insight: Make sure the sharp hooks are facing downward when handing these.

⚠ **CAUTION:** Care must be taken not to puncture gloves on the sharp point of the hook.

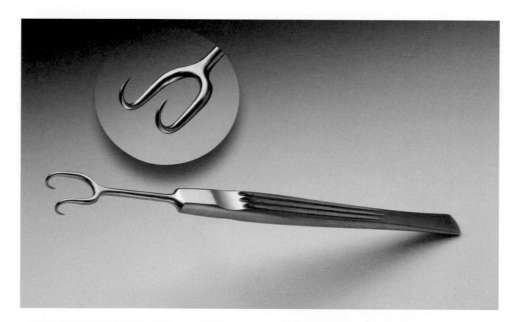

Instrument: DOUBLE COTTLE TENACULUM
Other Names: Tenaculum, hook
Category: Retracting and Exposing
Description: It is a sharp, double-hook retractor with a flattened ridged handle.
Use(s): It is used for retracting skin edges and deeper tissues of small incisions. Often used during nasal procedures.

Instrument Insight: Make sure the sharp hooks are facing downward when handing these.

⚠ **CAUTION:** Care must be taken not to puncture gloves on the sharp points of the hooks.

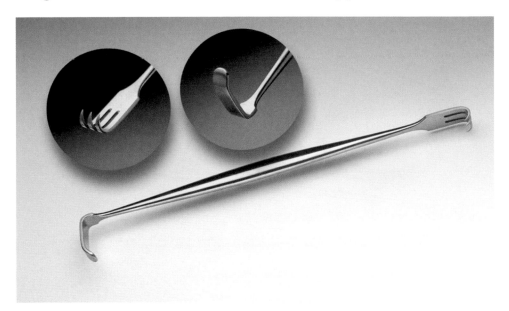

Instrument: MATHIEU RETRACTOR
Other Names: Cat paw retractor
Category: Retracting and Exposing
Description: The Mathieu retractor is a double-ended handheld retractor. One end has three sharp or blunt curved prongs, and the other end is a flat, laterally bent narrow strip.
Use(s): It is used for retracting skin edges and shallow wound edges.

Instrument Insight: The Mathieu retractor is often confused with the Senn retractor, but it is actually finer than the Senn. Make sure the sharp hooks are facing downward when handing these.

⚠ **CAUTION:** Care must be taken not to puncture gloves on the sharp points of the prongs.

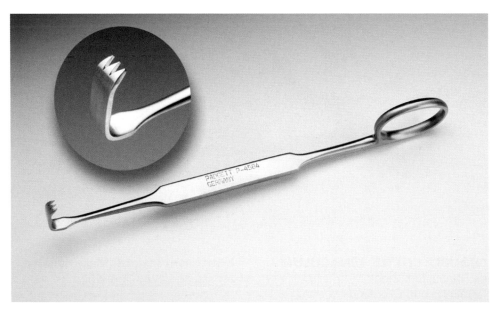

Instrument: MEYERDING FINGER RETRACTOR
Category: Retracting and Exposing
Description: It has a laterally bent narrow, flat end with a curved lip and a finger ring handle.

Use(s): It is used for retracting small wounds.

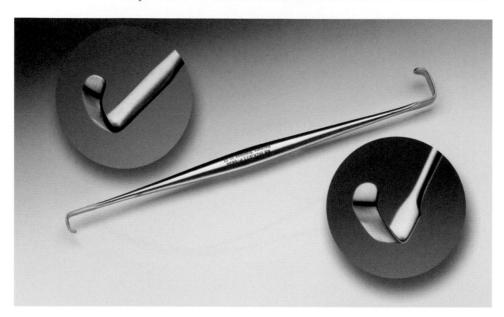

Instrument: RAGNELL RETRACTOR
Category: Retracting and Exposing
Description: It is a flattened, laterally curved, double-ended retractor with one end larger than the other.

Use(s): It is used to retract superficially and then deeper in a small wound.

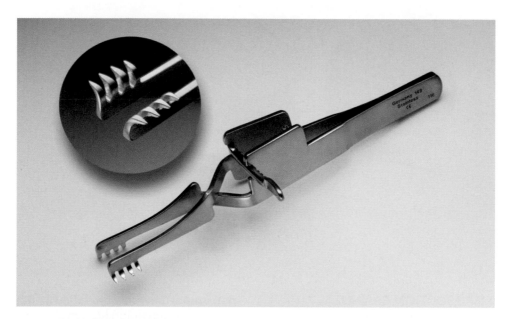

Instrument: HOLZHEIMER RETRACTOR
Other Names: Cricket retractor, finger retractor, Heiss retractor
Category: Retracting and Exposing

Description: It is a self-retaining retractor with four outward-curved claws.
Use(s): It is used for retracting a small, shallow wound edge.

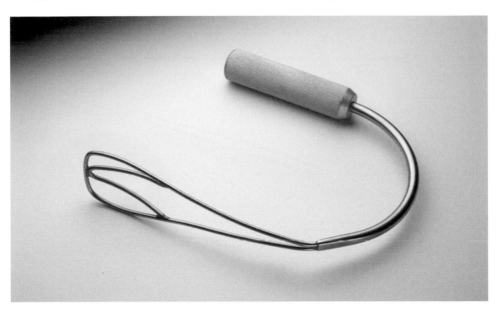

Instrument: BRIGGS MAMMOPLASTY RETRACTOR
Category: Retracting and Exposing
Description: It is a large curved retractor with a teardrop-shaped wire blade and a round grip handle.

Use(s): It is used for retracting breast tissues during a mammoplasty.

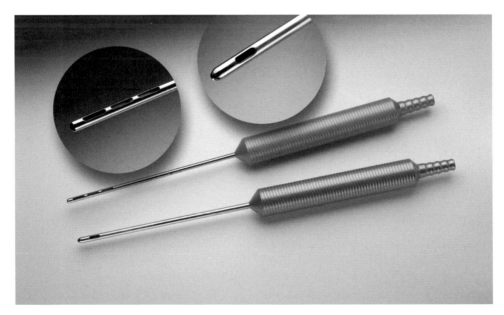

Instrument: LIPOSUCTION CANNULA
Category: Suctioning and Aspirating
Description: It is a rigid suction cannula with various lengths, sizes, and tips.
Use(s): It is used for aspirating adipose tissue during a liposuction procedure.

Instrument Insight: The cannulas attach to firm, large-bore suction tubing, which is then attached to a high-pressure suction unit.

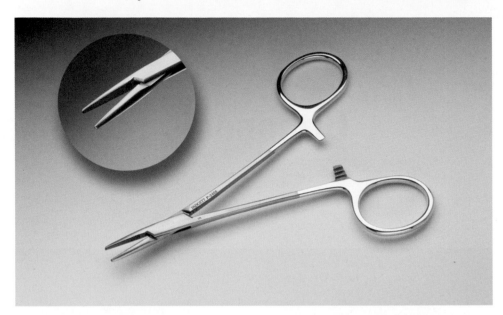

Instrument: WEBSTER NEEDLE HOLDER
Category: Suturing and Stapling
Description: It is a small fine-needle holder with carbide cross-hatch pattern serrations on the inner jaws.

Use(s): It is used for holding small suture needles during delicate procedures.

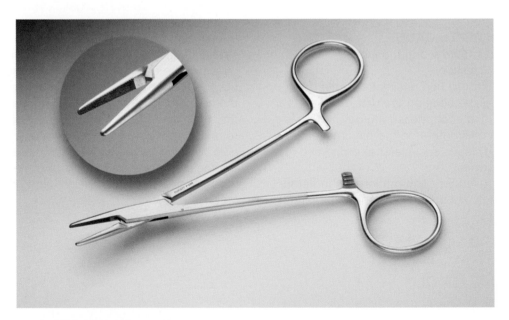

Instrument: HALSEY NEEDLE HOLDER
Category: Suturing and Stapling
Description: It is a small fine-needle holder with carbide cross-hatch pattern serrations on the inner jaws.

Use(s): It is used for holding small suture needles during delicate procedures.

13 Orthopedic Instruments

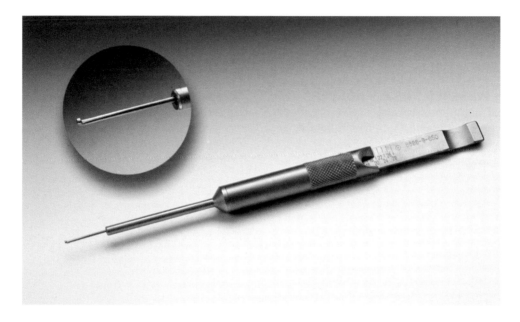

Instrument: DEPTH GAUGE
Other Names: Screw depth gauge
Category: Accessory
Description: It is a thin, stainless steel probe with a right-angle hook on the distal end and with a solid, flattened measuring device that is calibrated in millimeters on the proximal end. A sliding metal sleeve encircles the probe and measuring device.
Use(s): It is used for confirmation of the depth of the drill hole in bone to determine the length of the screw.

Instrument Insight: Always have the depth gauge available when placing bone screws. To measure the depth of a hole, the surgeon pushes the sleeve against the proximal side of the hole and extends the probe into and beyond the distal side of the hole; the surgeon then retracts the probe, finding the distal side of the hole with the hook. The surgeon reads the measurement of depth by examining the position of the proximal sleeve along the graduated scale.

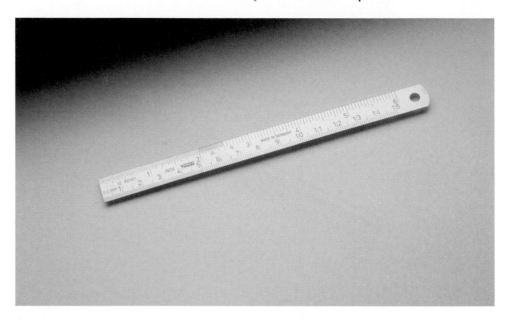

Instrument: RULER
Other Names: Measuring stick
Category: Accessory
Description: It is a stainless steel ruler that is calibrated in millimeters and inches.

Use(s): It is used for measuring structure and distances.
Instrument Insight: Rulers may also be made of plastic.

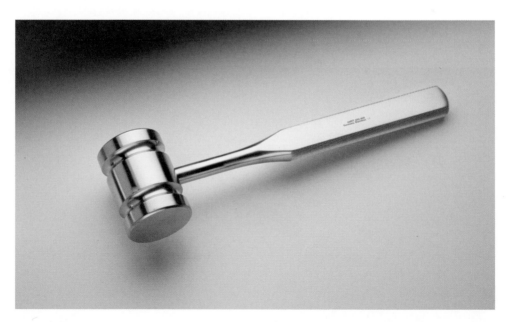

Instrument: MALLET
Other Names: Hammer
Category: Accessory
Description: It is a solid stainless steel hammer-like instrument or may also be brass-filled stainless steel. Weight is usually 1 to 3 pounds. Mallets are used in other specialties that involve bone work.

Use(s): It is used to impact and extract implants or exert force on osteotomes, chisels, gouges, tamps, and other specially designed instruments.
Instrument Insight: Make available after passing any osteotomes, chisels, tamps, etc.

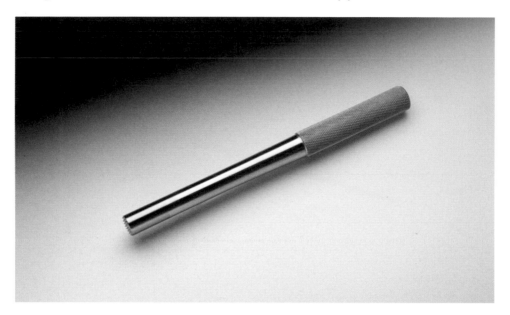

Instrument: BONE TAMP
Other Names: Tamp
Category: Accessory
Description: It is a solid stainless steel dowel with a grip handle and round, flattened working end with diamond cuts which prevent slipping.

Use(s): It is used to compact or wedge a structure into place (e.g., a bone wedge).
Instrument Insight: Hand to surgeon with a mallet.

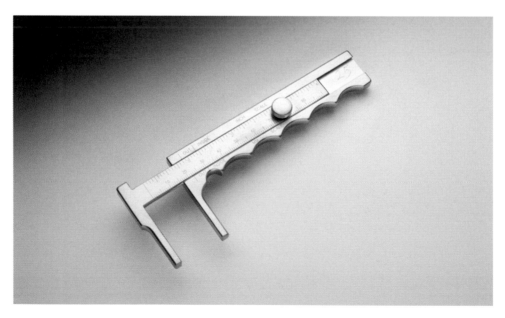

Instrument: TOWNLEY CALIPER
Other Names: Caliper
Category: Accessory
Description: It is a slide ruler that measures in millimeters and inches between the tips.

Use(s): It is used for measuring structures and distances. Commonly used for measuring the thickness of patella before cutting its undersurface during a total knee arthroplasty.

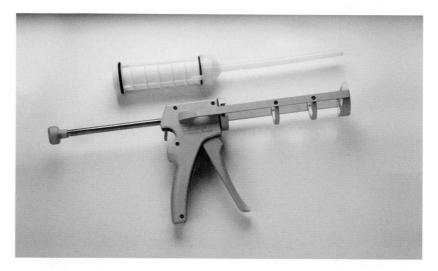

Instrument: BONE CEMENT INJECTOR
Other Names: Cement gun
Category: Accessory
Description: The proximal end of bone cement injector has a plunger-type disk that moves forward when the handles are compressed. This forces the glue through the chamber and out the tip, similar to a caulk gun.
Use(s): It is used for injecting polymethyl methacrylate (PMMA) bone cement during total joint procedures.

Instrument Insight: Setting time for PMMA is approximately 8 to 16 minutes after the prosthesis is positioned. The surgeon will need to know how the glue is setting; be sure to obtain a small amount of glue to test for heat and hardening and record the time when the glue was placed in the gun.

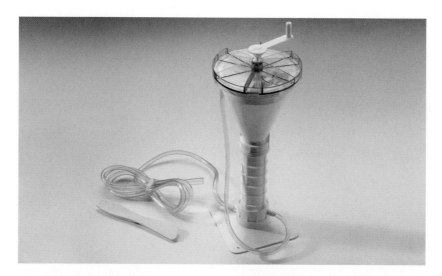

Instrument: BONE CEMENT SYSTEM
Category: Accessory
Description: It is a funnel-shaped mixing bowl that has a lockdown lid with attached stirring paddles on the underside and a crank handle on top. Screwed to the bowl is the injection cartridge with a removable supporting base. Attached to the base is the vacuum tubing. This system is a disposable closed vacuum system.
Use(s): It is used for mixing the liquid (monomer) and powder (polymer) to produce bone cement, also known as PMMA.

Instrument Insight: The manufacturer recommends double gloving when mixing cement. Nonlatex gloves are not recommended because the liquid monomer can be absorbed through gloves.

⚠ **CAUTION:** The liquid monomer is highly flammable; the electrosurgical pencil should never be used near the liquid or the uncured cement.

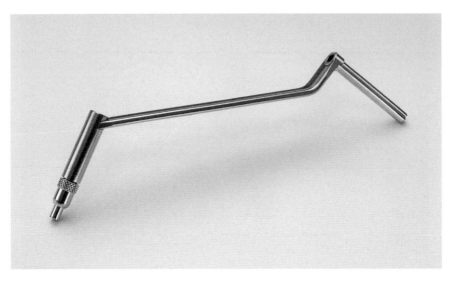

Instrument: DRILL GUIDE
Other Names: Drill sleeve, drill bit guide
Category: Accessory
Description: The working end of drill guide is a hollow tube called a sheath or cannula into which the drill bit slides. These can be single- or double-ended and may be straight or have angles of varying degrees. The rim of the sheath has V-shaped edges that seat the guide into the bone to prevent slipping.

Use(s): Drill guide provides a more precise drill hole. It is used to align the drill bit in the center of the hole in the plate, protects the soft tissue from damage, and prevents the drill from slipping and making a larger hole.
Instrument Insight: Some surgeons prefer that you slide the guide on the drill bit before handing the drill to them, while others prefer to place the guide first and then insert the drill bit into the guide.

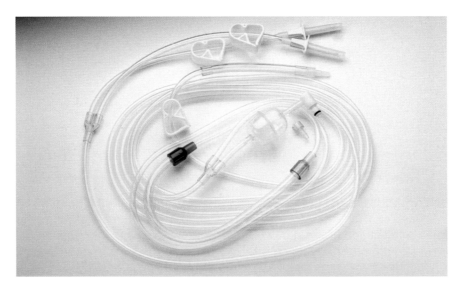

Instrument: PUMP TUBING
Category: Accessory
Description: It is a hollow tubing with bifurcated spike ports and tubing clamps on one end, and the pump attachment mechanism and a Luer-Lok attachment at the other end.

Use(s): It attaches irrigation fluid bags to pump at one end, with the other end attached to the arthroscopic irrigation cannula.

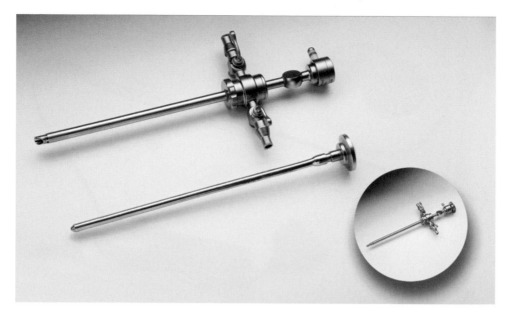

Instrument: 4-MM SHEATH WITH BLUNT OBTURATOR
Category: Accessory
Description: It is a hollow stainless steel sheath with a blunt-tipped obturator that fits inside.
Use(s): It creates a port into which the endoscope is introduced and exchanged through the sheath or cannula.

Instrument Insight: The blunt tip is less traumatic on the tissues. Tip can be various sizes, depending on the size of the joint.

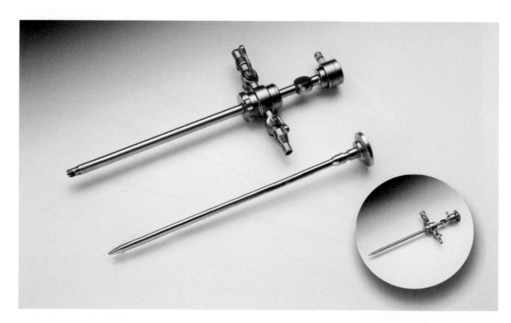

Instrument: 4-MM SHEATH AND SHARP OBTURATOR
Category: Accessory
Description: This is a hollow stainless steel sheath with a sharp-tipped obturator that fits inside. Tips are available in various sizes, depending on the size of the joint.

Use(s): It creates a port into which the endoscope is introduced and exchanged through the sheath or cannula.
Instrument Insight: The sharp tip is used to pass through tough tissue.

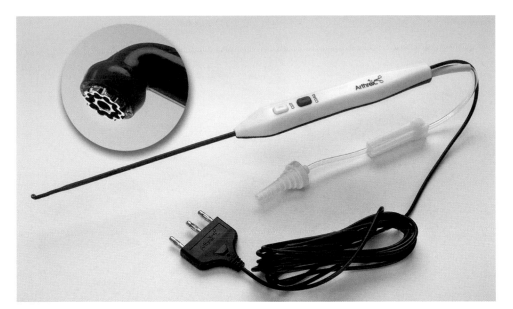

Instrument: ABLATION WAND
Other Names: Cool cut wand
Category: Accessory
Description: It is a radiofrequency ablation device with a white and blue plastic handle with buttons for cut and coagulation. A long insulated shaft advances from the handle, which leads to a 90-, 50-, or 30-degree tip. The working tip has two metal scalloped rings on it that facilitate the ablation.
Use(s): It is used to clean up and smooth out meniscus and articular surfaces during an arthroscopy.
Instrument Insight: This is a single-patient use item and is thrown away at the end of the procedure.

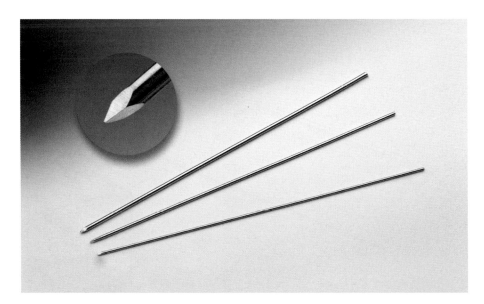

Instrument: KIRSCHNER WIRES
Other Names: K wires, metacarpal pins
Category: Accessory
Description: These are stainless steel wires are smooth or threaded with trocar and diamond points on one end or on both ends. K wires are available in sizes from 0.7 through 1.6 mm (0.028 through 0.062 inch).
Use(s): It is a steel wire used for fixation of bone fractures. These are often used on small bones such as phalanges, wrist, and ankle, and are often placed percutaneously.
Instrument Insight: Care should be taken when handling because these have very sharp points that can easily puncture skin.

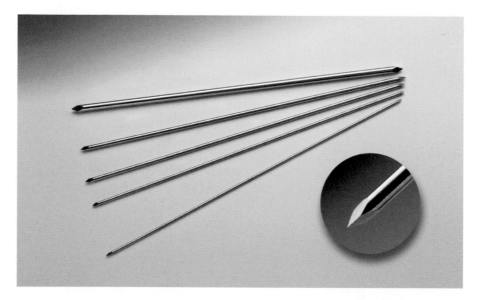

Instrument: SMOOTH STEINMANN PINS
Other Names: Smooth pins
Category: Accessory
Description: It is a smooth stainless steel pin with a trocar or diamond point. Steinmann pins are available in sizes from 2.0 through 4.8 mm (5/64 through 3/16 inch).
Use(s): These pins can be used for fixation of bone fractures, bone reconstruction, and as a guide pin when placing implants and placing skeletal traction. These are often used on larger bones.
Instrument Insight: Care should be taken when handling; these have very sharp points that can easily puncture skin.

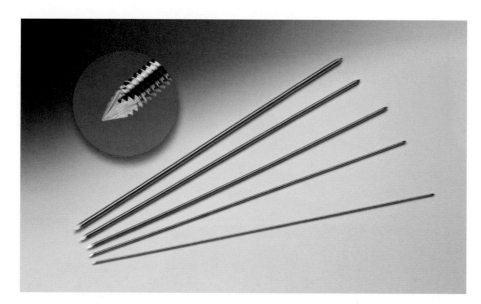

Instrument: THREADED STEINMANN PINS
Other Names: Threaded pins
Category: Accessory
Description: These are threaded stainless steel pins with a trocar or diamond point. Steinmann pins are available in sizes from 2.0 through 4.8 mm (5/64 through 3/16 inch).
Use(s): These pins can be used for fixation of bone fractures, bone reconstruction, and as a guide pin when placing implants and placing skeletal traction. These are often used on larger bones.
Instrument Insight: Care should be taken when handling; these have very sharp points that can easily puncture skin.

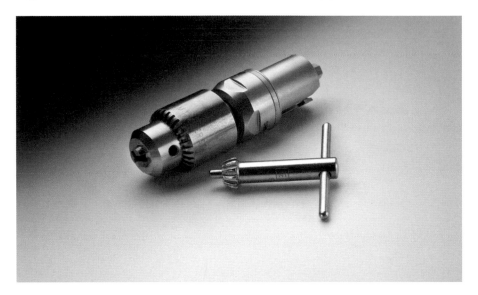

Instrument: JACOBS CHUCK AND KEY
Other Names: Drill chuck
Category: Accessory
Description: A chuck is a specialized type of clamp in which the jaws, which are arranged in a radially symmetric pattern like the points of a star, are used to hold a cylindric object.
Use(s): It is most commonly used to hold rotating devices, such as the drill bit or a pin in a power tool. Some chucks can also hold irregularly shaped objects and those that lack radial symmetry. Often the jaws will be tightened or loosened with the help of a chuck key, which is a wrench-like device made to tighten or loosen the jaws.

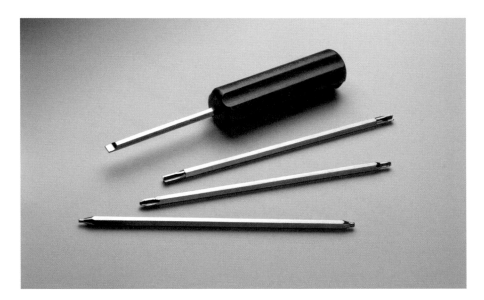

Instrument: UNIVERSAL SCREWDRIVER SET
Other Names: Screwdriver kit
Category: Accessory
Description: Universal screwdriver set consists of a handle that accommodates any of the four double-ended screwdriver bits and one each of small and large single-slot, cross and cruciate, 3.5-mm and 4.5-mm hex, and small and large Phillips heads.
Use(s): It is used during revision of total joint surgery in which screws were used, removal of bone plates, fracture fixation screws, or bone graft screws.
Instrument Insight: The set helps eliminate the opening of multiple sterile packs when a specific size or style of screwdriver is needed.

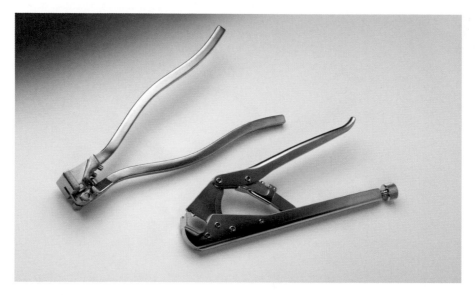

Instrument: PLATE-BENDING PLIERS
Other Names: Plate bender
Category: Accessory
Description: Pictured are large forceps. The plate is slid into the jaws and compressed to bend the plate. These come in various sizes and designs depending on the type of plating system that is being used and the size and type of bone that is being fixated.

Use(s): These are used during open reduction internal fixation (ORIF) to bend the plate to conform to the contour of the bone in which it is being implanted.
Instrument Insight: Often plate benders will be found in the fixation set that you are using.

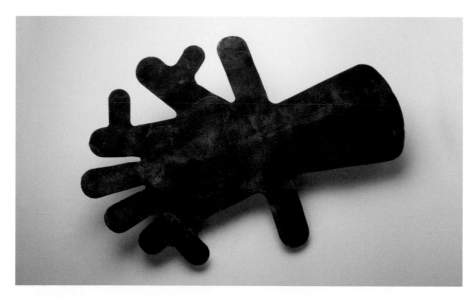

Instrument: LEAD HAND
Category: Accessory
Description: It is a hand-shaped malleable metal device with tabs.
Use(s): It is often used during hand procedures to position the hand open for exposure.

Instrument Insight: The patient's hand is generally laid onto the lead hand palm up. The metal fingers are bent up over the top of the patient's fingers to hold them down; then the tabs are molded around the wrist, index finger, and little finger to secure the hand open.

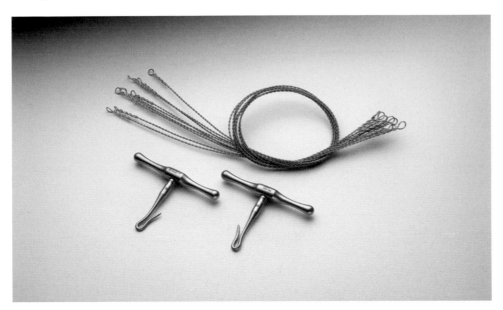

Instrument: GIGLI SAW

Category: Cutting and Dissecting

Description: It is a flexible, twisted wire cable with looped ends that affix to the hooks on the two T handles. The handles may also be oval or box shaped. The wire cable may be replaced after each use or when it becomes dull.

Use(s): It is a type of hand saw used for cutting bone. A back-and-forth movement of the T handle slides the cable over the bone, creating a notch that continues through the bone. Often used for amputations and can be used to open the skull for craniotomies.

⚠ **CAUTION:** Do not run fingers and/or hand along the blade; this could tear gloves and skin.

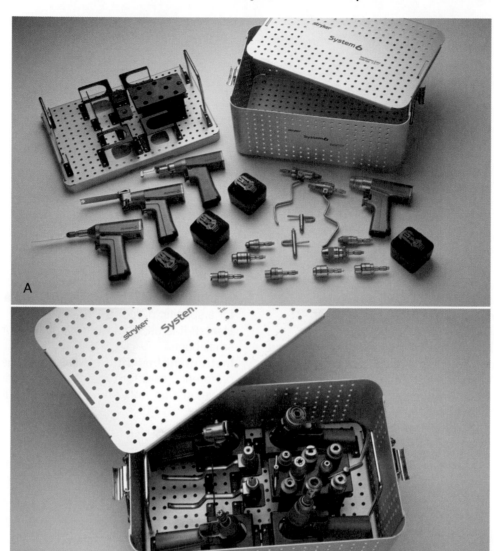

A

B

Instrument: STRYKER SYSTEM 6 POWER

Category: Cutting and Dissecting

Description: It is an all-in-one battery-powered system that consists of an oscillating saw, reciprocating saw, sternal saw, and a rotary handpiece. The rotary handpiece is used for reaming or drilling and has a variety of attachments and chucks that are used for a specific purpose.

Use(s): It is used for cutting, reaming, or drilling large bones.

Instrument Insight: Check batteries for a full charge. Check the surgeon's preference card for the appropriate saw blades. Power instruments should *never* be submerged in water.

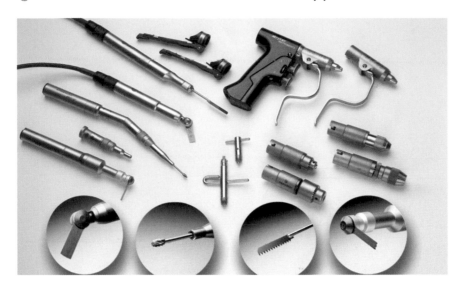

Instrument: STRYKER CORE SYSTEM
Other Names: TPS system
Category: Cutting and Dissecting
Description: It is an all-in-one electrical-powered system that consists of sagittal, oscillating, and reciprocating saws, microdrill, and a universal driver handpiece. The universal drivers are capable of pin and wire driving, sawing, drilling, tunneling, or reaming and have a variety of attachments, collets, and chucks that are used for a specific purpose.
Use(s): It is used for cutting, drilling, or burring small bones.
Instrument Insight: Refer to the surgeon's preference card for type of blades or burrs used. Power instruments should never be submerged in water.

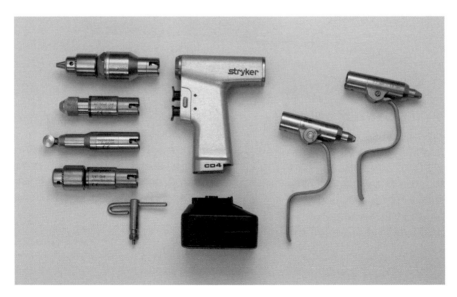

Instrument: CORDLESS DRIVER 4
Other Name: CD4 power system
Category: Cutting and Dissecting
Description: It is an all-in-one battery-powered system that consists of sagittal, oscillating, and reciprocating saws, microdrill, and universal driver handpiece. The universal drivers are capable of pin and wire driving, sawing, drilling, tunneling, or reaming and have a variety of attachments, collets, and chucks that are used for a specific purpose.
Use(s): It is used for cutting, drilling or burring bones.
Instrument Insight: Check batteries for a full charge. Check the surgeon's preference card for the appropriate saw blades. Power instruments should *never* be submerged in water.

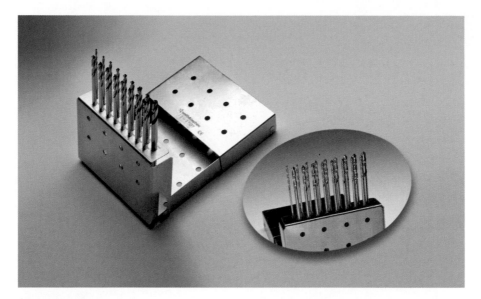

Instrument: DRILL BIT SET
Other Names: Drill box
Category: Cutting and Dissecting
Description: The drill bits in this case range from 1.6 to 4.7 mm.

Use(s): Drill bits are used to drill holes in bone, usually before the placement of a screw.

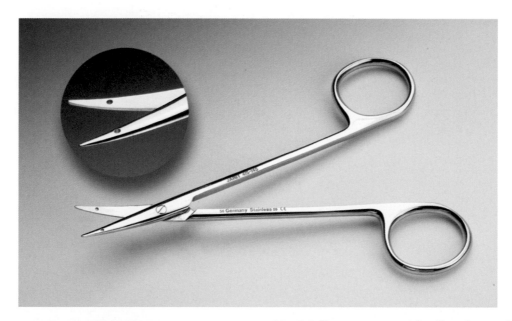

Instrument: LITTLER SCISSORS
Category: Cutting and Dissecting
Description: These are slightly curved, blunt-tipped, sharp blades. The holes on the blades serve to draw suture or muscle through a tunnel dissection.

Use(s): These are used for fine tissue dissection.
Instrument Insight: Use caution when passing because of sharp edges; only use on tissue—never use to cut drapes or sutures.

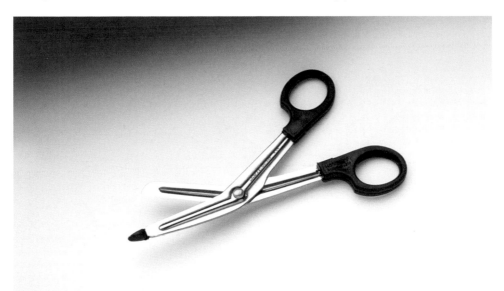

Instrument: UTILITY SCISSORS
Other Names: Bandage scissors
Category: Cutting and Dissecting
Description: These have serrated edge with a blunt tip on the lower jaw to prevent cutting tissue or skin.

Use(s): These are cut bandages, casting material, clothing, and other nonsterile items.
Instrument Insight: These are used to cut dressing, drapes cast material, etc. These scissors should never be used to cut tissues or suture.

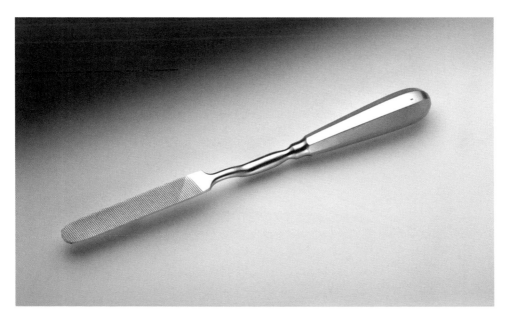

Instrument: BONE FILE
Other Names: Rasp
Category: Cutting and Dissecting
Description: A single-handle instrument with a flat end with serrations in a crisscross pattern.

Use(s): It is used for smoothing rough edges or surfaces of large bones.
Instrument Insight: This should always be available during total joint procedures to smooth bone surfaces.

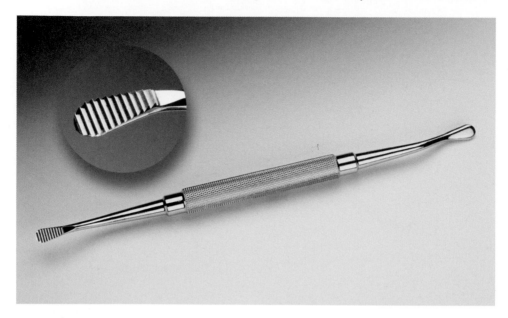

Instrument: MILLER RASP
Other Names: Small rasp
Category: Cutting and Dissecting
Description: It is a double-ended instrument with tear-shaped ends. One end has fairly thick ridges in parallel lines; the ridges on the other end are closer together.
Use(s): It is used for smoothing rough edges or surfaces of small bones.
Instrument Insight: This instrument is used to smooth bone surfaces in small areas or when the areas are hard to reach.

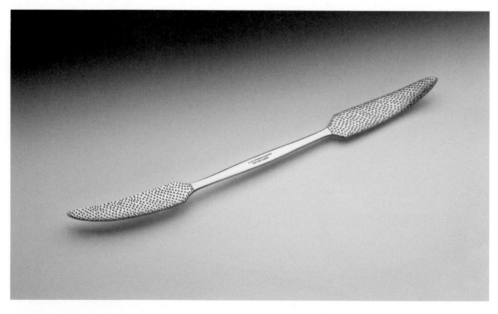

Instrument: PUTTI BONE RASP
Other Names: Putti-Platte rasp, rat tail
Category: Cutting and Dissecting
Description: It is a flattened, double-ended rasp with a rounded blade on one end and a half-rounded blade on the other end. The blade surfaces are covered with tiny spikes.
Use(s): It is used for smoothing rough edges or surfaces of large bones.
Instrument Insight: Immerse and gently stir the rasp in water to keep instrument surface clean between uses.

⚠ **CAUTION:** Do not run fingers and/or hand along the blade; this could tear gloves and skin.

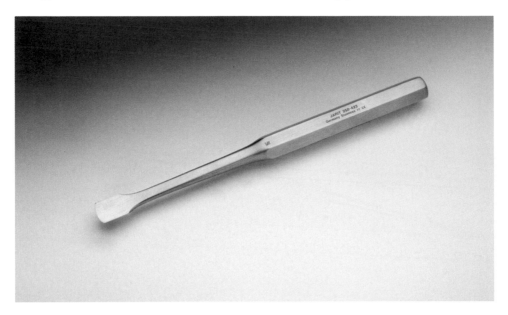

Instrument: KEY PERIOSTEAL ELEVATOR
Other Names: Key elevator
Category: Cutting and Dissecting
Description: It is a solid, smooth, octagonal handle with a squared, flat, and sharp working end that comes in a variety of sizes.

Use(s): It dissects or separates hard tissue (e.g., periosteum from bone).
Instrument Insight: Inspect edge before and after each use for nicks to ensure sharpness.

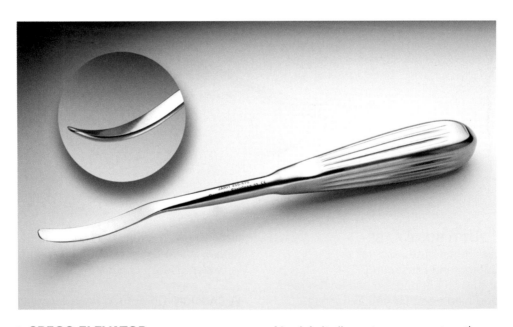

Instrument: CREGO ELEVATOR
Category: Cutting and Dissecting
Description: It has a thick handle with long, thin, curved, flat edge.

Use(s): It dissects or separates tissue; retracts tissue.
Instrument Insight: Inspect edge for nicks to ensure sharpness.

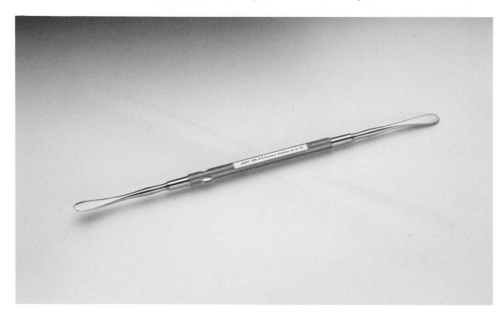

Instrument: FREER ELEVATOR
Category: Cutting and Dissecting
Description: It is a round handle with flattened, tear-shape tips at both ends; one end is sharper than the other.

Use(s): It lifts the periosteum from bone or retracts in confined spaces.
Instrument Insight: Small balls of bone wax are pressed onto the tip and then are smeared in bone edges for hemostasis.

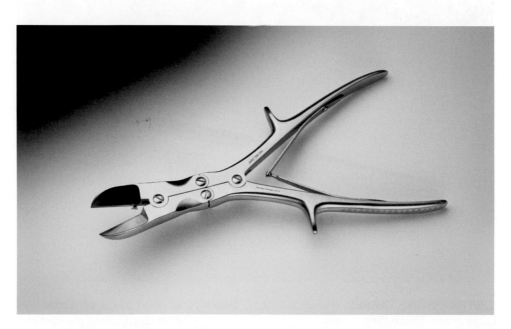

Instrument: LISTON BONE CUTTING FORCEPS
Other Names: Large bone cutters
Category: Cutting and Dissecting
Description: These are large double-action forceps with curved or straight blades that are rounded to the tip with sharp inner jaw edges.

Use(s): These are used for cutting large bones.
Instrument Insight: The double action gives the forceps more torque at the tip for better cutting action.

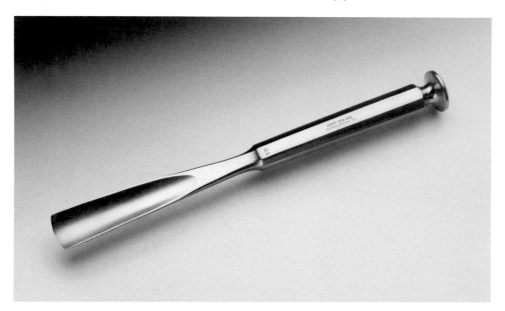

Instrument: STILLE BONE GOUGE
Category: Cutting and Dissecting
Description: It is a flat, round impaction platform with a solid octagonal handle that extends to a trough-like blade that has a sharp cutting edge. Gouges are available in cases or in sets with a variety of sizes.

Use(s): It is used to cut or scoop out a channel of bone.
Instrument Insight: Always hand the gouge to the surgeon with a mallet. Inspect edges for breaks or nicks to ensure precision, sharpness, and patient safety.

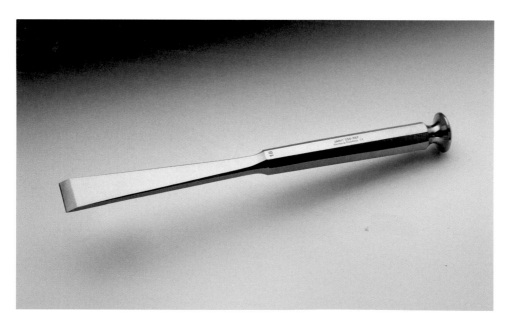

Instrument: STILLE BONE CHISEL
Category: Cutting and Dissecting
Description: It is a flat, round impaction platform with a solid octagonal handle that extends to a flattened, flared blade with a beveled edge. Chisels are available in cases or in sets with a variety of sizes.

Use(s): It is used to cut or shape bone. The chisel is often used when harvesting a bone graft.
Instrument Insight: Always hand the chisel to the surgeon with a mallet. Inspect edges for breaks or nicks to ensure precision, sharpness, and patient safety.

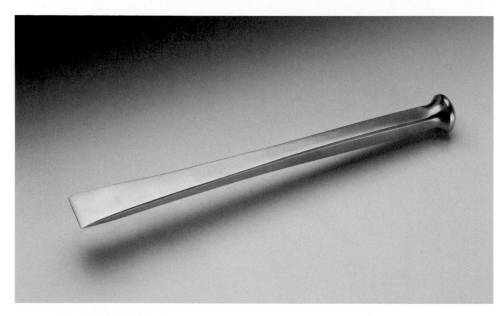

Instrument: STILLE BONE OSTEOTOME
Category: Cutting and Dissecting
Description: It is a flat, round impaction platform with a solid octagonal handle that extends to a flattened, flared blade. Osteotomes are available in cases or in sets with a variety of sizes.

Use(s): It is used to cut or shape bone. The osteotome is often used when harvesting a bone graft.
Instrument Insight: Always hand the osteotome to the surgeon with a mallet. Inspect edges for breaks or nicks to ensure precision, sharpness, and patient safety.

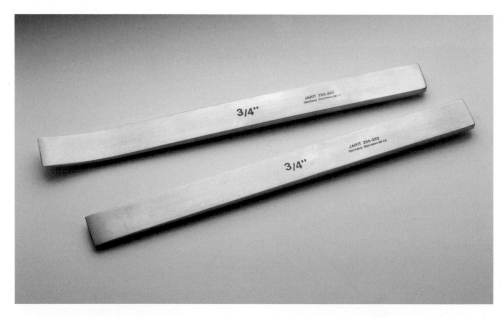

Instrument: LAMBOTTE OSTEOTOME
Category: Cutting and Dissecting
Description: It is a flattened stainless steel ribbon that tapers to a sharp cutting edge; osteotomes are available in widths of various sizes.
Use(s): It is used to cut or shape bone. An osteotome is often used when harvesting a bone graft.

Instrument Insight: Osteotomes may come in cases or sets with a variety of sizes and may be straight or curved. Inspect edges for breaks or nicks to ensure precision, sharpness, and patient safety.

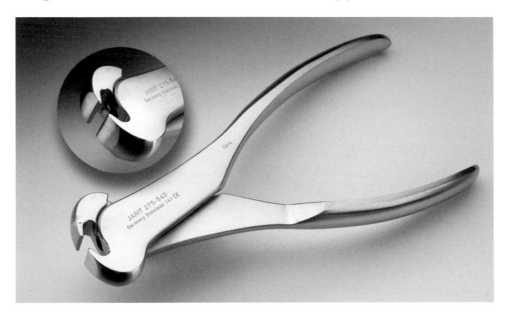

Instrument: **CANNULATED PIN CUTTER**
Other Names: Pin cutter
Category: Cutting and Dissecting
Description: It has heavy, curved handles with extremely curved jaws that meet flush against one another and have extremely sharp edges. There is a circular pin channel between the jaws that runs through the lock box and between the handles. The channel allows the pin to slide through the jaws so the proper length can be cut.
Use(s): It is used for cutting wire or small pins, such as Kirschner wires (K wires) or Steinmann pins.
Instrument Insight: Inspect jaw edges for breaks or nicks to ensure precision and sharpness.

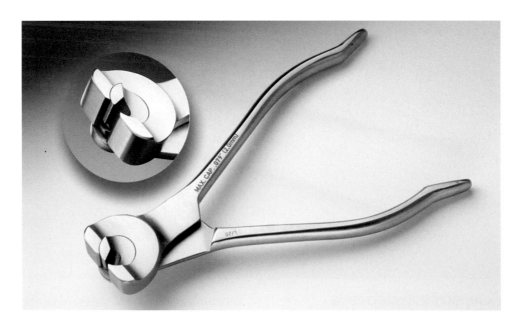

Instrument: **DIAMOND PIN CUTTER**
Other Names: Pin cutter
Category: Cutting and Dissecting
Description: It has heavy, curved handles with a guillotine-action tip. The working end has an angled channel that allows the pin to be placed into the jaw so the proper length can be cut.
Use(s): It is used for cutting wire or small pins, such as Kirschner wires (K wires) or Steinmann pins.
Instrument Insight: Double-action jaws allow for more power when cutting. Inspect for sharpness and smooth action of jaw and cutting surfaces.

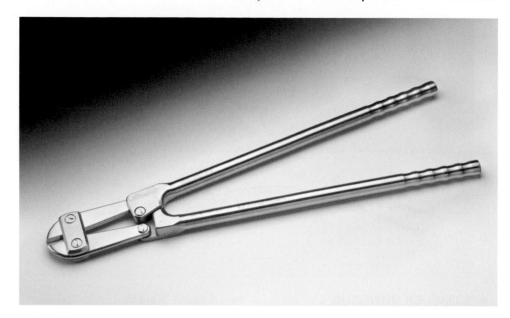

Instrument: LARGE PIN CUTTER
Other Names: Bolt cutter, rod cutter
Category: Cutting and Dissecting
Description: It has very long handles with double-action hinges and a sharp, small cutting surface.
Use(s): It is used for cutting heavy pins and rods.

Instrument Insight: A long handle with double action allows a great amount of force to be applied to the jaws.

⚠ **CAUTION:** When setting up, always check the screw to ensure it is tightened down and cannot fall out into the wound when in use.

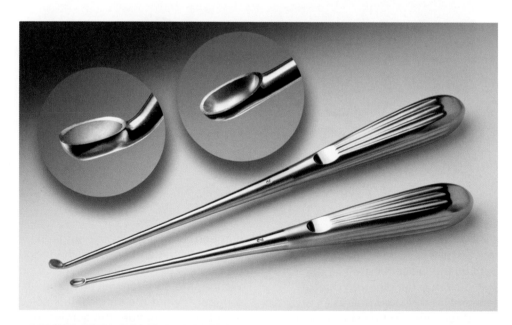

Instrument: BRUNS OVAL BONE CURETTES
Other Names: Curettes
Category: Cutting and Dissecting
Description: These are thick handles with a small scoop at one end; scoops have a variety of shapes and angles.

Use(s): These are used for scooping out tissue or material from small, tight areas.

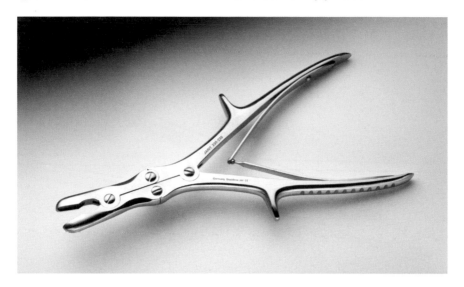

Instrument: STILLE-LUER RONGEUR
Other Names: Straight rongeur, large-mouthed rongeur
Category: Cutting and Dissecting
Description: It is a large-handled, double-action mechanism with large, oval cup-shaped jaws.
Use(s): It is used to grasp, bite, and detach large amounts of tissue.

Instrument Insight: It is a frequently used instrument for large cases that require significant dissection or cleaning of the area.

⚠ **CAUTION:** When setting up, always check the screw to ensure it is tightened down and not fall out into the wound when in use.

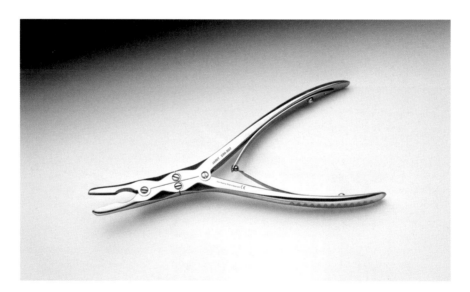

Instrument: ZAUFEL-JANSEN RONGEUR
Other Names: Small-mouthed rongeur
Category: Cutting and Dissecting
Description: It is a large handle with double-action mechanism and thin, sharp jaws.
Use(s): It is used for removing pieces of bone and the soft tissue surrounding the bone.
Instrument Insight: The double-action mechanism gives the rongeur more torque at the tip for better biting action. Always have a moistened sponge ready when handing the

surgeon a rongeur. As the surgeon works to remove tissue and/or bone, the rongeur has to be cleaned between uses. While focusing on the wound, the surgeon will point the tip of the rongeur toward the surgical technologist. Using a moistened sponge, the surgical technologist will clean the tissue from the jaws.

⚠ **CAUTION:** When setting up, always check the screw to ensure it is tightened down and cannot fall out into the wound when in use.

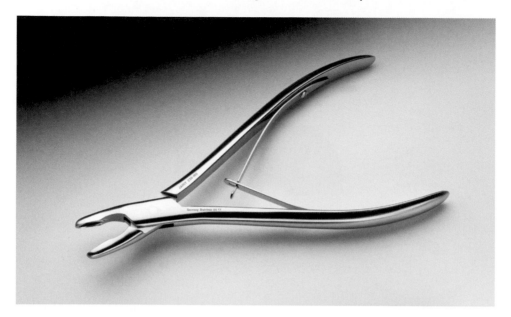

Instrument: **CUSHING RONGEUR**
Category: Cutting and Dissecting
Description: It is a medium-sized handle with a single hinge and short, oval, cup-shaped jaws.
Use(s): It is used for removing pieces of bone and the soft tissue surrounding the bone.
Instrument Insight: Always have a moistened sponge ready when handing the surgeon a rongeur. As the surgeon works to remove tissue and/or bone, the rongeur has to be cleaned between uses. While focusing on the wound, the surgeon will point the tip of the rongeur toward the surgical technologist. Using a moistened sponge, the surgical technologist will clean the tissue from the jaws.

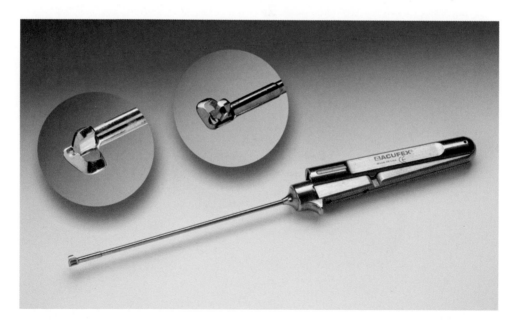

Instrument: **DUCKBILL RIGHT AND LEFT BITER**
Category: Cutting and Dissecting
Description: It is a thick handle with thumb lever that opens and closes the jaws. Has a square-shaped cutting tool on the right or left side of the instrument.
Use(s): It cuts and dissects tissue during arthroscopy procedures.
Instrument Insight: Before handing to the surgeon, hold this instrument by the handle with the cutting end away from you so that you may visualize what side the cutter is facing.

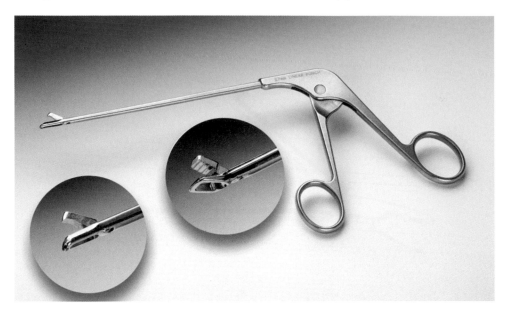

Instrument: DUCKBILL STRAIGHT BITER
Category: Cutting and Dissecting
Description: Ringed handles with a thin rod that has a rectangular-shaped cutter attached distally.

Use(s): It cuts and dissects tissue facing the surgeon.

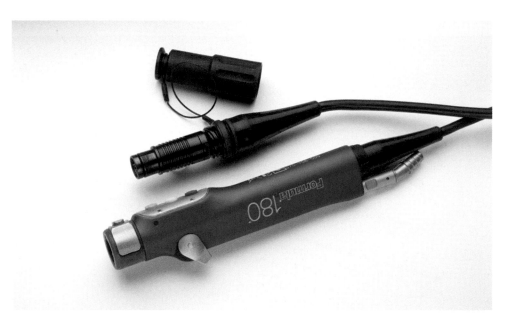

Instrument: SHAVER
Category: Cutting and Dissecting
Description: Motorized handpiece (pictured in blue) is an attachment for various burrs and blades that move at various speeds and directions. Suction tubing is connected to the adaptor next to the cord attachment. The black cord end is handed off the field and connected to the control panel. The shaver is activated by stepping on the foot pedal or with buttons on the handpiece.

Use(s): Houses various shaver attachments to remove, trim, or burr tissue and bone.

Instrument Insight: Shaver often gets clogged with debris. Remove shaver attachment, separate it into its two parts, and remove tissue. HINT: Strike the two parts together to remove tissue.

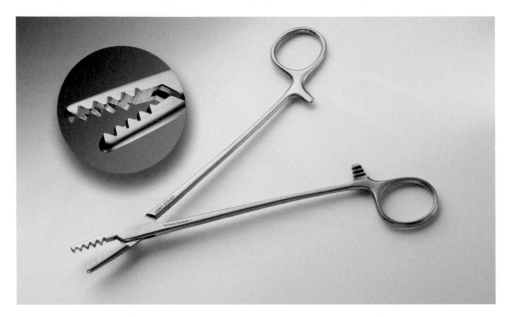

Instrument: MARTIN CARTILAGE CLAMP
Other Names: Meniscus clamp
Category: Grasping and Holding
Description: Ringed handles with large serrations placed in opposition.

Use(s): It is used for grasping heavy tissues and cartilage. The Martin clamp is often used to grasp the meniscus for dissection during total knee arthroplasty.

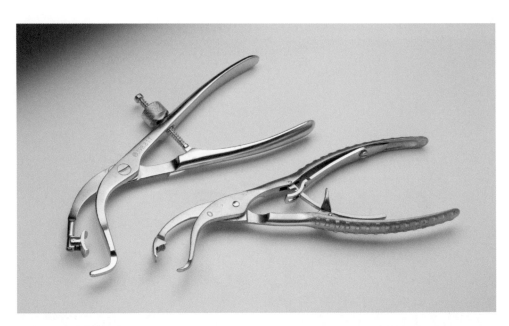

Instrument: PLATE FORCEPS
Other Names: Plate-holding forceps, plate holders, plate clamp
Category: Grasping and Holding
Description: These come in various sizes and designs depending on the type of plating system that is being used and the size and type of bone that is being fixated. The foot of the forceps fits into the counter of the plate, ensuring a firm grip of the plate and the back side of the bone. The foot often has the ability to swivel for precise positioning of the forceps onto the plate.
Use(s): During an ORIF, these are used to hold the plate in alignment while drilling and screw placement take place.

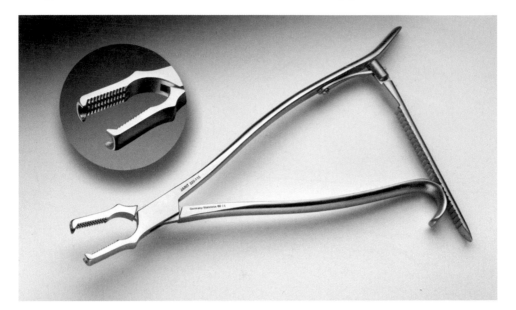

Instrument: KERN BONE HOLDING FORCEPS
Category: Grasping and Holding
Description: These are long, thin handles with a bar ratchet device between them to lock jaws in place. The inner jaws have four heavy tooth and heavy serrations that allow for secure grasping of the bone.
Use(s): These are used for manipulating bone fractures into place and for holding the fracture in alignment while plates and screws are placed. Also used during total joint procedures to grasp bone segments.
Instrument Insight: Hands and instruments should be kept away from the ratchet bar during the procedure to prevent inadvertently releasing it.

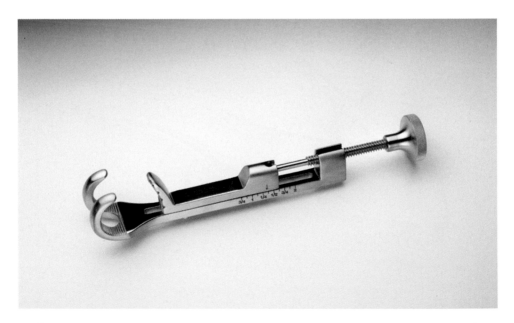

Instrument: LOWMAN BONE CLAMP
Category: Grasping and Holding
Description: It has three curved, grasping, blunt claws at the working end that are tightened into position by turning the screw mechanism at the proximal end.
Use(s): It is used for holding the fractured bone in alignment while plates and screws are placed.
Instrument Insight: Inspect the screw mechanism before surgery to ensure that it is working properly.

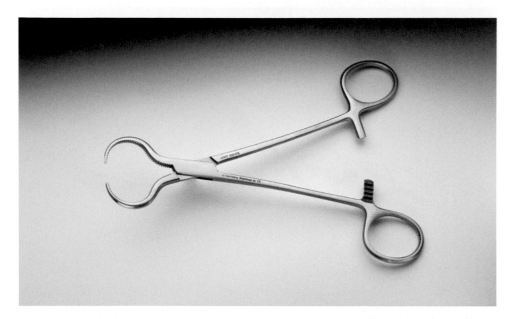

Instrument: LEWIN BONE HOLDING FORCEPS
Other Names: Joplin forceps
Category: Grasping and Holding
Description: These are ringed handles with very sharp double-curved graspers.
Use(s): These are used for manipulating bone fractures into place and for holding the fracture in alignment while plates and screws are placed. The Lewin forceps can also be used during a hip arthroplasty to punch holes in bone for passage of sutures when closing the joint.
Instrument Insight: Because of sharp ends, use extreme caution when handling.

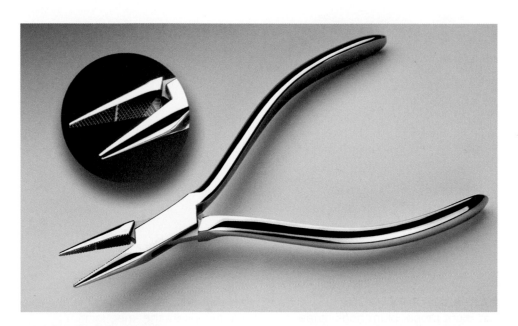

Instrument: NEEDLENOSE PLIERS
Category: Grasping and Holding
Description: These are thin, single-action handles with serrated jaws that narrow to a point.
Use(s): These are used to remove pins and hardware and twist wires.

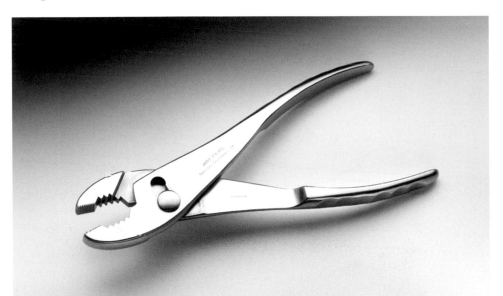

Instrument: PLIERS
Other Names: Channel locks
Category: Grasping and Holding
Description: These are thin, single-action handles with thin and thick serrations and rounded-end jaws. Hinge provides two opening sizes of the jaws.
Use(s): These are used to place or remove hardware and to grasp pointed trocar during drain insertion of deep wounds.

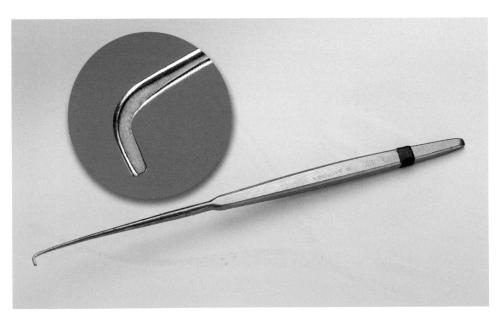

Instrument: ARTHROSCOPY PROBE
Other Names: Blunt probe, blunt hook, knee scope probe
Category: Probing and Dilating
Description: It is a right-angled blunt hook with a flattened handle.
Use(s): It is used to examine and move tissues around inside the knee joint.
Instrument Insight: Should be placed on the Mayo stand for every arthroscopy.

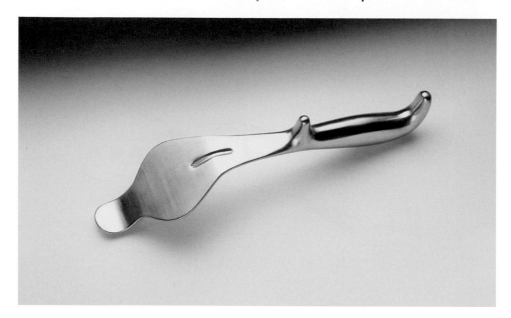

Instrument: BENNETT RETRACTOR
Category: Retracting and Exposing
Description: It is a smooth, solid grip type handle with a downward-curved, rounded, flared blade and a smaller upward-curved round lip.
Use(s): It is used for retracting tissues during procedures involving large bones (e.g., the proximal or midshaft of the femur).
Instrument Insight: The lip of the Bennett is slid behind and around the bone shaft for leverage when retracting tissues. There is no pulling needed when holding this retractor; once it is placed, simply hold the handle down or back.

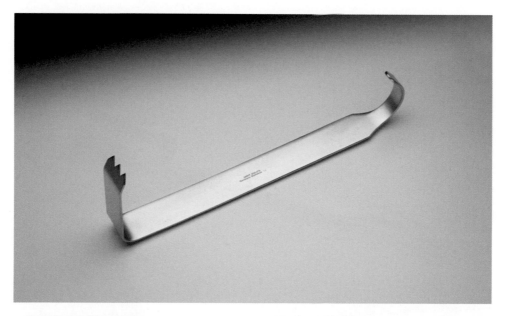

Instrument: HIBBS RETRACTOR
Category: Retracting and Exposing
Description: This is a flattened, double-ended retractor that has a laterally bent blade and slightly bent lip with V-shaped teeth on one end and a small, crescent-shaped blade on the other.
Use(s): This is a tissue retractor for either deep or superficial areas. The Hibbs retractor is often used in large bone cases.

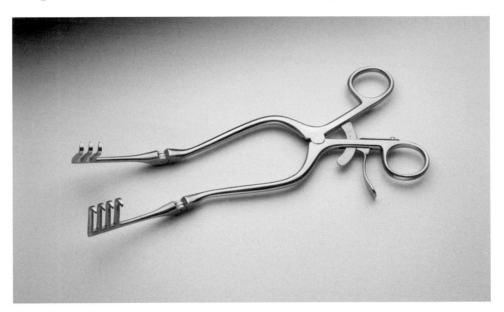

Instrument: BECKMAN RETRACTOR

Category: Retracting and Exposing

Description: It is a self-retaining, finger-ringed instrument with a ratcheted release device on the shanks. Two hinged arms extend from the shank to three outward-curved prongs on one side and four on the other. These prongs can be sharp or dull.

Use(s): It is used for retraction in procedures involving deep tissue, such as the spine, and in proximal femur fractures.

Instrument Insight: Always hand this retractor to the surgeon with the prongs pointing downward.

⚠ **CAUTION:** The prongs may be very sharp. Exercise care when handling sharp instruments to avoid puncture to gloves and/or skin.

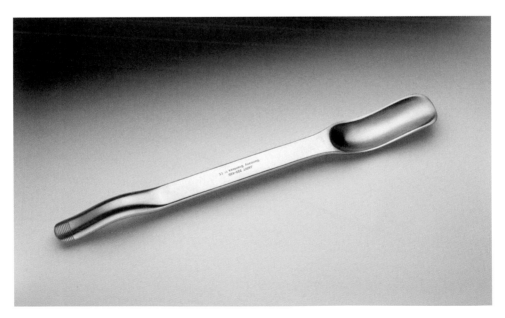

Instrument: MURPHY-LANE BONE SKID

Category: Retracting and Exposing

Description: It is double ended with large or small curved spoons at each end.

Use(s): It is used for removing the femoral head from the joint during total hip arthroplasty.

Instrument Insight: The size of the femoral head and the acetabulum will determine which end of the bone skid to use.

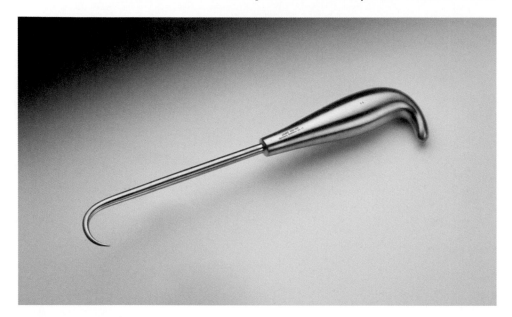

Instrument: BONE HOOK
Category: Retracting and Exposing
Description: It has a thick handle with an extremely sharp curved hook at the working end.
Use(s): It is used for retracting bone or heavy tissue.

Instrument Insight: Always hand the bone hook to the surgeon with the prongs pointing downward.

⚠ **CAUTION:** The prongs are very sharp. Exercise care when handling sharp instruments to avoid puncture to gloves and/or skin.

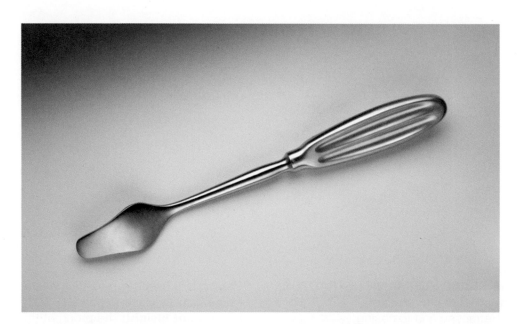

Instrument: CHANDLER RETRACTOR
Other Names: Chandler elevator
Category: Retracting and Exposing
Description: It is a thick handle with medium-curved, blunt blade.

Use(s): It is used for retracting bone and tissue.
Instrument Insight: This instrument is used to hold soft tissue away from bone, like a lever, when the surgeon is performing fixation.

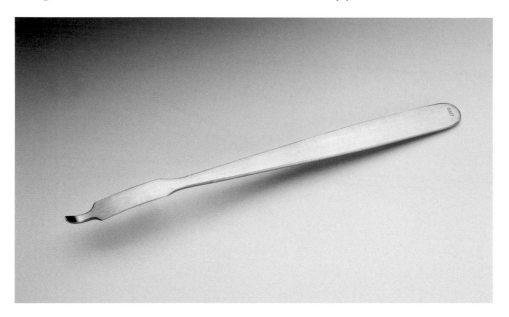

Instrument: MINI HOHMANN RETRACTOR
Category: Retracting and Exposing
Description: It is a flattened, smooth handle with thin, slightly curved blades and with a small, upward-curved, pointed tip. These come in different widths.
Use(s): It is used for retracting tissue or bone in tight, small areas. The mini-Hohmann retractor is often used during ORIF of the ankle.
Instrument Insight: The tip of the Hohmann retractor is slid behind and around the bone for leverage when retracting tissues. There is no pulling needed when holding this retractor; after it is placed, simply hold the handle down or back.

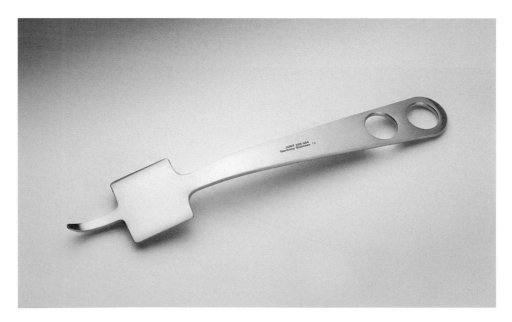

Instrument: SHARP HOHMANN RETRACTOR
Other Name: Hohmann retractor
Category: Retracting and Exposing
Description: It has a flat handle with two holes placed distally to aid in grasping the handle. The blade is shaped in a square with an upward, slightly curved prong at the end. These come in different widths.
Use(s): It is used for retracting a large area of tissue, usually close to bone.
Instrument Insight: The prong of the Hohmann retractor is slid behind and around the bone for leverage when retracting tissues. There is no pulling needed when holding this retractor; after it is placed, simply hold the handle down or back.

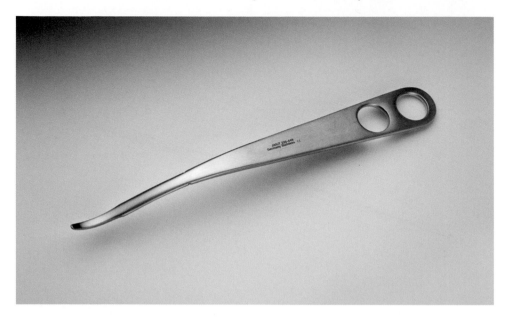

Instrument: BLUNT HOHMANN RETRACTOR
Category: Retracting and Exposing
Description: It is a flat handle with two holes placed distally. The blade is blunt, very thin, and slightly curved. There is no pulling needed when holding this retractor; after it is placed, simply hold the handle down or back. These come in different widths.
Use(s): It is used for retracting a small amount of tissue in a very tight area.

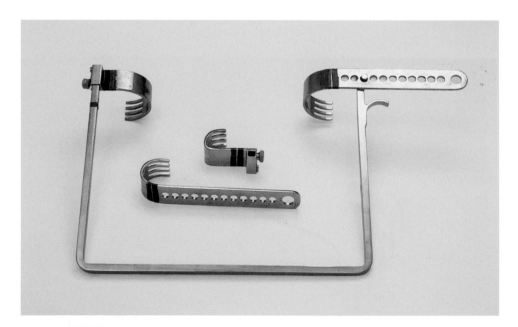

Instrument: CHARNLEY RETRACTOR
Other Names: Ortho Balfour retractor
Category: Retracting and Exposing
Description: It is a square-shaped frame with attachable blades.
Use(s): It is a self-retaining retractor often used during posterior hip surgeries to hold the wound open.

Instrument Insight: It comes with a cylinder weight with a chain that can be hooked to the frame to pull the retractor downward and out of the way.

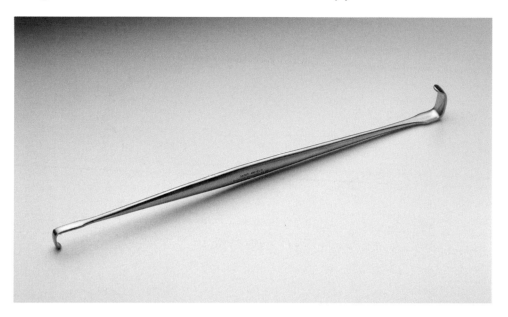

Instrument: RAGNELL RETRACTOR
Category: Retracting and Exposing
Description: It is double ended with right-angle blunt blades that are available in different sizes.

Use(s): It is used for retracting varying amounts of tissue at different depths in hand and wrist surgeries.

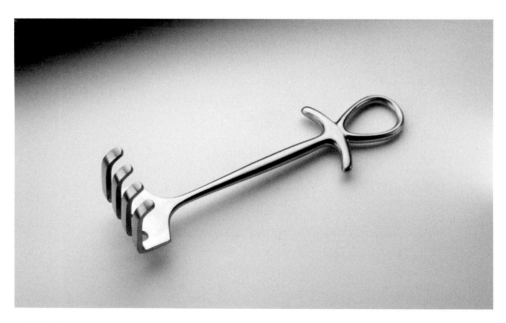

Instrument: ISRAEL RAKE RETRACTOR
Category: Retracting and Exposing
Description: The handle has a teardrop opening with two prongs on each side. It has four large claws that may be blunt or sharp.

Use(s): It is used for retracting large amounts of tissue that usually does not involve bone.
Instrument Insight: This instrument is also available with sharp prongs.

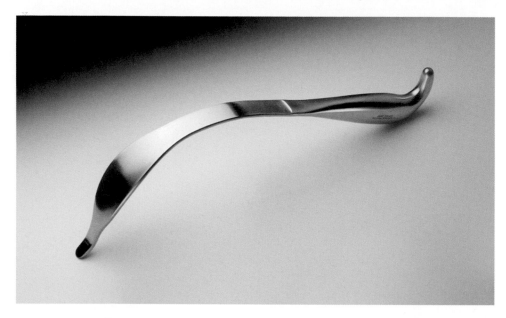

Instrument: COBRA RETRACTOR
Category: Retracting and Exposing
Description: This is a smooth, solid grip type handle with a downward-curved, flared blade and with a smaller upward-curved, round tip.
Use(s): It is used for retraction of large areas of tissue. The large bend in the blade allows tissue to be retracted far away from the field, allowing for better visualization.
Instrument Insight: There is no pulling needed when holding this retractor; after it is placed, simply hold the handle down or back.

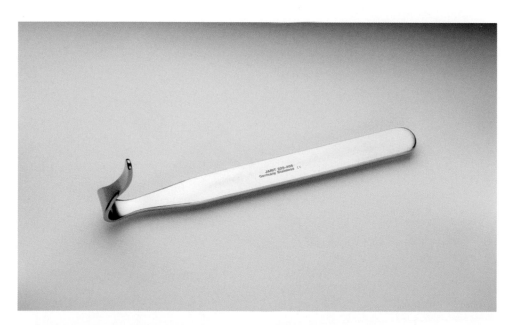

Instrument: BLOUNT KNEE RETRACTOR
Category: Retracting and Exposing
Description: It is a thin, flat handle with a blunt blade at a right angle and slightly curved.
Use(s): It is used for retracting tissue at a right angle.
Instrument Insight: It is often used as a lever to retract. There is no pulling needed when holding this retractor; after it is placed, simply hold the handle down or back.

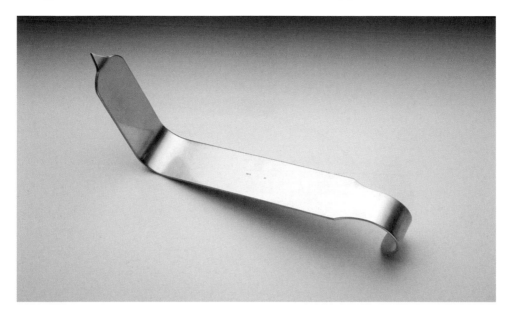

Instrument: TAYLOR HIP RETRACTOR
Category: Retracting and Exposing
Description: It is a thin handle with a curved, rounded end and blade at a right angle with a sharp tip.
Use(s): It is used for retracting tissue for exposure in total hip arthroplasties.

Instrument Insight: The sharp tip is placed next to or on the bone for leverage. There is no pulling needed when holding this retractor; after it is placed, simply hold the handle down or back.

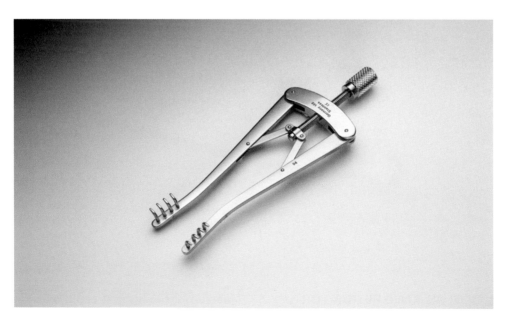

Instrument: ALM RETRACTOR
Category: Retracting and Exposing
Description: It is a self-retaining retractor. It has a thumb screw with flaring wings to open the arms of the retractor. It has four sharp prongs on each side.
Use(s): It is used for retracting in small areas.

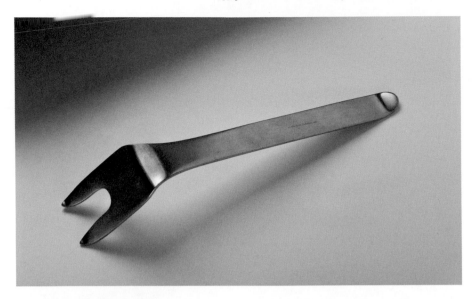

Instrument: HUMERAL HEAD RETRACTOR
Category: Retracting and Exposing
Description: It is an angled two-prong blade with a straight flat handle.

Use(s): It is placed between the glenoid and the humeral head to obtain exposure.

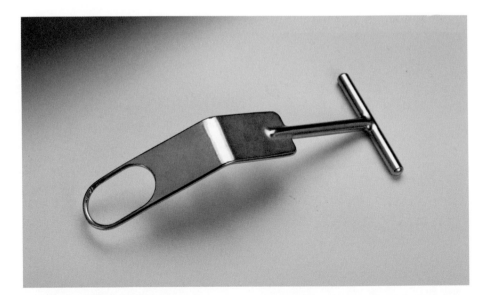

Instrument: FUKUDA HUMERAL HEAD RETRACTOR
Other Names: Humeral head retractor, Fukuda retractor
Category: Retracting and Exposing
Description: The Fukuda retractor is available in small and large sizes; it has a T-bar style handle with an angled blade and oval fenestration at the working end.
Use(s): It is used to retract the humeral shaft posteriorly and helping to expose the entire glenoid surface.

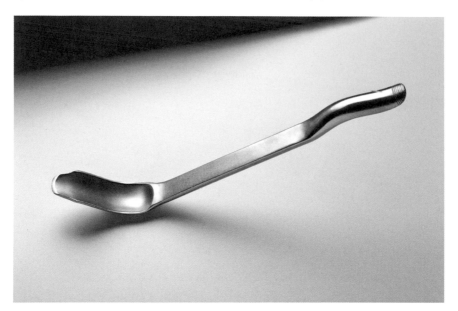

Instrument: LEVER SKID HUMERAL HEAD RETRACTOR
Other Names: Bone skid, shoulder skid
Category: Retracting and Exposing
Description: It is double ended with large and small curved spoons at each end.

Use(s): It is used for removal of the humeral head from the joint during a total shoulder arthroplasty.

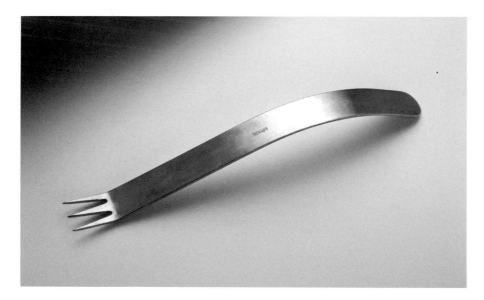

Instrument: CAPSULE RETRACTOR
Other Names: Fork retractor
Category: Retracting and Exposing
Description: It is a curved ribbon of steel with three angled sharp prongs at the working end. These come with one, two, or three prongs, which are designed to retract in different areas.

Use(s): The two- and three-prong retractors are designed to be placed medially along the scapular neck to retract the anterior capsule and labrum. The single-prong retractor is commonly used when retracting on the inferior rim of the glenoid.

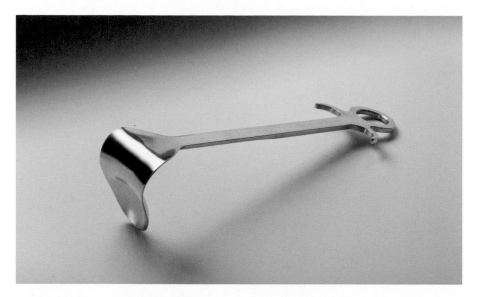

Instrument: BROWNE DELTOID RETRACTOR
Category: Retracting and Exposing
Description: The blade is concave and angled with a cup-like indentation at the working end. The handle is flat with a round opening and two curved prongs at each side of the distal end.
Use(s): It is placed to contour the humeral head for deltoid retraction to allow for exposure.

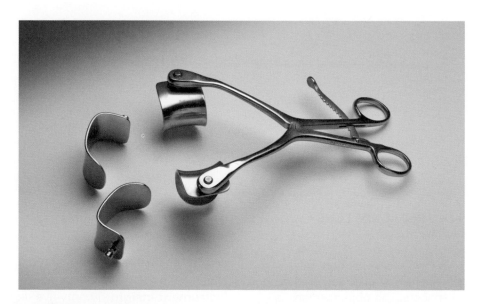

Instrument: KOLBEL SELF-RETAINING GLENOID RETRACTOR
Category: Retracting and Exposing
Description: It is a finger-ring, ratcheted self-retaining retractor that has exchangeable shallow to deep blades.
Use(s): It is used for retracting the capsule open during shoulder procedures.

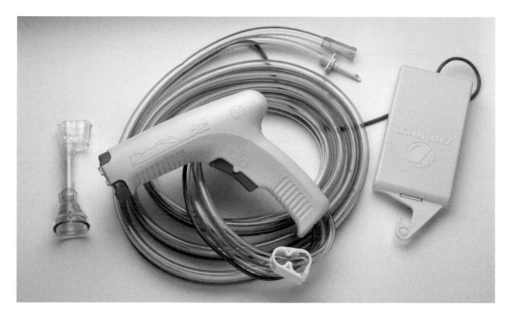

Instrument: **PULSAVAC**
Other Names: Pulse lavage
Category: Suctioning and Aspirating
Description: A battery pack provides power. The irrigation spike and the suction connection are handed off the sterile field. The Pulsavac gun has two speeds with controls on the handle. A barrel is attached to the gun with a funnel at the distal end of the gun.
Use(s): It is used for irrigation and debridement of tissues. The Pulsavac is commonly used for high-pressure irrigation during total joint arthroplasties.

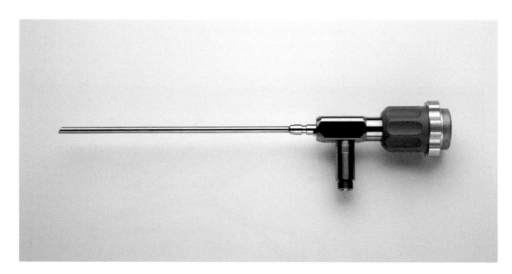

Instrument: **25-DEGREE, 4-MM LENS**
Other Names: Arthroscope
Category: Viewing
Description: It is a rigid stainless steel tube containing an optical chain of precisely aligned glass lenses and spacers. The objective lens is located at the distal tip of the scope. This determines the viewing angle. The stainless steel cylinder is called the optical element or the telescope, providing both images and light. The light connector allows attachment of the light cord to the telescope. At the proximal end is the eyepiece or ocular lens; this attaches to the camera coupler, or the surgeon may view the surgical field directly.
Use(s): It is used for viewing the inside of a joint.
Instrument Insight: Twenty-five degrees is the angle at which the objective lens views. The 25-degree endoscopes are very expensive and fragile. Care should be exercised when handling an endoscope; it should never be picked up by the distal telescope end, placed under heavy objects, or dropped.

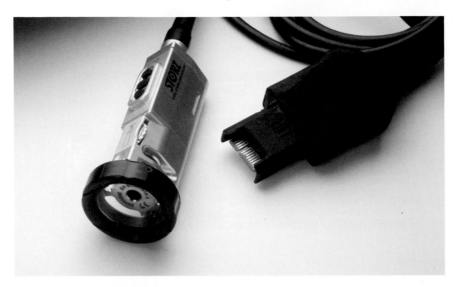

Instrument: ENDOSCOPIC CAMERA
Other Names: Arthroscope
Category: Viewing
Description: At the distal end of the camera is the coupler, which attaches the camera to the eyepiece of the rigid scope. The coupler is attached to the camera head, which provides the image quality. Attached to the camera head is the cord, which relays the images back to the video system.

Use(s): It is used for the transmission of images from the rigid or flexible endoscope to the video monitor.
Instrument Insight: Most camera failures are related to a damaged cord. Care should be exercised when handling the camera and cord. They should never be placed under a heavy object, dropped, twisted, or kinked. Also keep the distal end covered until it is ready to be plugged into the unit.

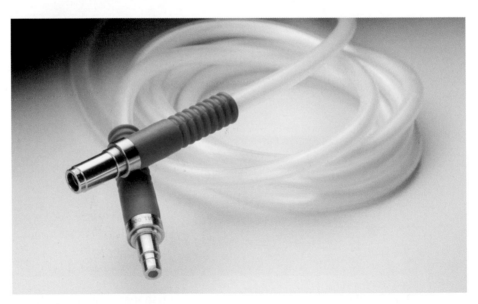

Instrument: FIBEROPTIC LIGHT CORD
Other Names: Light cord
Category: Viewing
Description: It is a 10-foot-long fiber-optic cable with an endoscope adaptor at the proximal end and a light source adaptor at the distal end.
Use(s): It is used for delivering high-intensity light to the endoscope for illumination during endoscopic procedures.
Instrument Insight: Exercise care when handling a fiber-optic cord; it should never be

placed under a heavy object, dropped, twisted, or kinked because the tiny fibers inside can be easily damaged.

⚠ **CAUTION:** When not in use, the light source must be placed on standby or turned off. The intense heat from the beam can cause the patient's drapes or any flammable vapors around the patient to ignite.

INSTRUMENT SETS

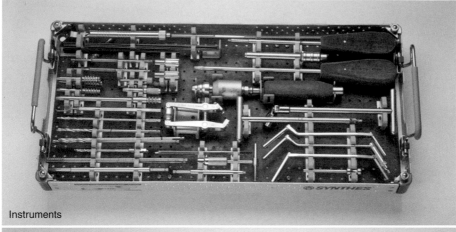

Instruments

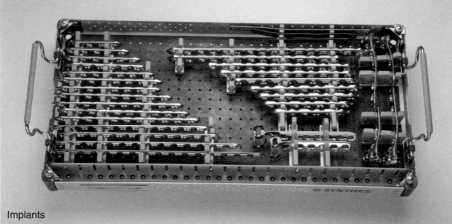

Implants

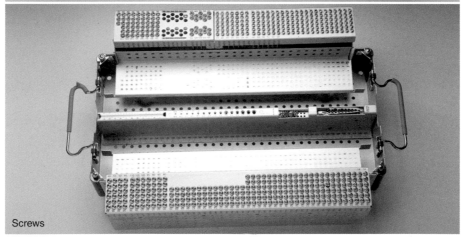

Screws

Instrument: LARGE FRAGMENT SET
Other Names: Large frag set
Category: Sets
Description: First tray (instruments): Different types of screwdrivers, depth gauge, variety of drill bits, taps, chuck, drill guides, and plate holders.

Second tray (implants): Narrow plates, broad plates, T-plates, and bending templates.

Third tray (screws): Variety of screws, locking screws, other implants, and screw forceps.

Use(s): These instruments, plates, and screws are used to secure fractures in large bones.
Instrument Insight: Check surgeon's preference card for type of screws, implants, drill bit sizes, and drill guides. Check each tray before use to determine that all instruments and sizes are in each tray. This is especially needed for screws because they are placed in the patient and not roused

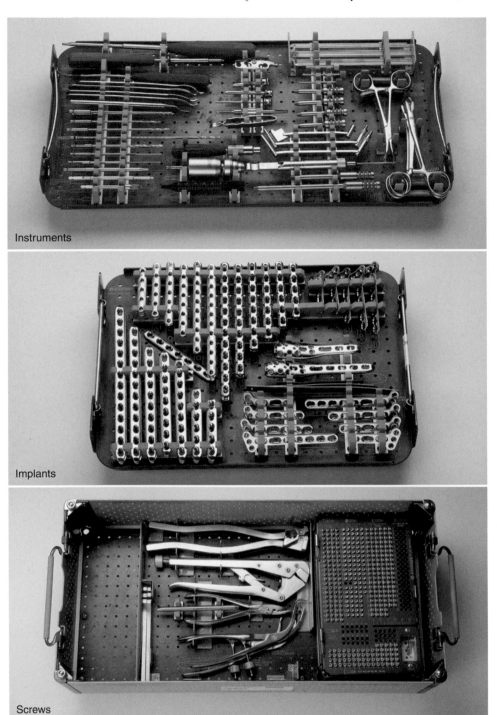

Instruments

Implants

Screws

Instrument: SMALL FRAGMENT SET
Other Names: Small frag
Description: First tray (instruments): variety of screwdrivers, drill bits, depth gauge, bone holding clamps, drill guides, small Hohmann retractors, k-wires, and screw retriever.

Second tray (plate implants): locking compression plates (LCP) plates, T-plates, one-third tubular, proximal humerus, straight reconstruction plates, curved reconstruction plates, and oblique, right angle plates and bending templates.

Third tray (screw implants): cortex, cancellous, shaft, and self-tapping; screws and washers also

in this tray are plate benders, plate holding and bone holding forceps.
Use(s): These instruments, implants, and screws are used to secure fractures in small bones.
Instrument Insight: Check surgeon's preference card for type of screws, implants, drill bit sizes, and drill guides. Check each tray before use to determine that all instruments and sizes are in each tray. This is especially needed for screws because they are placed in the patient and not reused.

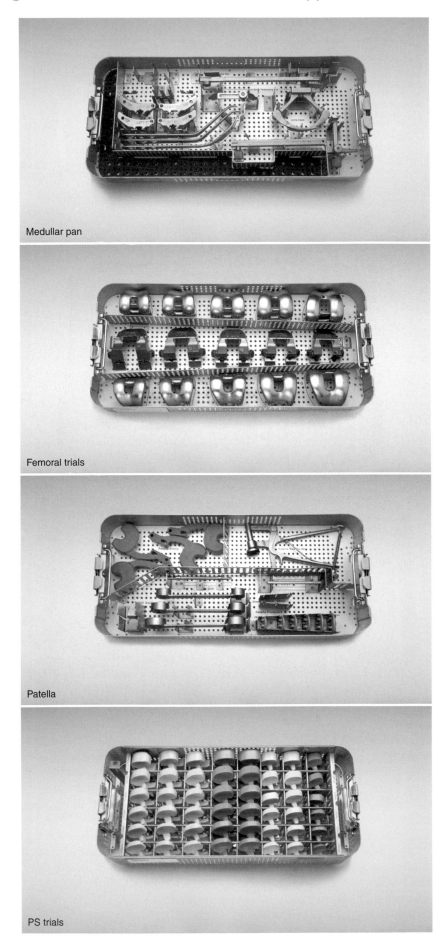

Medullar pan

Femoral trials

Patella

PS trials

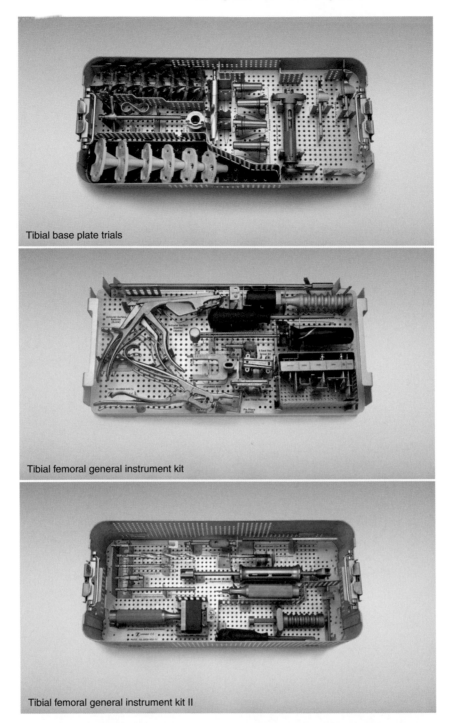

Tibial base plate trials

Tibial femoral general instrument kit

Tibial femoral general instrument kit II

Instrument: TOTAL KNEE INSTRUMENTS
Other Names: Knee arthroplasty set
Description: Several pans are opened to perform the arthroplasty. Shown here:
- Medullar pan
- Femoral trials
- Patella
- Posterior stabilization (PS) trials
- Tibial base plate trials
- Tibial femoral general instrument kit
- Tibial femoral general instrument kit II

Use(s): These are used to perform a total knee replacement (arthroplasty).
Instrument Insight: There are many different systems and companies that have their own systems. Total knee instrument pans are often set by the company sales representative for a specific surgeon or group of surgeons according to their preference; these systems will differ accordingly. These pictures were set up by a Zimmer representative for a specific surgeon. Sets can vary by facility.

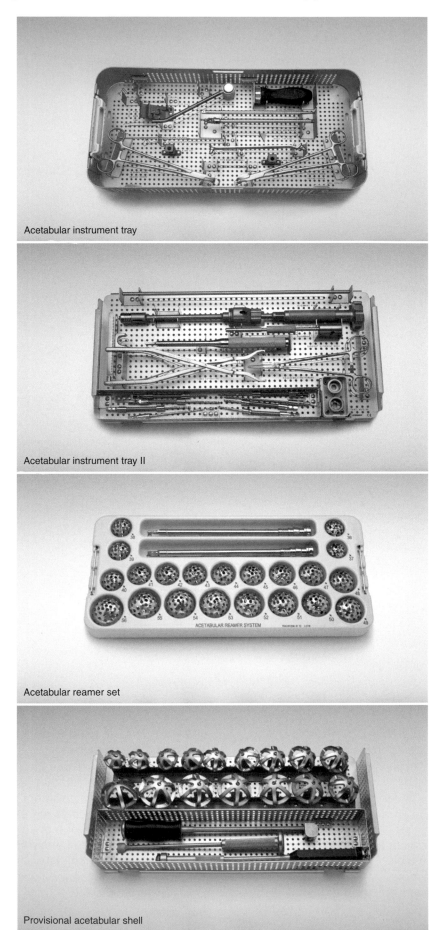

Acetabular instrument tray

Acetabular instrument tray II

Acetabular reamer set

Provisional acetabular shell

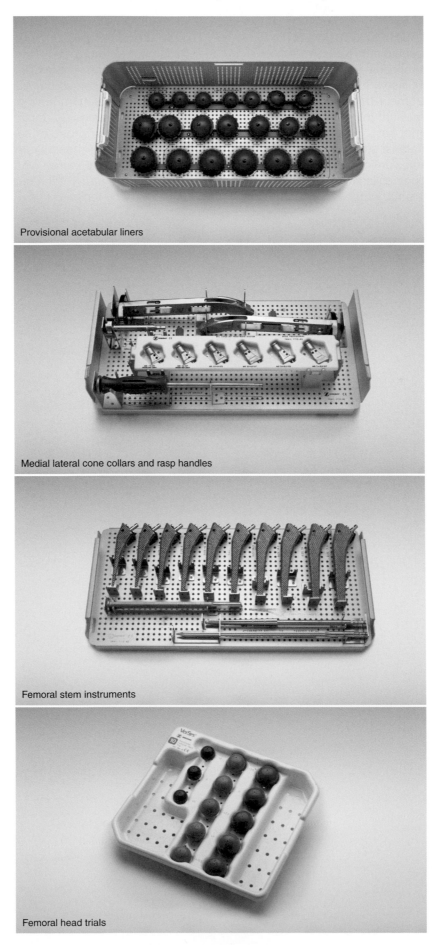

Provisional acetabular liners

Medial lateral cone collars and rasp handles

Femoral stem instruments

Femoral head trials

Instrument: TOTAL HIP INSTRUMENTS
Other Names: Total hip arthroplasty set
Description: Several pans are opened to perform the arthroplasty. Shown here:
- Acetabular instrument tray
- Acetabular instrument tray II
- Acetabular reamer set
- Provisional acetabular shell
- Provisional acetabular liners
- Medial lateral cone collars and rasp handles
- Femoral stem instruments
- Femoral head trials

Use(s): These are used to perform a total hip replacement (arthroplasty).
Instrument Insight: There are many different systems and companies that have their own systems. Total hip instrument pans are often set by the company sales representative for a specific surgeon or group of surgeons according to their preference; these systems will differ accordingly. These pictures were set up by a Zimmer representative for a specific surgeon. Sets can vary by facility.

14 Neurosurgical Instruments

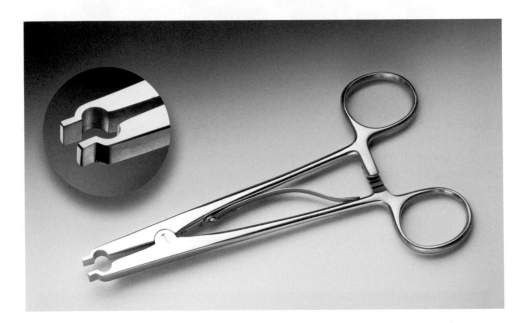

Instrument: RANEY CLIP APPLIER

Other Names: Scalp clip applier

Category: Accessory

Description: It is a finger-ringed ratcheted instrument with heavy, smooth jaws that have a crescent-shaped fenestration, which leads to a flattened tip. The jaws of the applier are spread apart when the instrument is ratcheted down and are brought together when the ratchet is released.

Use(s): It is used for applying Raney clips to scalp flap edges during a craniotomy.

Instrument Insight: To load a clip, the flattened tips of the applier are inserted into the opening on the back of the Raney clip. Upon compression of the ratchet, the jaws and clip open and are ready for application. Each clip controls bleeding only at the site on which it is applied. The length of the incision will determine the number required for hemostasis. Clips are placed along the incision edge with no more than a 1-cm gap between clips.

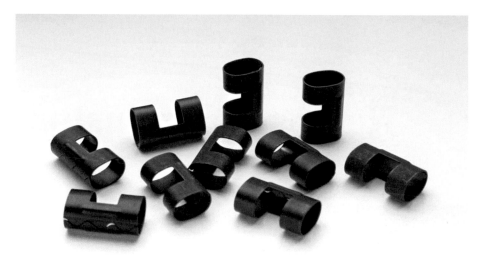

Instrument: RANEY CLIPS
Category: Accessory
Description: It is a disposable plastic or reusable metal spring-action clip with wave-like jaws on one side and a slot on the other.
Use(s): It is used to provide hemostasis by compressing the tissue layers of the scalp edges when turning a flap during a craniotomy.

Instrument Insight: The disposable clips are typically packaged in sets of 10 or 20. Several clips must be placed on each side of the incision, so multiple packages may be needed.

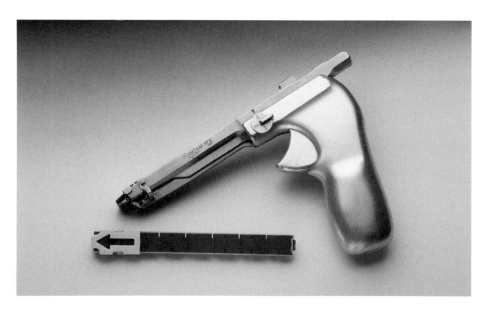

Instrument: SCALP CLIP GUN
Category: Accessory
Description: It is a reusable, gun-shaped device with disposable clip cartridges. The system components are a reusable clip gun, disposable scalp clip cartridges, and clip removal forceps.
Use(s): It is used for providing hemostasis by compressing the tissue layers of the scalp edges when turning a flap during a craniotomy.
Instrument Insight: With activation of the trigger, the clip is opened, closed, and released by the applier. The successive clip automatically slides into position and can be applied in the same manner. The disposable clip cartridge is packaged with 10 clips. Each clip controls bleeding only at the site on which it is applied. The length of the incision will determine the number required for hemostasis. Clips are placed along the incision edge with no more than a 1-cm gap between clips.

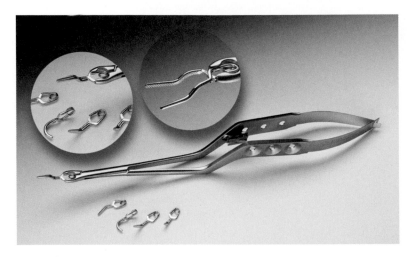

Instrument: ANEURYSM CLIP APPLIER AND CLIPS

Category: Accessory

Description: These are bayoneted spring-action forceps with slotted, inward-curving jaws that grasp around the clip. There are many different manufacturers and a variety of aneurysm clips available for use. Most of the clips are spring-loaded, made of titanium, and manufactured in an assortment of types, sizes, shapes, and lengths to accommodate the various needs of the aneurysms (e.g., location, dimension, form). Aneurysm clips are classified as permanent or temporary. Temporary clips are used to ensure proper position of the permanent clip or to clip the vessels that supply the aneurysm if rupture occurs or if the aneurysm is very large.

Use(s): It is used to clip the base or neck of an intracranial aneurysm to isolate it from normal circulation, thus causing it to deflate or obliterate.

Instrument Insight: There are many different aneurysm clip manufacturers (e.g., Sugita, Yasargil, Sundt, McFadden, Heifetz).

⚠ **CAUTION:** An aneurysm clip should never be compressed between the fingers or with any other device; this should only be done with the clip appliers. A clip that has been compressed open should never be used again. The closing force on a clip that has been opened, closed, and opened again can become sprung and unstable and endanger the patient.

⚠ **CAUTION:** Always have a temporary clip loaded in case a rupture occurs.

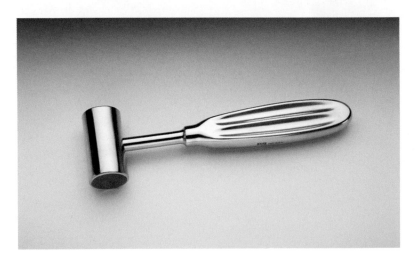

Instrument: MALLET

Category: Accessory

Description: It is a solid stainless steel or brass-filled stainless steel hammer-like instrument. Weight is 1 to 3 pounds. Mallets are used in other specialties that involve bone work.

Use(s): It is used to exert force on osteotomes, chisels, gouges, tamps, and other specially designed instruments. It is commonly used during spinal surgery to harvest the bone graft.

Instrument Insight: Make available after passing any chisel, tamp, etc.

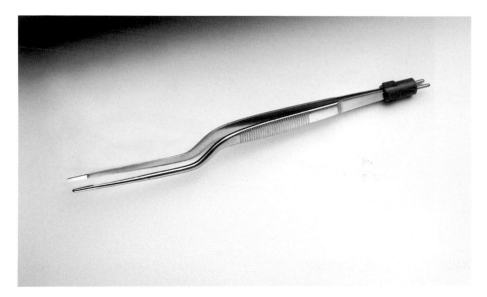

Instrument: CUSHING BIPOLAR FORCEPS
Other Names: BB forceps (bipolar bayonet)
Category: Accessory
Description: These are bayonet-style forceps with fine, smooth tips and a bipolar connection post at the end. Bipolar forceps can be either insulated or noninsulated.
Use(s): It is used for coagulating tissue that is grasped between the tips.
Instrument Insight: The bipolar forceps use a disposable cord that attaches to the post end and is then connected to the electrosurgical unit (ESU) generator located off the field. Stepping on a foot pedal activates the bipolar energy. The electricity travels from the ESU generator to one tip of the forceps, through the grasped tissue, into the other tip, and back to the generator. The current does not pass through the patient's body, so a dispersive electrode is not needed. The ESU bipolar forceps use less energy that travels a shorter pathway and is much safer than the monopolar forceps. Bayonet-shaped instruments are designed so that the user can see beyond their fingers.

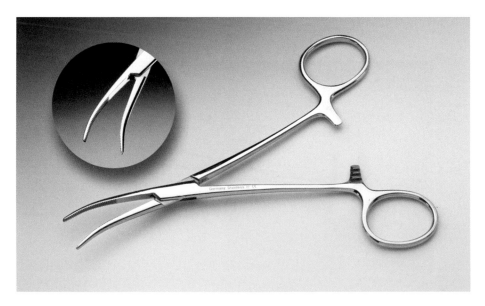

Instrument: DANDY FORCEPS
Other Names: Dandy clamp
Category: Clamping and Occluding
Description: These are sideways-curved forceps with horizontal serrations running halfway down the jaws.
Use(s): These are used for providing hemostasis on the scalp edges when lifting the flap during a craniotomy.

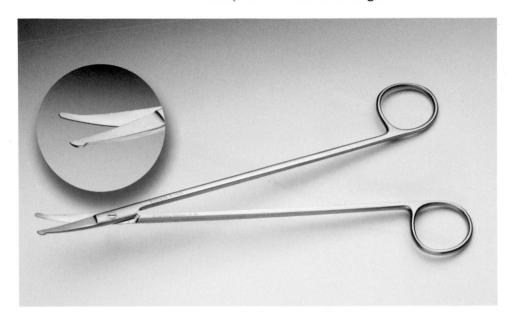

Instrument: STRULLY SCISSORS
Category: Cutting and Dissecting
Description: These are fine scissors with slightly curved blades and crescent-shaped probe tips.
Use(s): These are used for blunt and sharp dissection of delicate tissues.
Instrument Insight: The crescent-shaped tips are to protect underlying tissue from trauma during cutting (e.g., protecting brain tissue when cutting the dura).

⚠ **CAUTION:** When setting up, always check the screw to ensure it is tightened down and cannot fall out into the wound when in use.

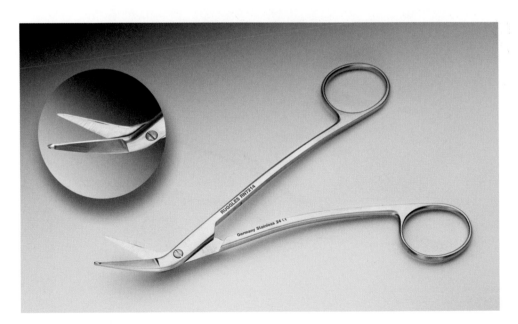

Instrument: TAYLOR DURAL SCISSORS
Other Names: Angled dura scissors
Category: Cutting and Dissecting
Description: These are angled, bladed scissors with a blunt tip on the lower blade to prevent damage to underlying tissue.
Use(s): These are used to extend the incision into the dura mater during a craniotomy.

⚠ **CAUTION:** When setting up, always check the screw to ensure it is tightened down and cannot fall out into the wound when in use.

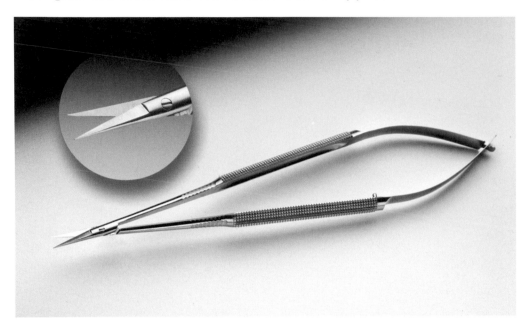

Instrument: RHOTON MICRO SCISSORS
Other Names: Micro scissors
Category: Cutting and Dissecting
Description: These are fine spring-operated scissors that may be curved or straight.

Use(s): These are used for microdissection of delicate tissue.

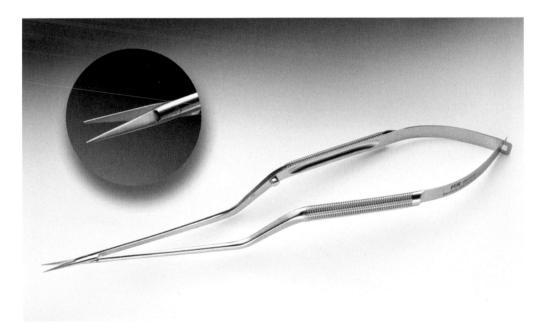

Instrument: RHOTON MICRO BAYONET SCISSORS
Category: Cutting and Dissecting
Description: These are bayonet-style spring action scissors that can have curved or straight blades.

Use(s): These are used for microdissection of delicate tissues.
Instrument Insight: Bayonet-shaped instruments are designed so that the user may see beyond his or her fingers.

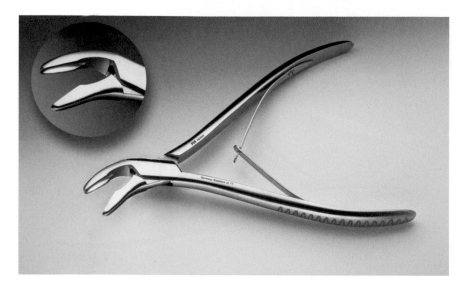

Instrument: BACON CRANIAL RONGEUR
Other Name: Bacon rongeur
Category: Cutting and Dissecting
Description: It is an angled rongeur with fine, oval-cupped jaws.
Use(s): It removes pieces of bone and the soft tissue surrounding the bone. The Bacon rongeur is often used to remove the jagged skull edges when drilling burr holes or creating a flap.

Instrument Insight: Always have a moistened sponge ready when handing the surgeon a rongeur. As the surgeon works to remove tissue and/or bone, the rongeur has to be cleaned between uses. While focusing on the wound, the surgeon will point the tip of the rongeur toward the surgical technologist. Using a moistened sponge, the surgical technologist will grasp the tissue from the jaws.

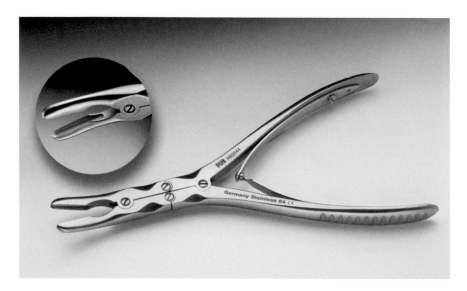

Instrument: BEYER RONGEUR
Category: Cutting and Dissecting
Description: It is a double-action, slightly angled rongeur with broad, elongated, trough-like jaws.
Use(s): It is used for removing pieces of bone and the soft tissue surrounding the bone.
Instrument Insight: The double action gives the rongeur more torque at the tip for better biting action. Always have a moistened sponge ready when handing the surgeon a rongeur. As the surgeon works to remove tissue and/or bone, the rongeur has to be cleaned between uses.

While focusing on the wound, the surgeon will point the tip of the rongeur toward the surgical technologist. Using a moistened sponge, the surgical technologist will clean the tissue from the jaws. All biting or gripping instruments should be inspected at the cups for chipping and sharpness.

⚠ **CAUTION:** When setting up, always check the screw to ensure it is tightened down and cannot fall out into the wound when in use.

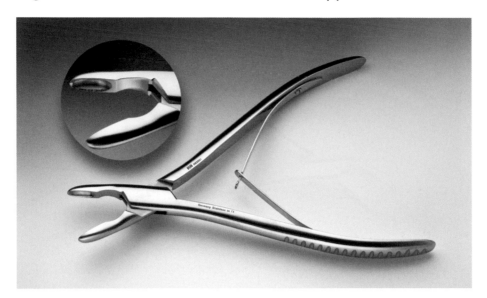

Instrument: ADSON CRANIAL RONGEUR
Category: Cutting and Dissecting
Description: It is a straight rongeur with oval cup jaws.
Use(s): It is used for removing pieces of bone and the soft tissue surrounding the bone.
Instrument Insight: Always have a moistened sponge ready when handing the surgeon a rongeur. As the surgeon works to remove tissue and/or bone, the rongeur has to be cleaned between uses. While focusing on the wound, the surgeon will point the tip of the rongeur toward the surgical technologist. Using a moistened sponge, the surgical technologist will grasp the tissue from the jaws.

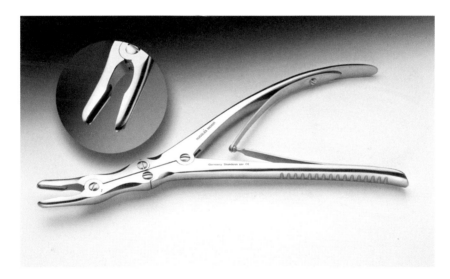

Instrument: LEKSELL RONGEUR
Category: Cutting and Dissecting
Description: It is a double-action, slightly angled rongeur with narrow, trough-like jaws.
Use(s): It is used for removing pieces of bone and the soft tissue surrounding the bone. The Leksell rongeur is often used in spinal surgery to remove the spinous process.
Instrument Insight: The double action gives the rongeur more torque at the tip for better biting action. Always have a moistened sponge ready when handing the surgeon a rongeur. As the surgeon works to remove tissue and/or bone, the rongeur has to be cleaned between uses. While focusing on the wound, the surgeon will point the tip of the rongeur toward the surgical technologist. Using a moistened sponge, the surgical technologist will grasp the tissue from the jaws.

⚠ **CAUTION:** When setting up, always check the screw to ensure it is tightened down and cannot fall out into the wound when in use.

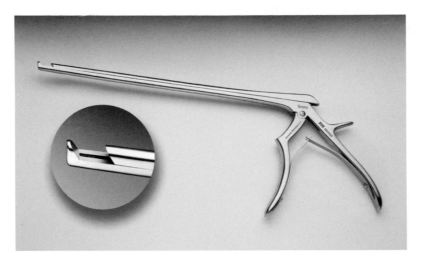

Instrument: KERRISON RONGEUR
Other Names: Upbiter
Category: Cutting and Dissecting
Description: These are compression handles that are attached to a long shaft with an angled guillotine-style action tip. The tips have a 40- or 90-degree angle and are either upbiting or downbiting, with the dimension of the bite ranging from 1 to 6 mm.
Use(s): It is used for removing pieces of bone and lamina during spinal procedures.
Instrument Insight: Always have a moistened sponge ready when handing the surgeon a rongeur. As the surgeon works to remove tissue and/or bone, the rongeur has to be cleaned between uses. While focusing on the wound, the surgeon will point the tip of the rongeur toward the surgical technologist. Using a moistened sponge, the surgical technologist will grasp the tissue from the jaws.

⚠ **CAUTION:** When setting up, always check the screw to ensure it is tightened down and cannot fall out into the wound when in use.

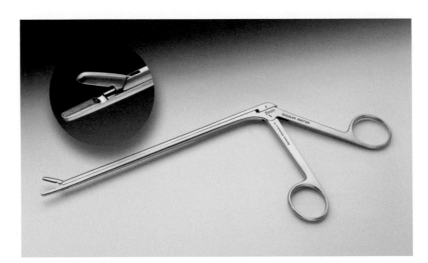

Instrument: CUSHING PITUITARY RONGEUR
Other Names: Pituitary forceps, bean rongeur
Category: Cutting and Dissecting
Description: It is a finger-ringed instrument with a long shaft that extends to narrow, elongated, oval cup jaws. The jaws may be straight, up-angled, or down-angled.
Use(s): It is used for removing herniated disc fragments when performing a discectomy.
Instrument Insight: Always have a moistened sponge ready when handing the surgeon a rongeur. As the surgeon works to remove tissue, the rongeur has to be cleaned between uses. While focusing on the wound, the surgeon will point the tip of the rongeur toward the surgical technologist. Using a moistened sponge, the surgical technologist will grasp the tissue from the jaws.

⚠ **CAUTION:** When setting up, always check the screw to ensure it is tightened down and cannot fall out into the wound when in use.

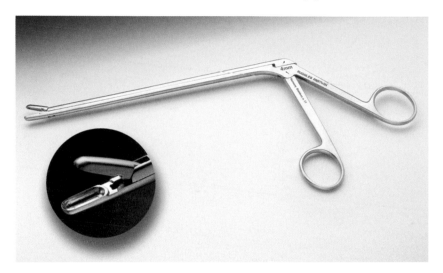

Instrument: SPURLING RONGEUR (STRAIGHT)

Category: Cutting and Dissecting

Description: It is a finger-ringed instrument with a long shaft that extends to oval cup jaws. The jaws may be straight, up-angled, or down-angled.

Use(s): Used for removing herniated disc fragments when performing a discectomy.

Instrument Insight: Always have a moistened sponge ready when handing the surgeon a rongeur. As the surgeon works to remove tissue, the rongeur has to be cleaned between uses. While focusing on the wound, the surgeon will point the tip of the rongeur toward the surgical technologist. Using a moistened sponge, the surgical technologist will grasp the tissue from the jaws.

⚠ **CAUTION:** When setting up, always check the screw to ensure it is tightened down and cannot fall out into the wound when in use.

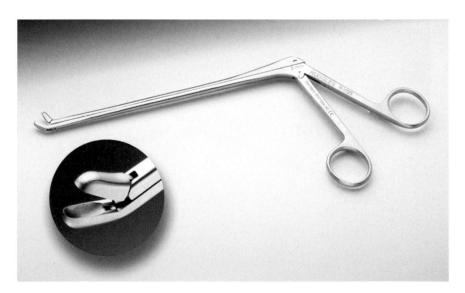

Instrument: PEAPOD RONGEUR

Category: Cutting and Dissecting

Description: It is a finger-ringed instrument with a long shaft that extends to upward-bent, oval cup jaws.

Use(s): It is used for removing herniated disc fragments when performing a discectomy.

Instrument Insight: Always have a moistened sponge ready when handing the surgeon a rongeur. As the surgeon works to remove tissue and/or bone, the rongeur has to be cleaned between uses. While focusing on the wound, the surgeon will point the tip of the rongeur toward the surgical technologist. Using a moistened sponge, the surgical technologist will grasp the tissue from the jaws.

⚠ **CAUTION:** When setting up, always check the screw to ensure it is tightened down and cannot fall out into the wound when in use.

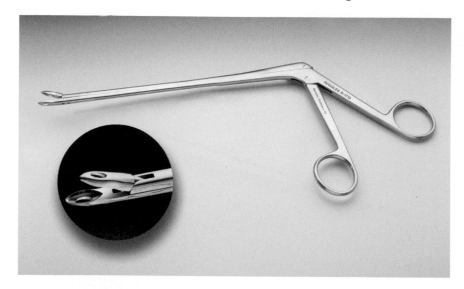

Instrument: WILDE RONGEUR
Other Names: Fenestrated
Category: Cutting and Dissecting
Description: It is a finger-ringed instrument with a long shaft that extends to eye-shaped, fenestrated, cupped jaws. The jaws can be straight or up-angled.
Use(s): It is used for removing herniated disc fragments when performing a discectomy.
Instrument Insight: Always have a moistened sponge ready when handing the surgeon a rongeur. As the surgeon works to remove tissue and/or bone, the rongeur has to be cleaned between uses. While focusing on the wound, the surgeon will point the tip of the rongeur toward the surgical technologist. Using a moistened sponge, the surgical technologist will grasp the tissue from the jaws.

⚠ **CAUTION:** When setting up, always check the screw to ensure it is tightened down and cannot fall out into the wound when in use.

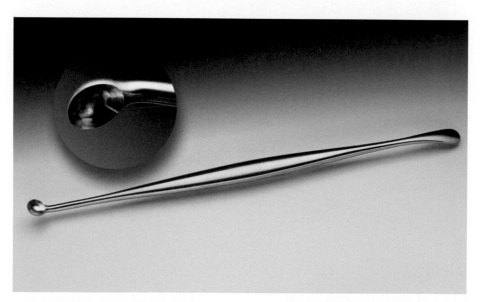

Instrument: NO. 1 PENFIELD DISSECTOR
Category: Cutting and Dissecting
Description: It is a double-ended instrument with a broad, curved dissector at one end and a sharp, round spoon at the other end.
Use(s): It is used for retracting, manipulating, and dissecting nerves, vessels, bone, and tissues during craniotomies, carotid endarterectomies, and spinal procedures.

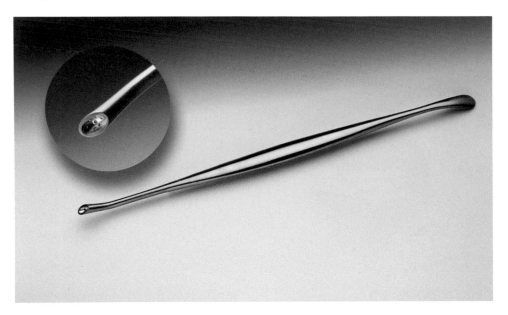

Instrument: NO. 2 PENFIELD DISSECTOR
Category: Cutting and Dissecting
Description: It is a double-ended instrument with a slightly curved dissector at one end and a wax packer at the other end.

Use(s): It is used for retracting, manipulating, and dissecting nerves, vessels, bone, and tissues during craniotomies, carotid endarterectomies, and spinal procedures.

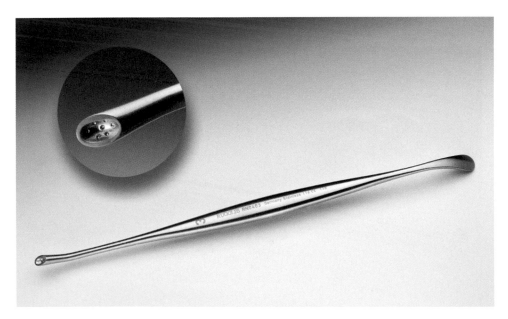

Instrument: NO. 3 PENFIELD DISSECTOR
Category: Cutting and Dissecting
Description: It is a double-ended instrument with a full curved dissector at one end and a wax packer at the other end.

Use(s): It is used for retracting, manipulating, and dissecting nerves, vessels, bone, and tissues during craniotomies, carotid endarterectomies, and spinal procedures.

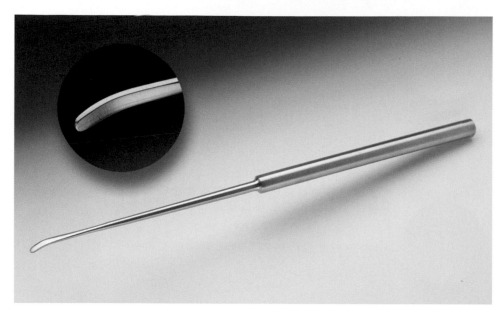

Instrument: NO. 4 PENFIELD DISSECTOR
Category: Cutting and Dissecting
Description: It has a solid round handle with a slightly curved dissector at the working end.
Use(s): It is used for retracting, manipulating, and dissecting nerves, vessels, bone, and tissues during craniotomies, carotid endarterectomies, and spinal procedures. The Penfield no. 4 dissector is commonly used to remove arterial plaque from the walls of the carotid artery.
Instrument Insight: Small balls of bone wax are pressed onto the tip and then are smeared on the cranial edges for hemostasis.

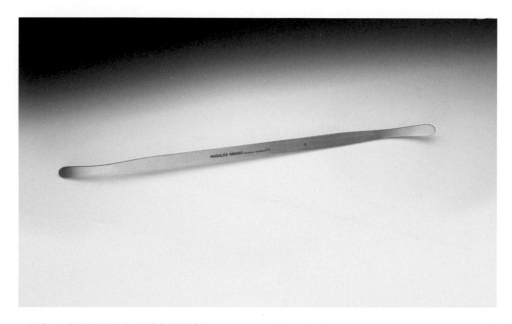

Instrument: NO. 5 PENFIELD DISSECTOR
Category: Cutting and Dissecting
Description: It is a double-ended flattened dissector with a full curved dissector at one end and a slightly curved blunt dissector at the other end.
Use(s): It is used for retracting, manipulating, and dissecting nerves, vessels, bone, and tissues during craniotomies, carotid endarterectomies, and spinal procedures.

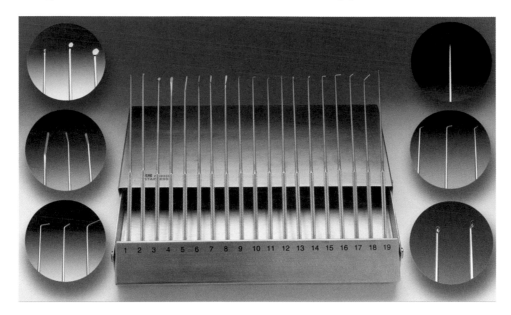

Instrument: RHOTON DISSECTOR EXTENDED SET
Category: Cutting and Dissecting
Description: These are extremely precise and delicate micro dissecting instruments. The Rhoton set contains round and spatula micro dissectors, micro hooks, micro curettes, micro needlepoint, and micro elevators.

Use(s): It is used for manipulation and dissection of very fine nerves, tissues, and tumors of the brain when performing a craniotomy.
Instrument Insight: These instruments should be wiped clean after every use with a moistened sponge. They are very delicate and should be handled with extreme care.

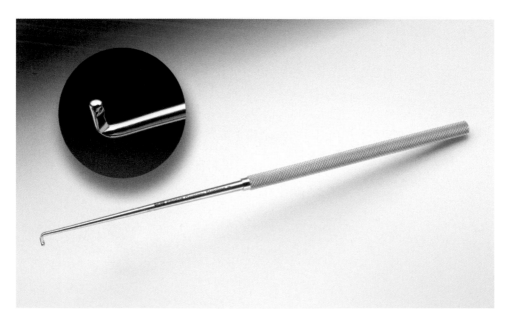

Instrument: MICRO KNIFE
Category: Cutting and Dissecting
Description: It is a round grip handle with a right hook at the distal end that has a sharp edge on the inner side.

Use(s): It is used for dissection of very fine nerves, tissues, and tumors of the brain when performing a craniotomy.

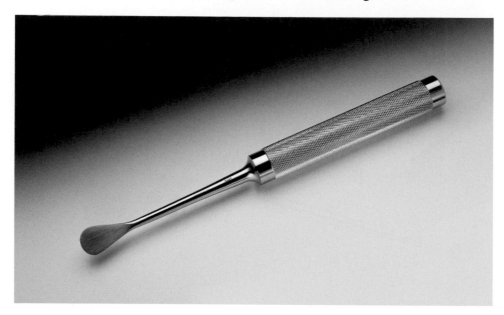

Instrument: COBB ELEVATOR
Category: Cutting and Dissecting
Description: It is an elongated, solid, rounded grip handle that extends to a narrowed, smooth shaft that terminates with a flat, broad, tear-shaped, sharp working end.
Use(s): It is used for stripping the paraspinous muscles and the periosteum off the laminae.

This is done when performing a laminectomy during spinal surgeries.
Instrument Insight: As the area is stripped, Raytex sponges that have been opened are packed along the side of the spine to compress bleeding.

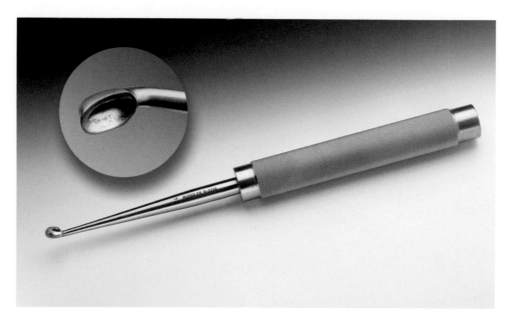

Instrument: COBB CURETTE
Category: Cutting and Dissecting
Description: It is an elongated, solid, round grip handle that extends to a narrowed, smooth shaft that terminates with a sharp-edged, oval-scooped working end. The tips may be straight, angled, or reverse-angled.
Use(s): It is used for scraping bone during spinal surgery.

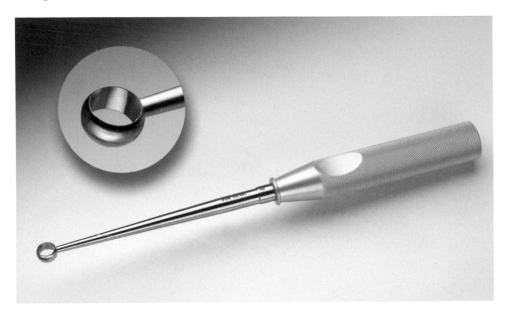

Instrument: COBB RING CURETTE
Category: Cutting and Dissecting
Description: It is an elongated, solid, round grip handle that extends to a narrowed smooth shaft that terminates with a sharp ring-shaped working end.
Use(s): It is used to strip muscle and the periosteum off bone.

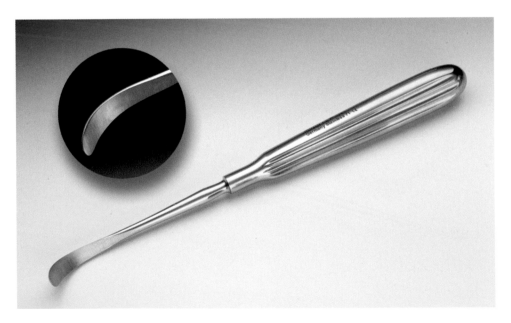

Instrument: ADSON PERIOSTEAL ELEVATOR
Other Names: Joker
Category: Cutting and Dissecting
Description: It is a narrowing handle that leads to a flattened, curved, rounded tip.
Use(s): It is used for elevating the skull off the dura when turning a flap or for scraping the periosteum off bone.

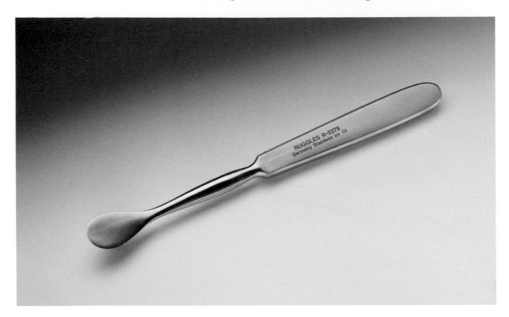

Instrument: HOEN PERIOSTEAL ELEVATOR
Category: Cutting and Dissecting
Description: It is a smooth, elongated handle that extends to a narrowed, smooth shaft that terminates with a flattened, broad, rounded, sharp working end.

Use(s): It is used for reflecting the scalp flap off the skull and/or scraping the periosteum off the skull when creating a bone flap during a craniotomy procedure.

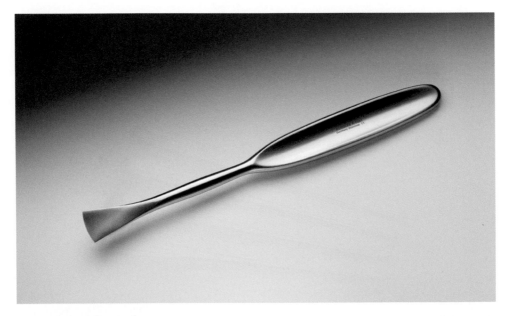

Instrument: LANGENBECK PERIOSTEAL ELEVATOR
Category: Cutting and Dissecting
Description: It is a smooth, elongated, concave handle that extends to a narrowed, smooth shaft that terminates with a flattened, fan-shaped, sharp working end.

Use(s): It is used for reflecting the scalp flap off the skull and/or scraping the periosteum off the skull when creating a bone flap during a craniotomy procedure.

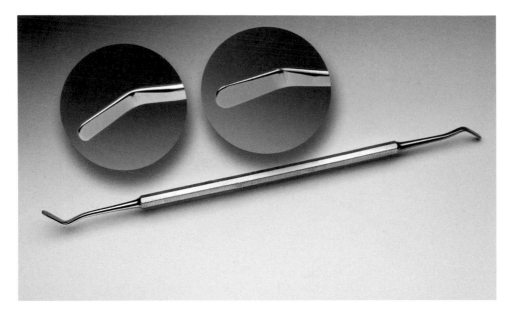

Instrument: WOODSON ELEVATOR
Category: Cutting and Dissecting
Description: It is a double-ended instrument with slightly angled, rounded spatula ends, with one end being wider than the other.
Use(s): It is used for separating the dura from the cranium when creating a burr hole or turning a bone flap.

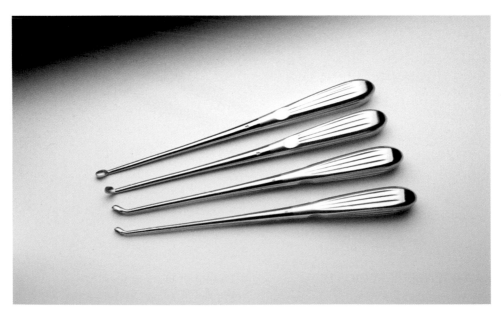

Instrument: SPINAL CURETTE
Category: Cutting and Dissecting
Other Names: Brun curette
Description: This is a small spoon-like instrument with sharp edges. The tips can be straight, angled, or reverse-angled. They come in a variety of sizes.
Use(s): It is used to scrape out bone and tissue.

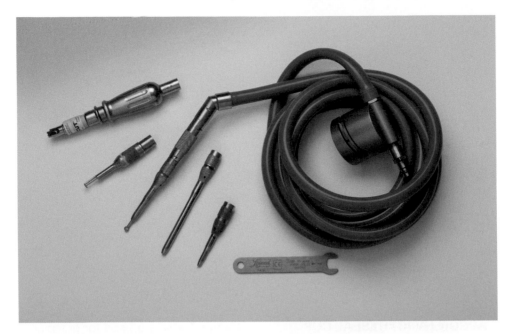

Instrument: MIDAS REX DRILL
Other Names: Craniotome, perforator
Category: Cutting and Dissecting
Description: This is a high-speed pneumatic drill that is activated by a foot pedal. The handpiece has multiple attachments with disposable burrs and blades.

Use(s): It is used for perforating the skull when creating burr holes or for turning a bone flap during a craniotomy.
Instrument Insight: As the burr holes and/or flap are prepared, the bit of the drill should be irrigated with saline to reduce the heat and bone dust that is generated from the friction.

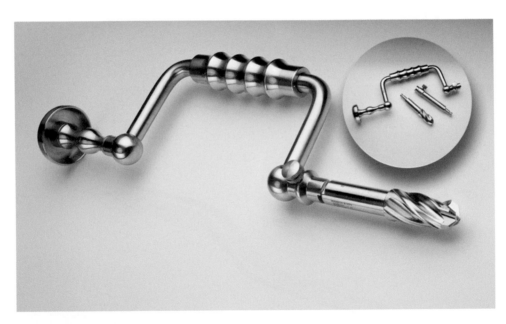

Instrument: HUDSON HANDHELD DRILL
Other Names: Hudson brace
Category: Cutting and Dissecting
Description: It is a handheld drill with a stabilizing handle on the proximal end that is in succession with a handle that rotates in a circle. The distal end has a thumb screw chuck, which locks the bits in place. The bits come in a variety of shapes and sizes.

Use(s): It is used for perforating the skull when creating burr holes.
Instrument Insight: The perforator bit has a sharp cutting point that is designed to penetrate the skull. The burr bits are rounded and are used to enlarge the hole made by the perforator.

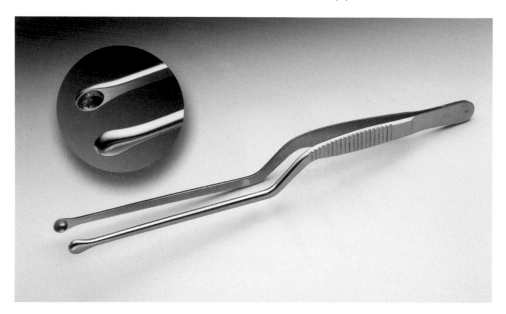

Instrument: ADSON HYPOPHYSEAL CUP TISSUE FORCEPS
Other Names: Baskin Robin cup forceps, cup forceps, scoop forceps
Category: Cutting and Dissecting
Description: These are bayonet-shaped grasping forceps with smooth cup tips.

Use(s): These are used for grasping and removing tumors.
Instrument Insight: Bayonet-shaped instruments are designed so that the user may see beyond his or her fingers. Tissue is removed from the cups with a moistened sponge.

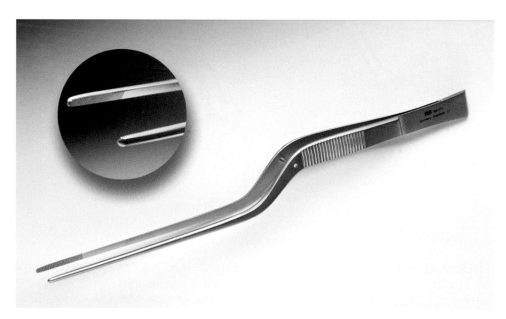

Instrument: CUSHING BAYONET TISSUE FORCEPS
Category: Grasping and Holding
Description: These are bayonet-shaped grasping forceps with serrated blunt tips.

Use(s): These are used for grasping delicate tissues.
Instrument Insight: Bayonet-shaped instruments are designed so that the user may see beyond his or her fingers.

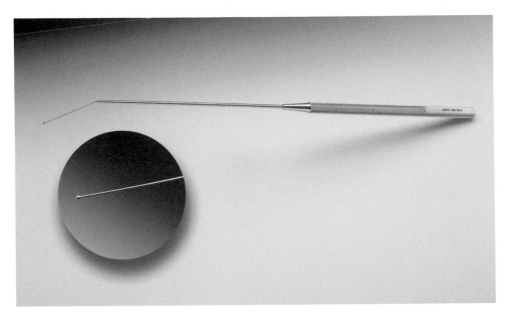

Instrument: BALL TIP PROBE
Category: Probing and Dilating
Description: It has a round handle with a straight probe that leads to an angled wire with a solid ball tip.

Use(s): It is used for manipulating and probing blood vessels, nerves, and brain tissues.

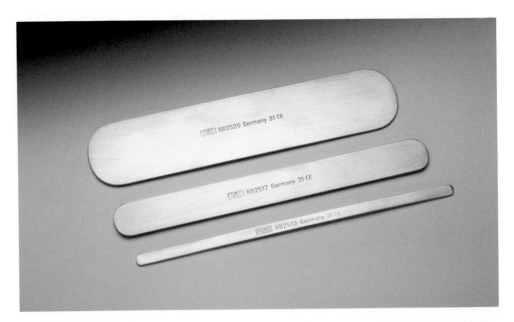

Instrument: DAVIS BRAIN SPATULAS
Other Names: Baby ribbons
Category: Retracting and Exposing
Description: These are small, handheld, malleable, smooth, flat metal ribbons with rounded ends. The widths vary from $1/4$ inch to $1\frac{1}{2}$ inches.

Use(s): It is used to retract the brain and tissues during a craniotomy.
Instrument Insight: An assortment of sizes should be included in the set. Brain spatulas should always be moistened before being placed on the brain.

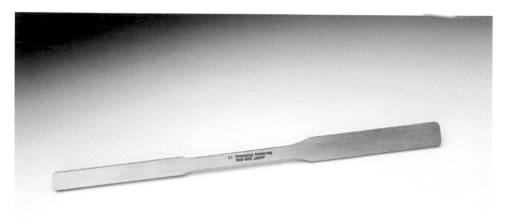

Instrument: SCOVILLE BRAIN SPATULA
Category: Retracting and Exposing
Description: These are small, handheld, double-ended, malleable, flat retractors with squared, blunt ends. One end is larger than the other end.

Use(s): It is used to retract the brain and tissues during a craniotomy.
Instrument Insight: Brain spatulas should always be moistened before being placed on the brain.

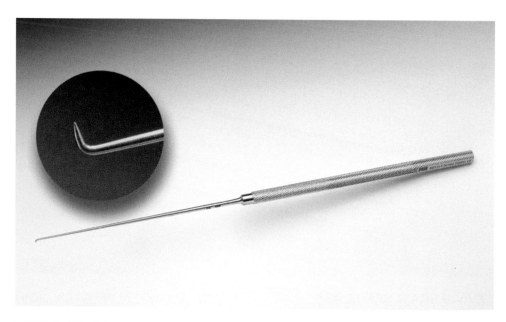

Instrument: DURA HOOK
Category: Retracting and Exposing
Description: It is a sharp right-angle hook with a round handle.
Use(s): It is used for elevating the dura.

Instrument Insight: Exercise care when handling this sharp hook because it can easily compromise the integrity of your gloves or those of the surgeon.

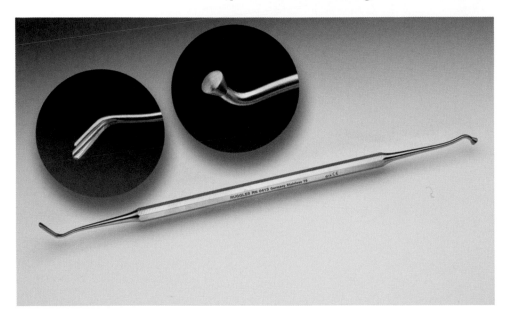

Instrument: WOODSON DURA SEPARATOR
Category: Retracting and Exposing
Description: It is a double-ended instrument with a slightly angled, rounded spatula on one end and a blunt probe on the other end.

Use(s): It is used to separates the dura from the cranium when creating a burr hole or turning a bone flap.

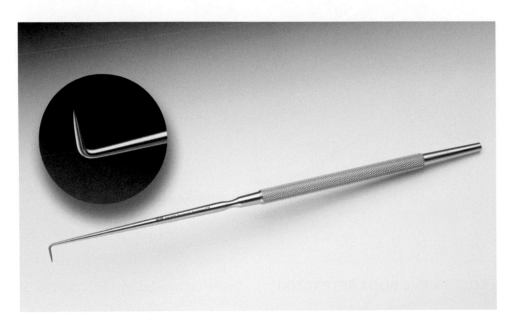

Instrument: ADSON HOOK, SHARP
Category: Retracting and Exposing
Description: It is a sharp, right-angle, elongated hook with a round handle.
Use(s): It is used for elevating the dura.

Instrument Insight: Exercise care when handling this sharp hook because it can easily compromise the integrity of your gloves or those of the surgeon.

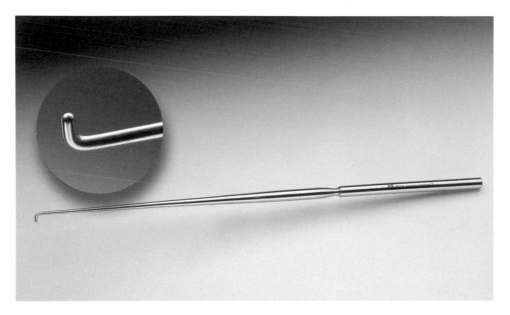

Instrument: DANDY NERVE HOOK
Category: Retracting and Exposing
Description: It is a blunt right-angle hook with a round handle.

Use(s): It is used for manipulation, probing, and dissection of very fine nerves, tissues, and vessels.

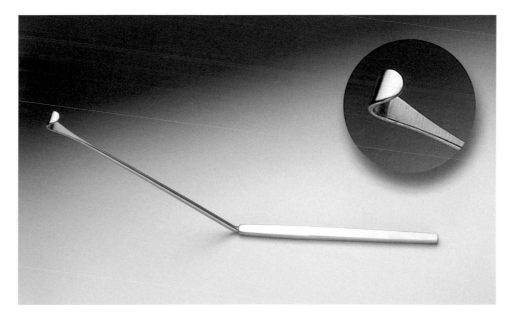

Instrument: LOVE NERVE ROOT RETRACTOR (ANGLED)
Category: Retracting and Exposing
Description: It is a flattened handle that extends to a long round shaft with a smooth, cup-shaped, curved blade with a crescent-shaped lip. The shaft of the retractor can be straight or angled.

Use(s): It is used for retracting the dura and the nerve root.
Instrument Insight: To prevent damage to the nerve root, the retractor should not be moved after it has been placed by the surgeon. Because of the delicate nature of the tissue, care should be taken to not pull on the retractor but simply hold it in place.

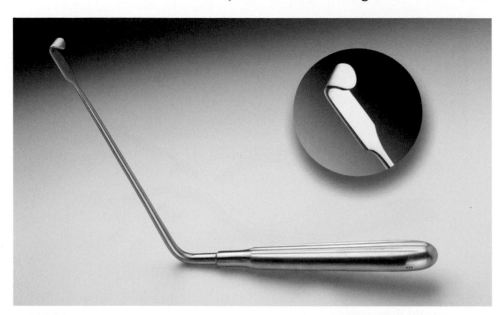

Instrument: SCOVILLE NERVE ROOT RETRACTOR (ANGLED)
Category: Retracting and Exposing
Description: It is a round tapered handle that extends to a long round shaft with a smooth, flattened, elongated blade with a crescent-shaped lip. The shaft of the retractor can be straight or angled.

Use(s): It is used for retracting the dura and the nerve root.
Instrument Insight: To prevent damage to the nerve root, the retractor should not be moved after it has been placed by the surgeon. Because of the delicate nature of the tissues, care should be taken to not pull on the retractor but simply hold it in place.

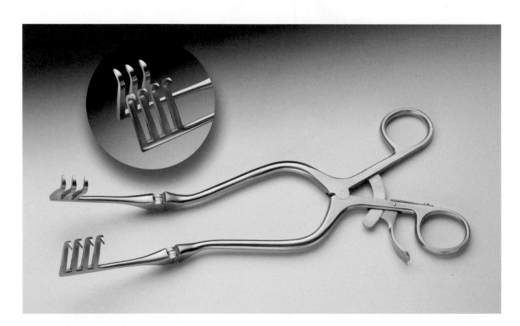

Instrument: BECKMAN RETRACTOR
Category: Retracting and Exposing
Description: It is a self-retaining, finger-ringed instrument with a ratcheted release device on the shanks. Two hinged arms extend from the shank to three outward-curved prongs on one side and four on the other. These prongs can be sharp or dull.

Use(s): It is used for retracting the wound edges during spinal surgery.
Instrument Insight: Always hand this retractor to the surgeon with the prongs pointing down.

⚠ **CAUTION:** The prongs may be very sharp. Exercise care when handling sharp instruments to avoid puncture to gloves and/or skin.

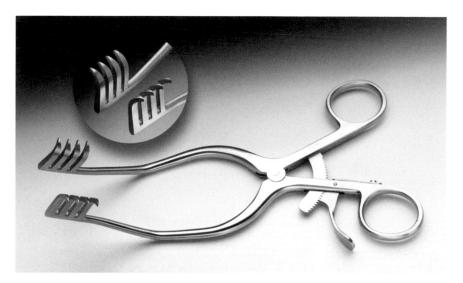

Instrument: CEREBELLAR RETRACTOR
Category: Retracting and Exposing
Description: It is a self-retaining, finger-ringed instrument with a ratcheted release device on the shanks. Two arms extend from the shank to four outward-curved prongs on each arm. These prongs can be sharp or dull.

Use(s): It is used for retracting the scalp flap.
Instrument Insight: Always hand this retractor to the surgeon with the prongs pointing down.

⚠ **CAUTION:** The prongs may be very sharp. Exercise care when handling sharp instruments to avoid puncture to gloves and/or skin.

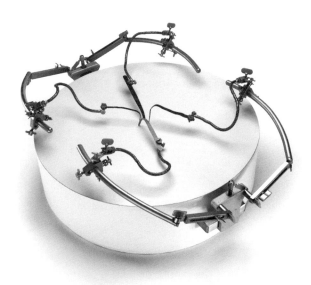

Instrument: LEYLA RETRACTOR
Other Names: Fukushima retractor, Leyla-Yasargil retractor
Category: Retracting and Exposing
Description: It is a self-retaining, table-mounted retractor. This retractor has table clamps, U bars, C clamps, and snake arms. The flexible snake arms consist of a series of small metal tubes joined by a ball and socket. They are held together by a tension cable running through the middle of them, which is tightened by turning the knob on the distal end. When the cable is tightened, the

numerous metal components become rigid, thus maintaining the position in which they were placed. The brain spatulas are attached to the distal end of these flexible arms. At the proximal end the arms are fixed to a C clamp, which allows the arms to be slid onto the U bar.
Use(s): It is used to sustain gentle retraction of brain and neural tissues.

⚠ **CAUTION:** Care should be taken not to inadvertently bump the retractor after it is placed.

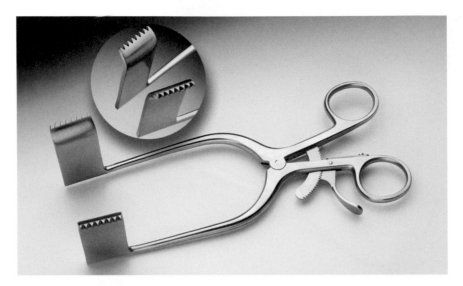

Instrument: **MEYERDING LAMINECTOMY RETRACTOR**
Category: Retracting and Exposing
Description: It is a self-retaining, finger-ringed instrument with a ratcheted release device on the shanks. Two arms extend from the shank to two outward-curved blades with multiple V-shaped teeth on each.
Use(s): It is used for deep retraction during spinal surgery.
Instrument Insight: Always hand this retractor to the surgeon with the teeth pointing down.

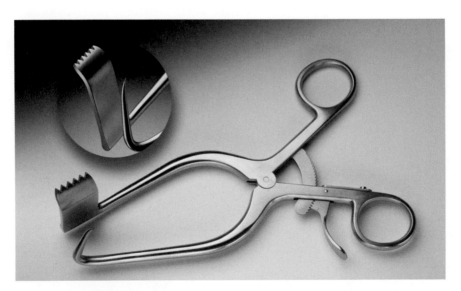

Instrument: **WILLIAMS HEMILAMINECTOMY RETRACTOR**
Other Names: Meyerding hemilaminectomy retractor
Category: Retracting and Exposing
Description: It is a self-retaining, finger-ringed instrument with a ratcheted release device on the shanks. Two arms extend from the shank to an outward-curved blade with multiple V-shaped teeth on one side; the other arm has a sharp, angled prong. The blade will be on the right or left side.
Use(s): It is used for deep retraction during spinal surgery. It is used when the lamina is being removed on one side of the spine only.
Instrument Insight: The surgeon will ask for a right or left Williams retractor. Right or left is determined by which side contains the blade.

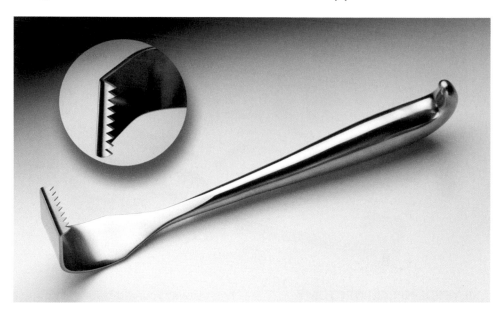

Instrument: MEYERDING HANDHELD RETRACTOR
Category: Retracting and Exposing
Description: It has a smooth-grip handle with a lateral-curved blade with multiple V-shaped teeth on the lip.

Use(s): It retracts wound edges.

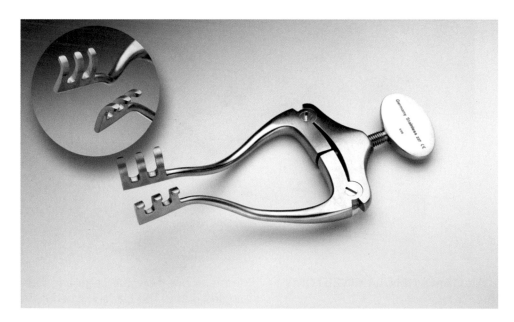

Instrument: DAVIS SCALP RETRACTOR
Category: Retracting and Exposing
Description: It is a small self-retaining retractor with a screw-locking mechanism that has two elongated downward-curving arms with three outward (dull) curved prongs at each tip.

Use(s): It is used for retracting the scalp when creating burr holes.

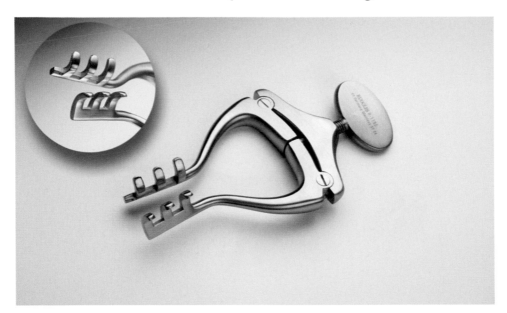

Instrument: JANSEN SCALP RETRACTOR
Category: Retracting and Exposing
Description: It is a small self-retaining retractor with a screw-locking mechanism that has two arms with three outward-curved (dull) prongs at each tip.
Use(s): It is used for retracting the scalp when creating burr holes.

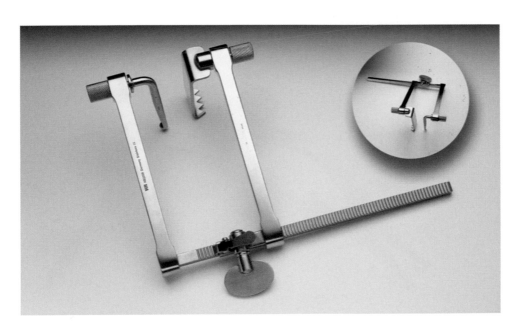

Instrument: SCOVILLE RETRACTOR
Other Names: Scofield-Meyerding self-retaining retractor
Category: Retracting and Exposing
Description: This is a key-ratcheted self-retaining frame with an interchangeable blade mechanism at the end of each arm. The interchangeable blades come in various sizes and styles.
Use(s): It is used for retracting wound edges during lumbar procedures.

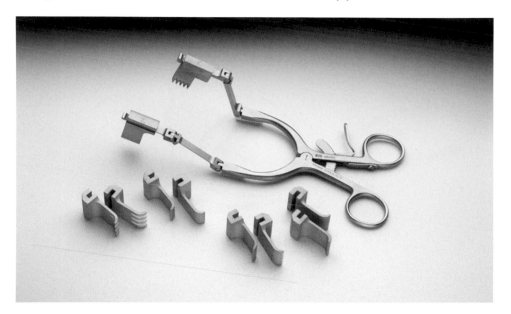

Instrument: ANTERIOR CERVICAL FUSION RETRACTOR
Other names: ACF retractor
Category: Retracting and Exposing
Description: It is a self-retaining retractor with two different style frames and a variety of interchangeable blades.

Use(s): It retracts wound edges during an anterior cervical discectomy and fusion.

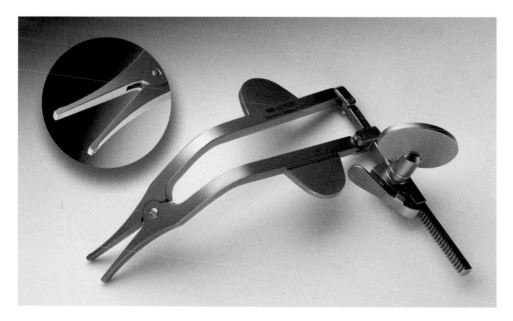

Instrument: CLOWARD VERTEBRA SPREADER
Category: Retracting and Exposing
Description: This is a key-ratcheted device that has downward angle shanks with smooth, slightly outward-bending jaws. The inner jaws are smooth, and they square off at the tips. On the outer edge is a small, criss-crossed grip patch.
Use(s): It is used for opening the vertebral space.

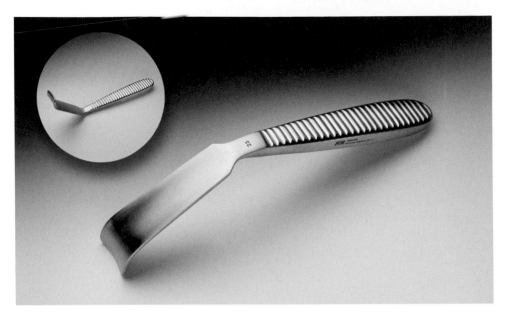

Instrument: CLOWARD CERVICAL RETRACTOR
Category: Retracting and Exposing
Description: It is a solid grip handle with a smooth, elongated 45-degree angle blade that has a crescent-shaped lip.

Use(s): It is used for retracting the wound during a cervical discectomy and fusion.

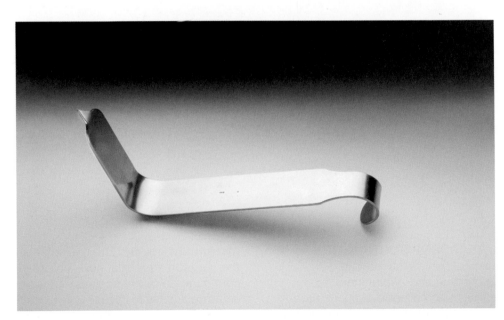

Instrument: TAYLOR SPINAL RETRACTOR
Category: Retracting and Exposing
Description: This is a flat, stainless-steel strip with a lateral-curved blade and a sharp V-shaped tip on the end. The width and length vary according to need.
Use(s): It is used for wound retraction during lumbar spinal procedures.

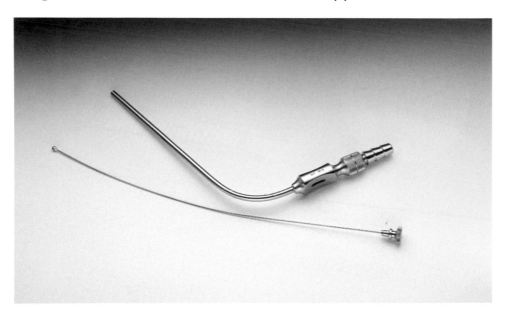

Instrument: POPPEN SUCTION TIP
Category: Suctioning and Aspirating
Description: It is an angled, malleable, cylindric tube with a relief opening/hole on the handgrip. The diameter of the suction tube is measured on the French (F) scale and ranges from 6F to 12F.
Use(s): It is used for suctioning in confined spaces such as the nasal cavity and during lumbar and cervical procedures or craniotomies.

Instrument Insight: It is usually packaged with a metal stylet, which fits inside the cylinder. The stylet is used to maintain patency of the suction tube by relieving tissue, debris, blood, and other materials that may be caught inside the tube during suctioning. The suction is increased by covering the relief opening/hole.

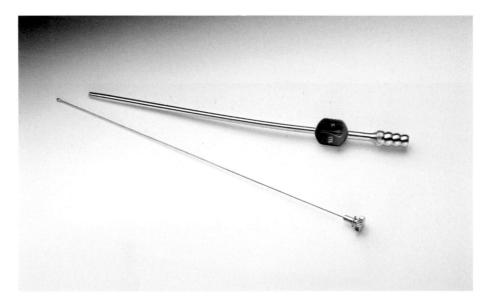

Instrument: TEARDROP SUCTION TIP
Other Names: Fukushima suction tip
Category: Suctioning and Aspirating
Description: This is a malleable cylindric tube with a teardrop-shaped control relief opening/hole on the handgrip. The diameter of the suction tube is measured on the French scale and ranges from 3F to 12F.
Use(s): It is used for suctioning of tissue, especially in hard-to-reach areas.

Instrument Insight: The malleable shaft gives the surgeon additional flexibility to adjust the configuration of the suction tube as necessary, allowing access in cases where difficult patient anatomy or tumor location may prevent the use of standard suction tubes. The suction is increased by covering the relief opening/hole.

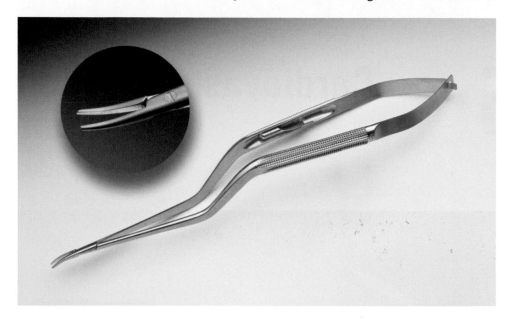

Instrument: RHOTON MICRO NEEDLE HOLDERS
Category: Suturing and Stapling
Description: It is a bayonet-style spring-locking needle holder with curved or straight fine jaws.

Use(s): It is used for holding very fine suture needles during microsurgical procedures.
Instrument Insight: Bayonet-shaped instruments are designed so that the user may see beyond his or her fingers.

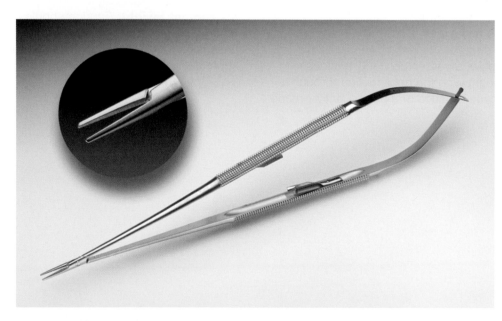

Instrument: JACOBSEN NEEDLE HOLDER
Category: Suturing and Stapling
Description: It is a spring-locking needle holder with curved or straight fine jaws.

Use(s): It is used for holding very fine suture needles during microsurgical procedures.

Cardiovascular Thoracic Instruments

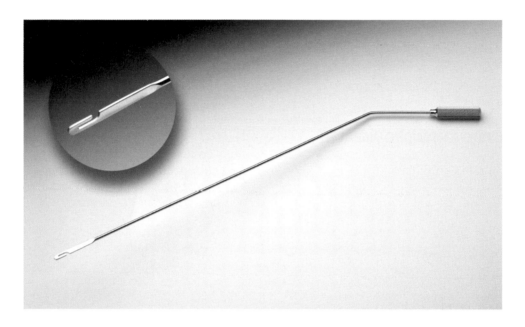

Instrument: RUMEL TOURNIQUET HOOK (STYLET)

Category: Accessory

Description: This instrument has a hook or eyelet at the distal end.

Use(s): The surgeon encircles a vessel with umbilical tape or a vessel loop, and the loose ends are caught with the hook, pulled through a red rubber catheter shod or a plastic factory-made tubing tourniquet, and held taut with a hemostat to control flow in the vessel. Purse strings are also "snagged" this way when placing a cannula.

Instrument Insight: Caution should be used when pulling the strings through the tourniquet because some tissues, such as an atrial appendage, are very fragile.

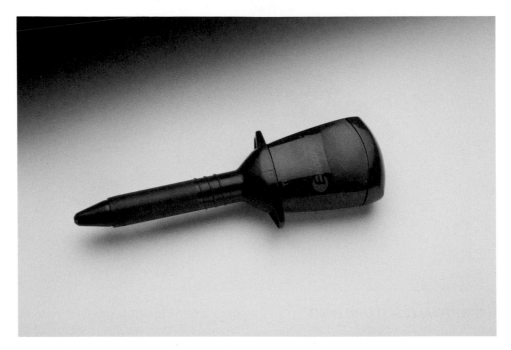

Instrument: ENDOPATH THORACIC TROCAR
Other Names: Thoracoport, Flexipath
Category: Accessory
Description: This trocar has a round-tipped obturator and a thoracic sleeve with stability threads.
Use(s): The thoracic trocar sleeve is used for an access port to internal organs in thoracoscopic procedures and other minimally invasive procedures that do not require insufflation.
Instrument Insight: There are many different manufacturers of these types of trocars, so there may be a variety of different styles.

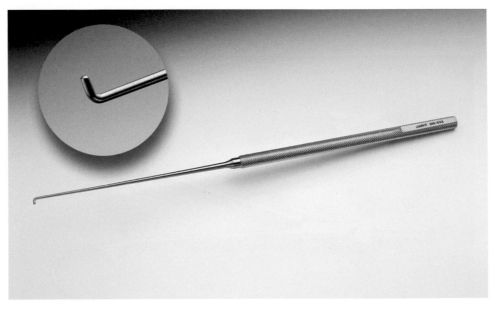

Instrument: BLUNT HOOK
Other Names: Nerve hook
Category: Accessory
Description: This instrument has a right-angled hook.
Use(s): It is used for "snagging" tangled or knotted fine sutures. Also used for manipulating the leaflets in valve surgeries.
Instrument Insight: This instrument can also be used to retract strings during placement of sutures during anastomosis.

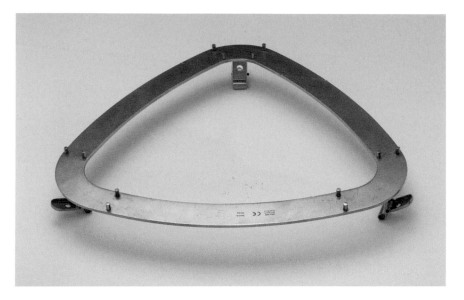

Instrument: GRUNWALD SUTURE RING
Other Names: Suture guide holder, Suture ring
Category: Accessory
Description: The holder is a stainless steel rigid frame with a center opening for access to the incision area. The frame rests directly on the arms of the chest retractor and is secured to the drapes by the clips on the underside of the frame. The studs on the top side of the ring receive the suture guides, securing the guides in position. It is used with Gabbay-Frater type suture guides.
Use(s): It is used for keeping numerous sutures properly arranged during cardiac valve replacement procedures.

Instrument Insight: The Grunwald holder provides a level, secure surface for the suture guides and aids in faster suture placement by eliminating the use of multiple towel clips that can tend to get in the way when suturing.

⚠ **CAUTION:** Care should be taken when attaching the guide to the drapes to ensure that the patient's skin is not pinched in the clips.

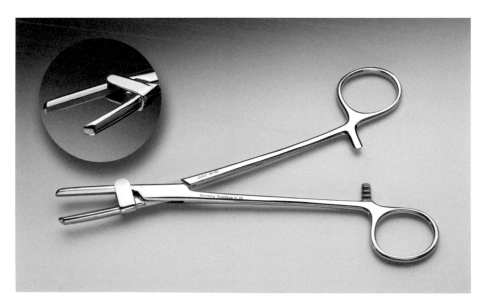

Instrument: VORSE TUBING OCCLUDING CLAMP
Other Names: Tube clamp
Category: Clamping and Occluding
Description: It is a heavy instrument with ratchet handles and nonslip jaws.

Use(s): This clamp is used to clamp off tubing and cannulas.
Instrument Insight: Perfusionists use these on the heart-lung machine during bypass surgery; tube clamps are also used on the sterile field.

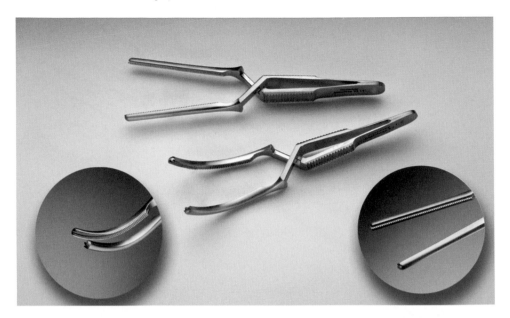

Instrument: DEBAKEY BULLDOG CLAMP
Other Names: Bulldog clamp
Category: Clamping and Occluding
Description: This is a cross-action clamp. The jaws vary in length and can be straight or curved.

Use(s): It is used for clamping off the flow in a vessel. The jaws are serrated with the DeBakey design.
Instrument Insight: This is often used to mark the end of a vein graft to specify flow direction.

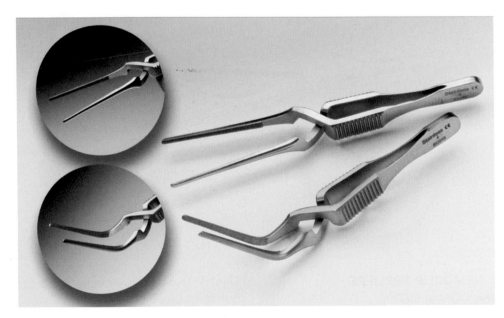

Instrument: DIETHRICH BULLDOG CLAMP
Category: Clamping and Occluding
Description: This is a fine cross-action clamp. It can be straight or angled
Use(s): This small clamp is used to impede the flow in a vessel.

Instrument Insight: This is used more often than the heavier bulldog clamp because there is less trauma to the vessel.

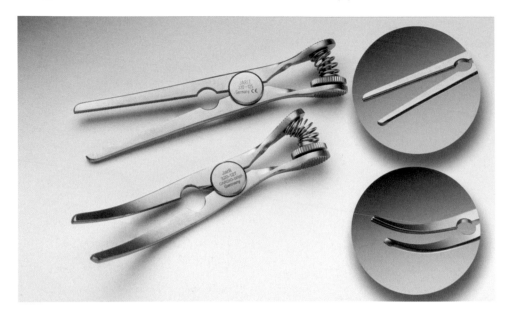

Instrument: GLOVER BULLDOG CLAMP
Category: Clamping and Occluding
Description: This clamp is available in a variety of lengths. Serrations in the jaws are of the Cooley design.

Use(s): This is used to stop flow in a vessel and to clamp vessel loops encircling a vessel.
Instrument Insight: This is seldom used because the Cooley jaws are more crushing.

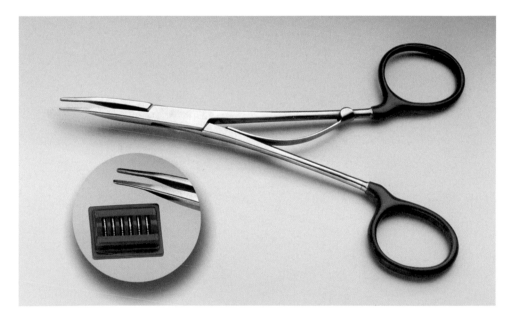

Instrument: HEMOCLIP APPLIERS
Other Names: Ligaclip applier
Category: Clamping and Occluding
Description: These appliers are available in small, medium, medium/large, and large sizes. They can also have an angled end. The clip bars that hold the actual clips come in red, blue, green, and orange, and the applier handles have the same color.

Use(s): This instrument is used to clip side branches on vessels instead of tying with suture material.
Instrument Insight: "Load" by pushing instrument jaws onto the clip and lifting. The surgeon "fires" the clip by squeezing the handles.

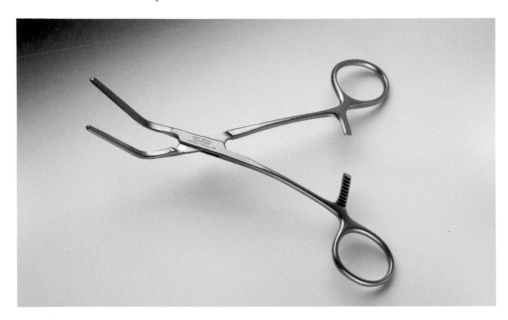

Instrument: COOLEY CLAMP
Other Names: Angled clamp
Category: Clamping and Occluding
Description: This instrument has ratcheted handles and jaws. The angle is 45 or 55 degrees. Serrations are of the Cooley design.

Use(s): It is used for total occlusion of a vessel.
Instrument Insight: The ratchets allow the surgeon to adjust the clamp according to the blood pressure inside the vessel. They also allow gradual increase or decrease of blood flow.

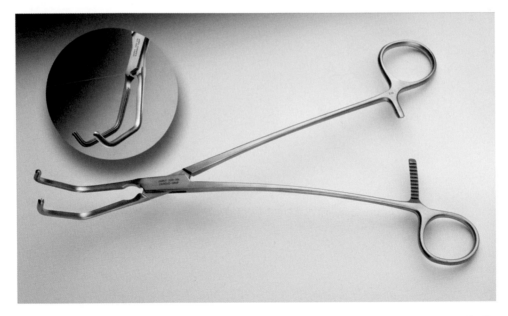

Instrument: SATINSKY VENA CAVA CLAMP
Other Names: Satinsky partial occlusion clamp
Category: Clamping and Occluding
Description: This is a partial occlusion clamp. The clamp comes in a variety of lengths, with noncrushing jaws of the DeBakey design and ratchet handles.

Use(s): It is used for partially occluding vessels.
Instrument Insight: This clamp is sometimes used to encircle the superior or inferior vena cava before placement of umbilical tape around the vessel. It is also sometimes used to clamp the atrial appendage.

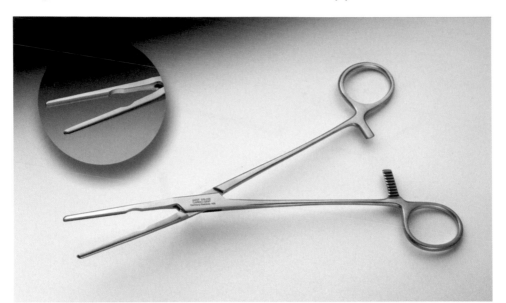

Instrument: GLOVER PATENT DUCTUS CLAMP
Category: Clamping and Occluding
Description: This clamp is straight or angled slightly. It has ratcheted handles and DeBakey design serrated jaws.

Use(s): This clamp can have a variety of uses and is a total occlusion clamp.
Instrument Insight: Ratchets allow the surgeon to adjust the clamp according to the blood pressure inside the vessel. They also allow gradual increase or decrease of blood flow.

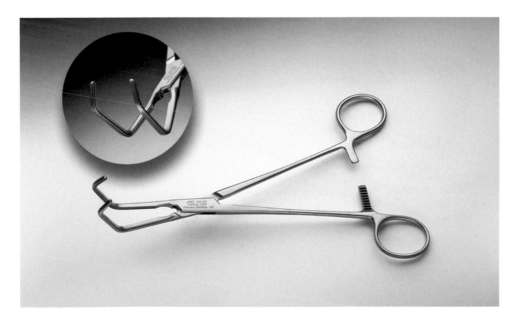

Instrument: BECK AORTIC CLAMP
Other Names: Pedicle clamp
Category: Clamping and Occluding
Description: This clamp comes in varying sizes, as do the jaws. It has the DeBakey design jaw serrations.

Use(s): This is a partial occlusion clamp used in deep areas; it can also be used as a total occlusion clamp on larger vessels.

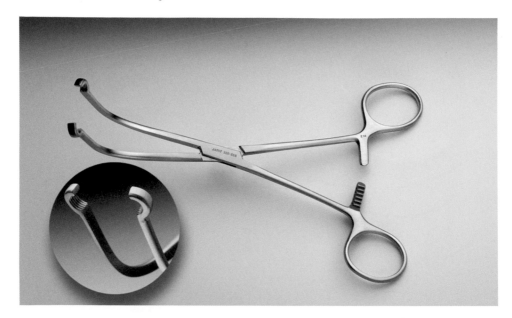

Instrument: JAVID CAROTID ARTERY CLAMP
Other Names: Javid carotid shunt clamp
Category: Clamping and Occluding
Description: It is a ratcheted angled clamp in which the tip of each jaw is a half-circle that clamps around the artery and the shunt to hold it in place.

Use(s): It is used during a carotid endarterectomy procedure to secure the Javid shunt in the carotid artery when diverting the blood flow away from the operative site.
Instrument Insight: This can be used with other shunts as well as for holding introducers in place during endovascular procedures.

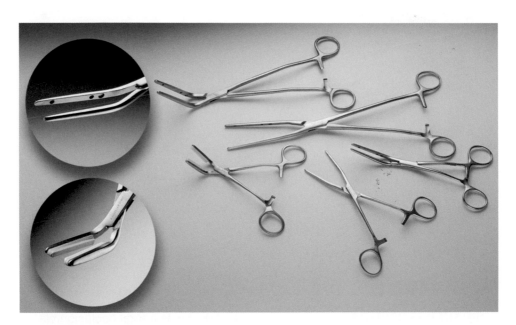

Instrument: FOGARTY CLAMP WITH JAW INSERTS
Other Names: Hydragrip clamp, softjaw clamp
Category: Clamping and Occluding
Description: These clamps can be angled or straight. The inserts come in a pair, with one as a hydrajaw and one as a traction jaw.
Use(s): This is a vascular clamp with soft jaws for vessels as well as graft material.
Instrument Insight: These clamps are used in vascular, pulmonary, cardiac, and gastrointestinal procedures.

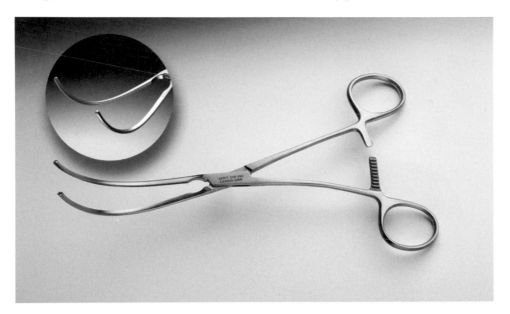

Instrument: DEBAKEY AORTIC CLAMP
Category: Clamping and Occluding
Description: This clamp has curved shanks with DeBakey design serrations in the jaws.

Use(s): This is a multiple-use clamp. It can be used for partial occlusion or total occlusion. It is also used to tunnel under the tissues to pull a graft through to its distal anastomosis.

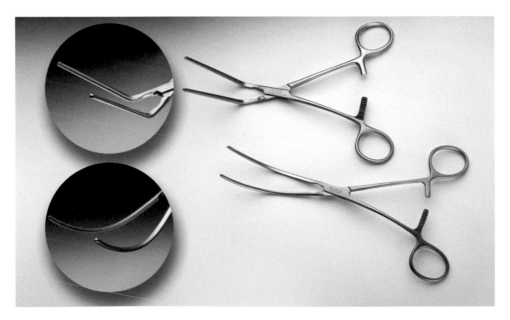

Instrument: DEBAKEY PERIPHERAL VASCULAR CLAMP
Other Names: Angled or sometimes referred to by degree, such as a 35- or 45-degree clamp.
Category: Clamping and Occluding
Description: It is a ratcheted clamp with straight, curved, or various angled jaws that have DeBakey style serrations.

Use(s): This is a total occlusion clamp.
Instrument Insight: Ratchet handles allow the surgeon to adjust the clamp according to the blood pressure inside the vessel. They also allow gradual increase or decrease of blood flow.

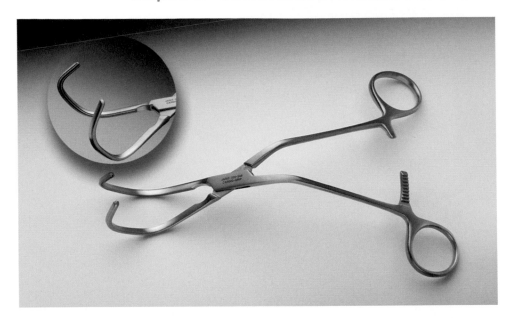

Instrument: LAMBERT-KAY AORTA CLAMP
Other Names: Side biter
Category: Clamping and Occluding
Description: This clamp has DeBakey design serrations in the jaws.

Use(s): This is a partial occlusion clamp.
Instrument Insight: This is often used to partially occlude the aorta for proximal-end anastomosis of saphenous vein grafts in coronary artery bypasses.

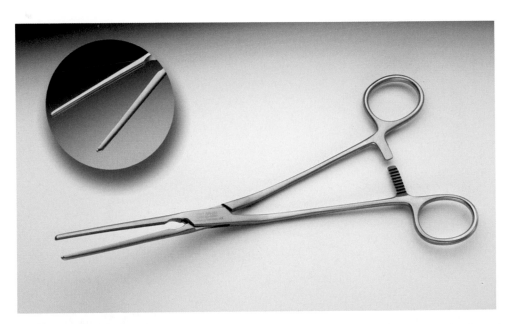

Instrument: DEBAKEY COARCTATION CLAMP
Other Names: Patent ductus clamp
Category: Clamping and Occluding
Description: This clamp is slightly angled. The jaw has DeBakey design serrations.
Use(s): This clamp is used on the iliac and femoral arteries during abdominal aortic aneurysm (AAA) repair.
Instrument Insight: This clamp is often used to occlude more than one vessel at a time, such as the femoral and profunda femoris arteries.

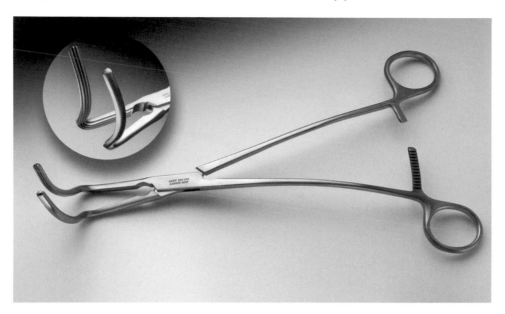

Instrument: DEBAKEY SIDEWINDER AORTA CLAMP
Other Names: Subramanian clamp
Category: Clamping and Occluding
Description: The clamp is angled and the jaws are curved.

Use(s): This is an aortic occlusion clamp.
Instrument Insight: This clamp is often used on the aorta during AAA repair when there is limited room for a cross-clamp.

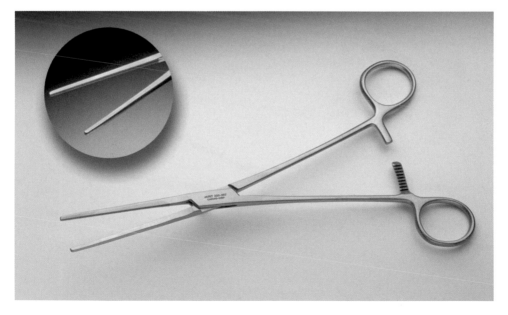

Instrument: COOLEY COARCTATION CLAMP
Other Names: Straight clamp
Category: Clamping and Occluding
Description: It is a total occlusion clamp that has straight cardio-grip jaws.

Use(s): This is often used when clamping deep anatomic vessels.

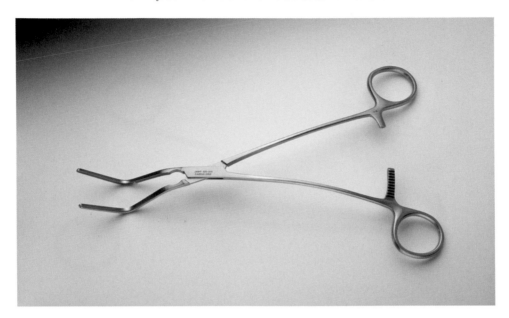

Instrument: LEE BRONCHUS CLAMP
Category: Clamping and Occluding
Description: This clamp has 90-degree angle tips.
Use(s): This clamp is used for total occlusion of the bronchus during lung procedures.

Instrument Insight: This instrument is often used for occlusion of structures during lung procedures.

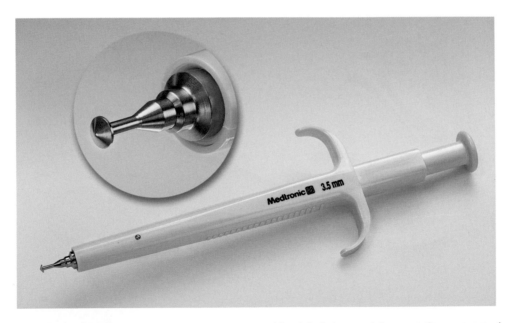

Instrument: AORTIC PUNCH
Other Names: Punch
Category: Cutting and Dissecting
Description: Aortic punch composed of a plastic outer body and stainless steel punch and cutting head to produce precise circular or oval openings. It ranges in diameter from 2.7 to 6.0 mm.

Use(s): It is used for creating an opening in the wall of the aorta or other selected vessels to prepare a site for vein graft anastomosis in a coronary artery bypass procedure.
Instrument Insight: The aortic punch is single-patient use and is disposable.

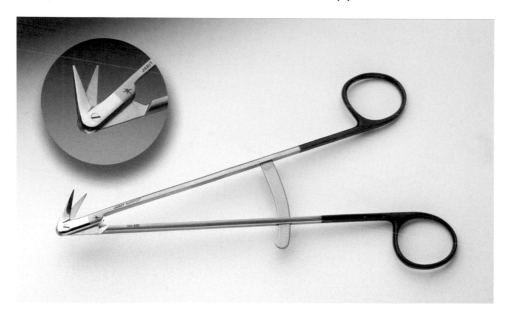

Instrument: DIETHRICH SCISSORS
Other Names: Ducks scissors
Category: Cutting and Dissecting
Description: These scissors vary in degrees of angles; they have a stabilizing bar on the handles, and the blades have a sharp point.

Use(s): These scissors are used to extend an opening in an artery or vein.
Instrument Insight: These are considered a delicate instrument and should never be used for anything except opening a vessel. Wipe clean after each use with a damp sponge.

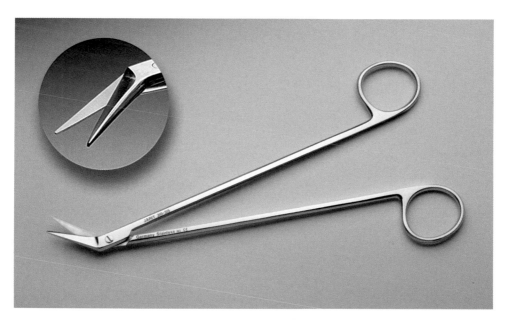

Instrument: POTTS-SMITH SCISSORS
Other Names: Potts scissors
Category: Cutting and Dissecting
Description: These scissors come in a variety of degrees of angles. They are heavier than Diethrich scissors yet are still considered a delicate instrument.

Use(s): These scissors are used to extend an opening in an artery or vein.
Instrument Insight: These scissors are to be used on vessels only. They are heavier and can cut through calcified plaque.

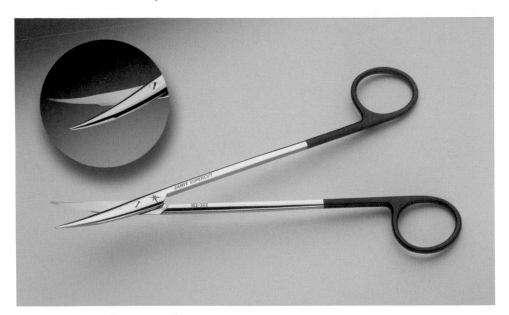

Instrument: JAMISON SCISSORS
Other Names: Tenotomy scissors
Category: Cutting and Dissecting
Description: These are fine scissors with sharp points and curved blades. They are available in a variety of lengths.
Use(s): These scissors are used to dissect plaque out of an artery and to cut arterial branches when taking the mammary down. They are fine dissection scissors.
Instrument Insight: These delicate scissors should not be used to cut sutures. The tips should be protected while sterilizing and packaging.

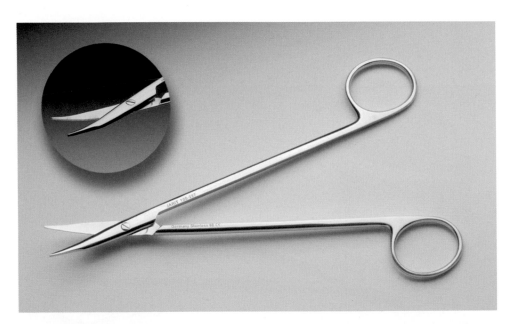

Instrument: REYNOLDS SCISSORS
Other Names: Jameson scissors
Category: Cutting and Dissecting
Description: These scissors are available in a variety of lengths.
Use(s): These are fine dissection scissors and are often used to bevel the vein when making an anastomosis.
Instrument Insight: Jameson, Reynolds, and tenotomy scissors are often indistinguishable. Reynolds scissors are delicate scissors and should be wiped clean after each use with a damp sponge. The tips should also be protected during sterilization and packaging.

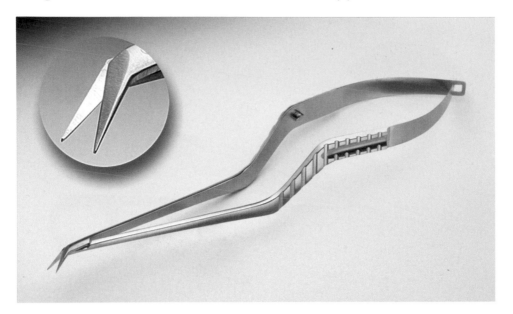

Instrument: YASARGIL SCISSORS
Other Names: Yasar scissors
Category: Cutting and Dissecting
Description: These are delicate, bayonet-type, spring-handled scissors.
Use(s): These scissors are used to extend an arteriotomy, usually in deep or hard-to-reach vessels such as a circumflex coronary artery.

Instrument Insight: These delicate scissors should be cleaned after each use with a damp sponge, and the tips should be protected during sterilization and packaging.

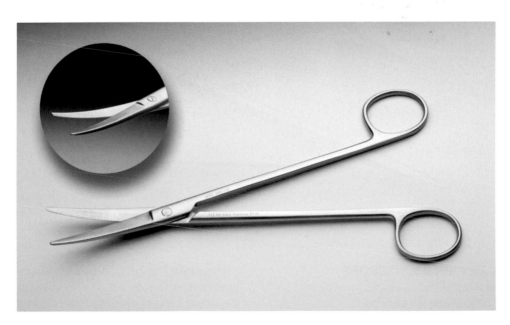

Instrument: COOLEY SCISSORS
Category: Cutting and Dissecting
Description: These scissors have curved Mayo-type blades.

Use(s): These are versatile scissors with many uses. They dissect tissue, cut sutures, and can be used to cut grafts.

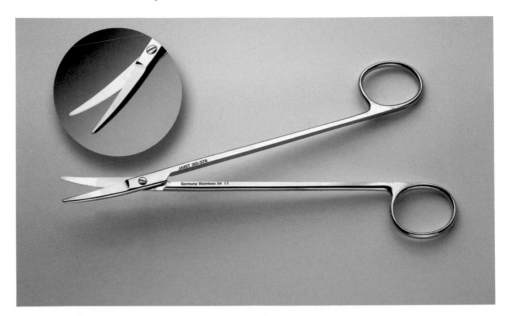

Instrument: LILLY SCISSORS
Category: Cutting and Dissecting
Description: These scissors have blunt, pointed, slightly curved blades.

Use(s): These scissors are used for dissection of soft tissues.
Instrument Insight: These scissors are similar to Metzenbaum scissors.

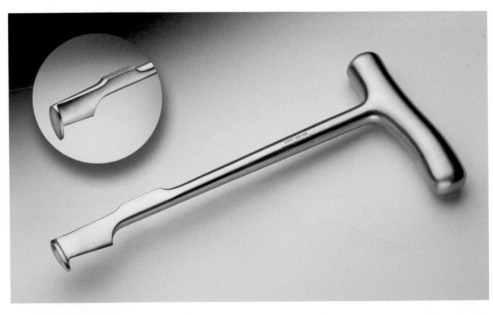

Instrument: LEBSCHE KNIFE
Other Names: Sternal knife
Category: Cutting and Dissecting
Description: This is a heavy instrument with a flat, smooth distal end to protect the pericardium. The blade sits just above the flat end.

Use(s): It is used for opening the sternum lengthwise.
Instrument Insight: This is only used when a power saw is unavailable or during a power outage. Use it with a mallet. It may also be used in a trauma situation.

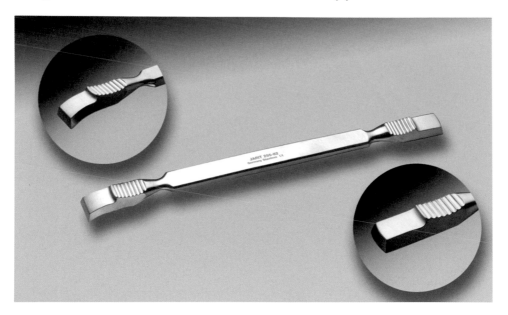

Instrument: FARABEUF RASP
Other Names: Alexander rasp
Category: Cutting and Dissecting
Description: This is a heavy double-ended instrument with a blade. One end is curved and the other is straight.

Use(s): It is used for scraping periosteum from rib bone.
Instrument Insight: Care should be taken to protect the edges of the blades against chipping or gouging.

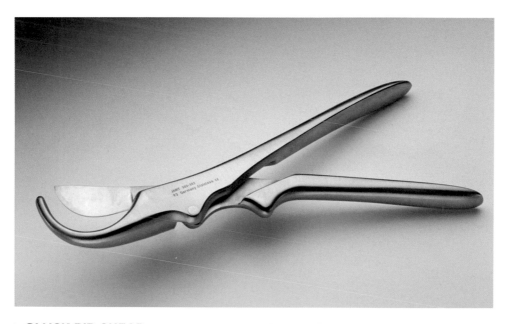

Instrument: GLUCK RIB SHEAR
Other Names: Rib cutter
Category: Cutting and Dissecting
Description: This is a heavy shear. The outside blade encircles the rib and the inside blade cuts down.

Use(s): It is used for resecting ribs.
Instrument Insight: Patient anatomy as well as which rib is being excised dictates which rib cutter is preferred.

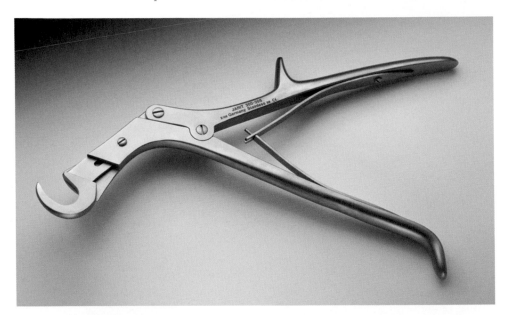

Instrument: STILLE-GIERTZ RIB SHEAR
Other Names: Shoemaker rib shear
Category: Cutting and Dissecting
Description: This shear is heavy. The distal end encircles the rib, and squeezing the handle brings the blade down, much like a guillotine, to cut the rib. The double-action handle allows for increased cutting pressure.

Use(s): It is used for resecting ribs.
Instrument Insight: Patient anatomy as well as which rib is being excised dictates which rib shear is preferred. Inspect the blade for nicks or gouges before use.

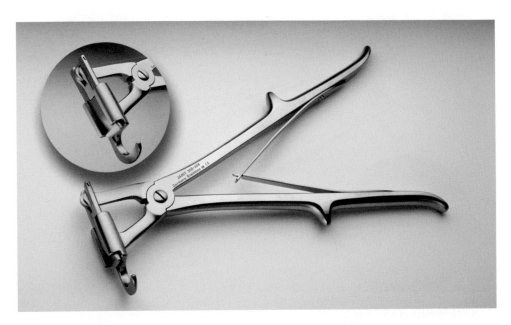

Instrument: SAUERBRUCH RIB RONGEUR
Other Names: Rib cutter
Category: Cutting and Dissecting
Description: This rib shear is heavy. The working element encircles the rib, and squeezing the handles slides a blade out to cut the rib.

Use(s): Used for resecting ribs.
Instrument Insight: Patient anatomy, rib location, and surgeon's preference dictate which rib shear is used. Inspect the blade for nicks or gouges before use.

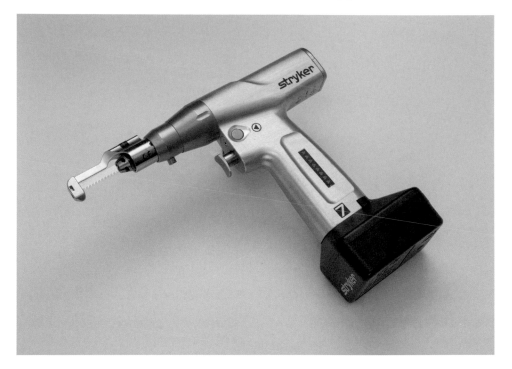

Instrument: STERNAL SAW
Other Names: Stryker sternal saw
Category: Cutting and Dissecting
Description: This is a reciprocating-action saw with a disposable blade and a snap-on battery.
Use(s): This is used to create a median sternotomy; it opens the chest by sawing through the sternum.

Instrument Insight: Depending on the surgeon's preference, the blade is loaded with the teeth up when sawing from the xiphoid to the sternal notch and the teeth down when sawing from the sternal notch to the xiphoid.

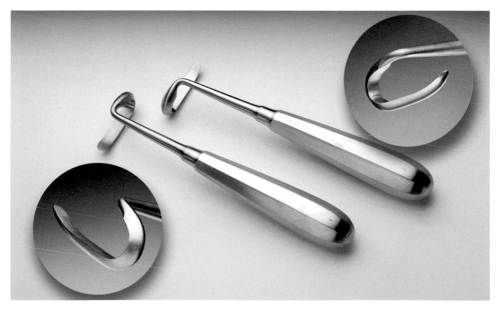

Instrument: DOYEN RIB RASPATORIES
Other Names: Doyen elevator and stripper
Category: Cutting and Dissecting
Description: It is a solid, tapering handle attached to a straight shaft that leads to an outward C-shaped curve at the distal end. The inside of the C shape is flattened and has sharp edges.

Use(s): This pair of instruments is used to scrape periosteum from rib bones before cutting.
Instrument Insight: The distal end encircles the rib and slides the length of rib to be excised, stripping the periosteum from the bone. Both right and left raspatories are available.

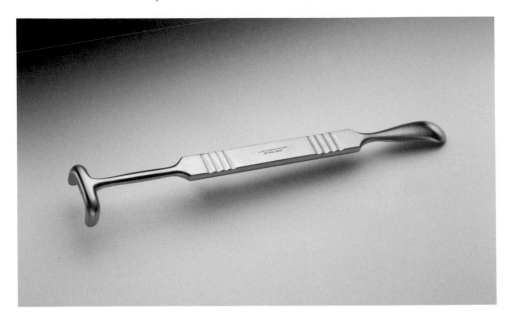

Instrument: MATSON RIB STRIPPER AND ELEVATOR
Other Names: Stripper
Category: Cutting and Dissecting
Description: This is a double-ended instrument with a flattened, tear-shaped elevator on one end and a U-shaped, sharp rib stripper on the other.

Use(s): It is used for scraping periosteum from rib bone before cutting with a shear.
Instrument Insight: Before use, inspect the ends for gouges or nicks.

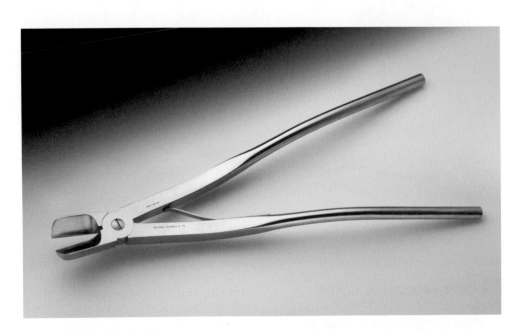

Instrument: BETHUNE RIB SHEARS
Category: Cutting and Dissecting
Description: This heavy shear has straight cutting blades.

Use(s): It is used for resecting ribs.
Instrument Insight: The long handles provide greater force when cutting bone.

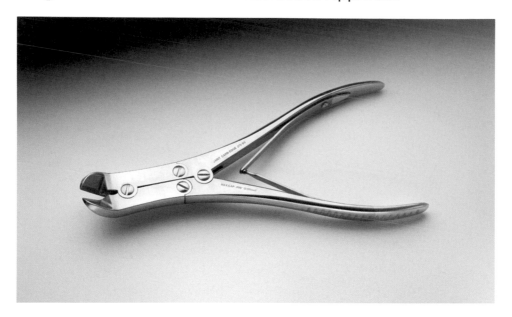

Instrument: HEAVY WIRE CUTTER
Other Names: Pin cutter
Category: Cutting and Dissecting
Description: This wire cutter has double-action, angled blade tips.

Use(s): This wire cutter is used to cut sternal wires.
Instrument Insight: Double action provides extra strength.

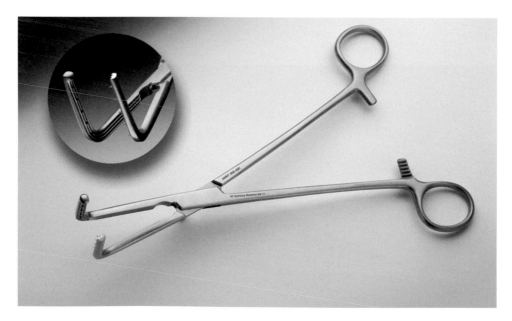

Instrument: SAROT BRONCHUS CLAMP
Category: Grasping and Holding
Description: These clamps come in a set of two: right and left, curved or angled. They have longitudinal serrations with holes on one side of the jaws and pegs on the opposite jaw to match up and hold the tissue stable.

Use(s): During lung procedures, this clamp is used to hold and occlude the bronchus while stapling.
Instrument Insight: Take care not to snag gloves on pegs.

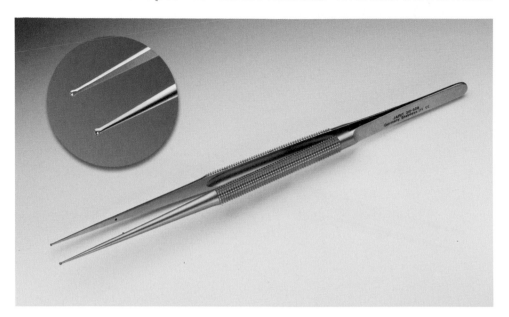

Instrument: MILLS-DENNIS MICRO RING TISSUE FORCEPS

Category: Grasping and Holding

Description: These are very fine forceps with Barraquer-style handle and tiny ring tips with serrations.

Use(s): These forceps are used to take down the mammary from the chest wall and also to hold the mammary during anastomosis in bypass surgery.

Instrument Insight: These forceps are very fine, with tiny serrations. The tips of these forceps should be protected during packaging and sterilization.

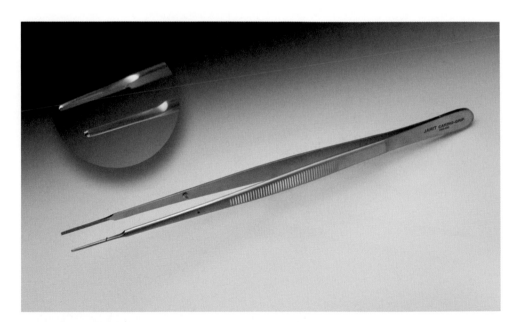

Instrument: GERALD TISSUE FORCEPS

Other Names: Mammary forceps

Category: Grasping and Holding

Description: These forceps have very fine, narrowed tips with horizontal serrations.

Use(s): It is often used during a coronary artery bypass procedure to manipulate the vessel and tissues while taking down the mammary artery from the chest wall and to grasp the coronary artery and graft during the anastomosis.

Instrument Insight: These forceps are delicate and should be protected during sterilization and packaging. They are also used for opening the lumen of a vein and holding it open for suture placement.

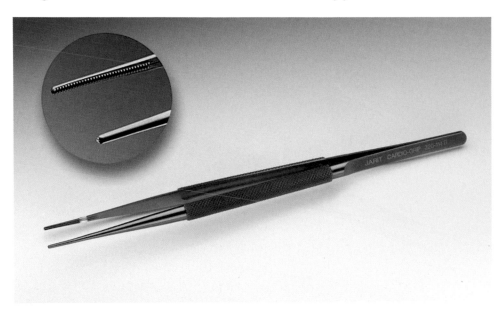

Instrument: DEBAKEY-DIETHRICH TISSUE FORCEPS
Other Names: Titanium forceps
Category: Grasping and Holding
Description: These fine forceps have Barraquer-style handles and noncrushing jaws of the DeBakey design.

Use(s): These are used for holding the vein during bypass surgery.
Instrument Insight: These forceps are delicate, and the tips should be protected during sterilization and packaging.

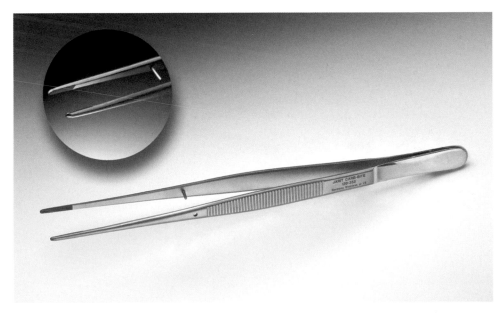

Instrument: POTTS-SMITH TISSUE FORCEPS
Other Names: Walter forceps, Goldie forceps
Category: Grasping and Holding
Description: These forceps have fine, serrated, carbide tips.
Use(s): These are used to hold and grasp tissue and vessels.

Instrument Insight: These are very sturdy forceps that are often used when the surgeon is suturing because the jaws do not bend or damage the needle.

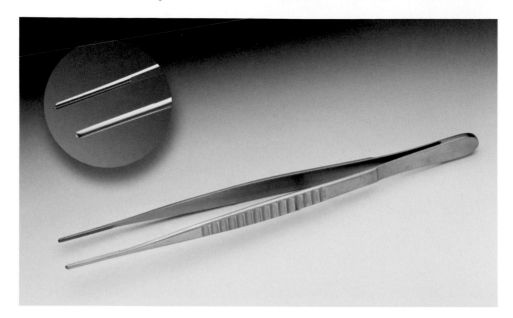

Instrument: DEBAKEY VASCULAR TISSUE FORCEPS
Other Name: Fine Debakey
Category: Grasping and Holding
Description: They come in a variety of lengths, and the jaws are of the DeBakey design.

Use(s): These forceps are used for holding and grasping tissue.
Instrument Insight: The 7- and 8-inch DeBakey forceps are the most commonly used tissue forceps and are often used in other specialties.

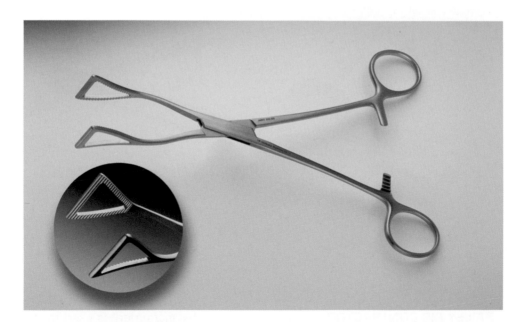

Instrument: DUVAL LUNG FORCEPS
Other Names: Lung clamp
Category: Grasping and Holding
Description: These are angled or straight forceps with triangular fenestrated tips that have horizontal serrations.

Use(s): These are used to grasp and hold lung tissue.
Instrument Insight: These clamps are used for lung tissue but can be used on other friable tissue as well.

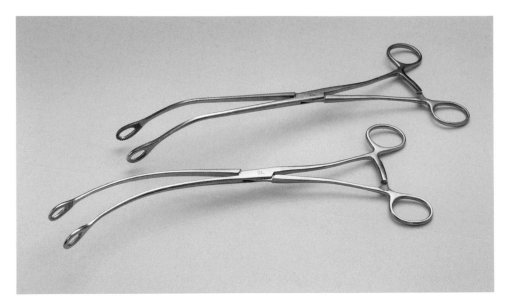

Instrument: THORACIC RING FORCEPS
Other Names: Curved ring forceps
Category: Grasping and Holding
Description: These are long forceps that have different degrees of curves. The tips are oval rings with horizontal serrations.

Use(s): These are often used to grasp the lung during thoracoscopy.

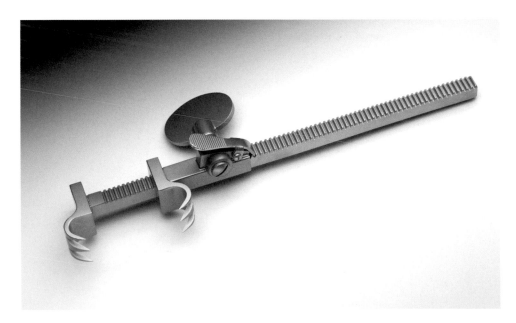

Instrument: BAILEY RIB CONTRACTOR
Other Names: Rib approximator
Category: Grasping and Holding
Description: This instrument has claws facing each other on a serrated post and a "paw" mechanism to tighten the claws, approximating the ribs.

Use(s): This instrument is used to approximate the ribs and hold them until sutures can be placed and secured after a thoracotomy.
Instrument Insight: When handling the Bailey rib contractor, care must be taken; the jaws are sharp and may snag gloves, and it should be handed to the surgeon with the jaws closed.

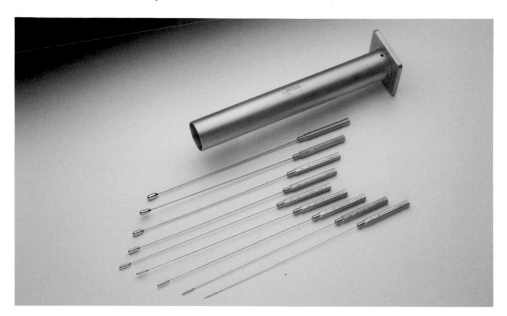

Instrument: GARRETT VASCULAR DILATORS
Category: Probing and Dilating
Description: These come in a set of nine and have tips of varying sizes. This instrument has an oval, solid, stainless steel tip that attaches to a narrowed malleable stem, which extends to a solid, smooth handle.

Use(s): These are used to dilate vessels gradually.
Instrument Insight: The set comes in its own container or box to hold them in order of size. They are malleable but after a lot of use can actually break, so let the surgeon do the bending.

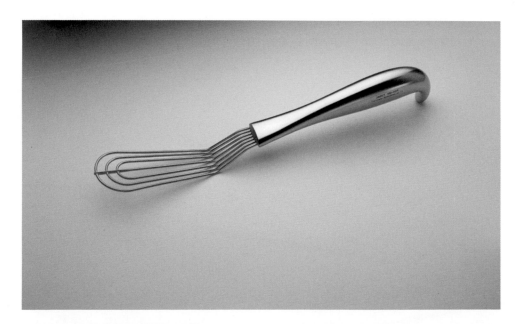

Instrument: ALLISON LUNG RETRACTOR
Other Names: Whisk
Category: Retracting and Exposing
Description: It is a solid-grip handle that leads to multiple heavy wires that form a rounded spatula shape.

Use(s): This is used to retract lung tissue.
Instrument Insight: This retractor is not pulled but simply held in place.

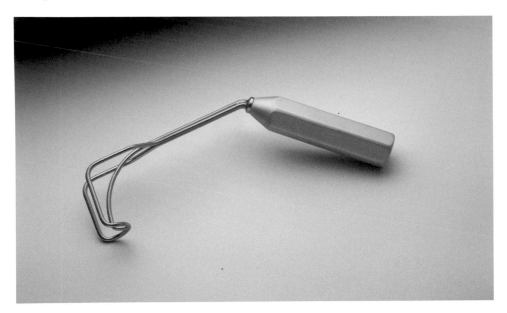

Instrument: COOLEY ARTERIAL RETRACTOR
Other Names: Mitral valve retractor
Category: Retracting and Exposing
Description: It is a solid octagonal handle that leads to a rod-like shaft that trifurcates to create a curved, open blade.

Use(s): It is used to retract the atrium during mitral valve procedures.
Instrument Insight: This retractor is seldom pulled but is placed and held in position.

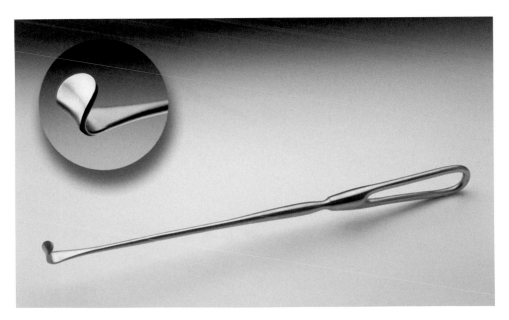

Instrument: CUSHING VEIN RETRACTOR
Category: Retracting and Exposing
Description: This retractor has a plain, smooth, upward-curved end and should be categorized as a retracting and exposing instrument.

Use(s): It is used for retracting vessels and tissues for exposure.
Instrument Insight: Vein retractors should always be in your set.

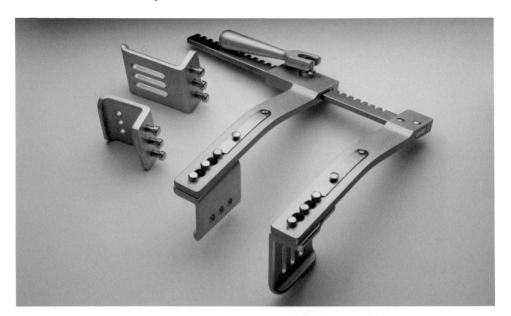

Instrument: BURFORD RIB SPREADER
Other Names: Chest spreader, Burford-Finochietto rib spreader
Category: Retracting and Exposing
Description: It is a crank-ratcheted, self-retaining frame with interchangeable blades that attach to the end of each arm.

Use(s): This instrument is used to retract ribs for lung procedures and to spread the sternum in cardiac procedures.
Instrument Insight: This chest spreader is lightweight. Both the blades and the arms are marked "R" and "L" to aid in assembly.

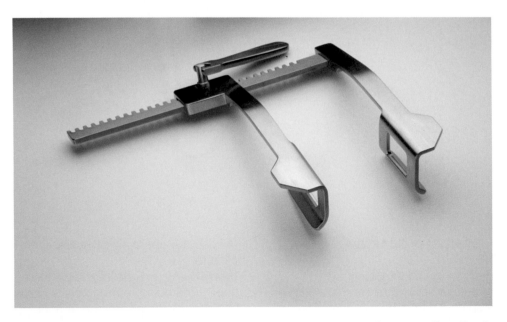

Instrument: FINOCHIETTO RIB SPREADER
Other Names: Chest or rib spreader
Category: Retracting and Exposing
Description: This self-retaining retractor has curved and straight blade arms, and the blades do not detach.

Use(s): It is used for spreading ribs for exposure of the chest cavity.

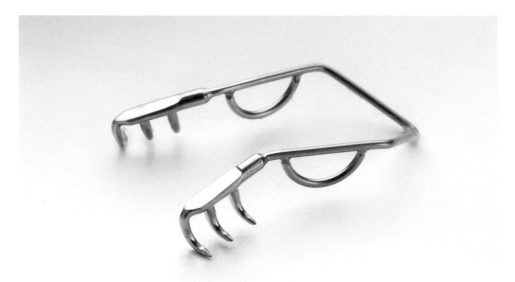

Instrument: **PARSONNET EPICARDIAL RETRACTOR**
Category: Retracting and Exposing
Description: This is a tiny, very light, self-retaining retractor that fits between the fingertips to place.
Use(s): This is used to expose coronary arteries in adipose tissue during bypass surgery.
Instrument Insight: This is a delicate instrument and should be sterilized and packaged with care and protection.

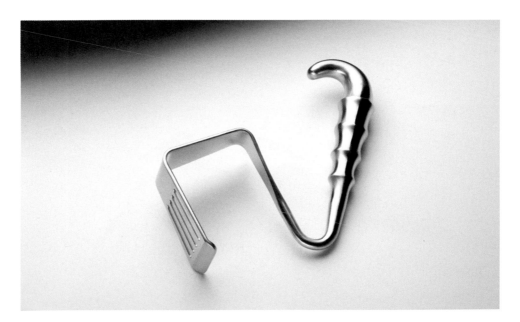

Instrument: **DAVIDSON SCAPULA RETRACTOR**
Category: Retracting and Exposing
Description: It is a heavy retractor that resembles a spatula that is bent in the shape of an S.
Use(s): It is used for retracting the scapula to expose the ribs during thoracic entry and closure.
Instrument Insight: This retractor is used for a short time during entry into the chest and sometimes during closure. It does not require pulling.

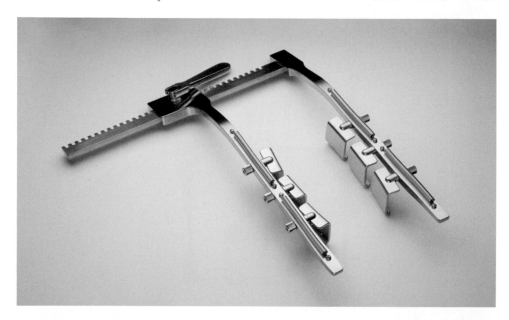

Instrument: ANKENEY RETRACTOR
Other Names: Chest spreader
Category: Retracting and Exposing
Description: This is a self-retaining retractor with six blades that each screw onto the arms of the retractor. The blades come in two depth lengths.

Use(s): It is used to spread the sternum open following a sternotomy during cardiac procedures.
Instrument Insight: Retractor should be closed completely when handing it to the surgeon.

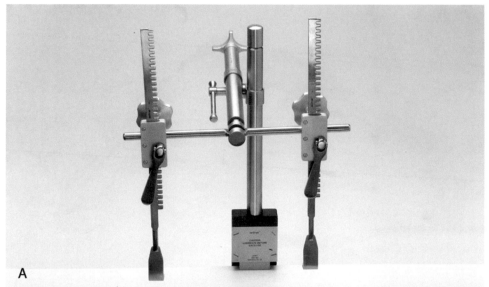

A

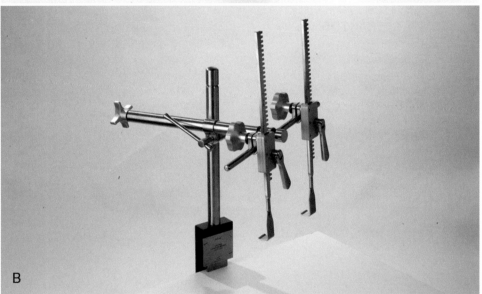

B

Instrument: INTERNAL MAMMARY RETRACTOR

Other Names: Mammary retractor, Favaloro retractor

Category: Retracting and Exposing

Description: The support bar clamps to the side rail of the operating table. Rake retractors are positioned on the sternum, and the ratchet assembly lifts the arms of rakes to the desired position or height that the surgeon needs to take down the mammary.

Use(s): It is used for lifting up one side of the chest wall after a sternotomy to facilitate internal mammary dissection.

Instrument Insight: An unsterile person clamps the support bar to the bed and unclamps it after mammary dissection.

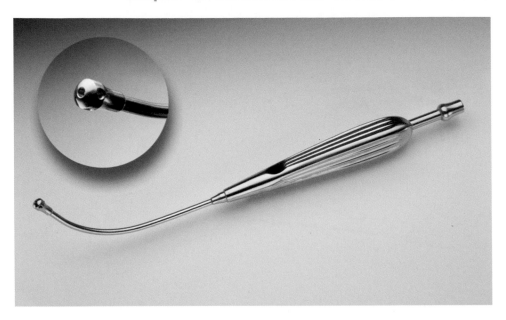

Instrument: ANDREWS-PYNCHON SUCTION TIP
Other Names: CV suction tip, baby Yankauer suction tip
Category: Suctioning and Aspirating
Description: This is a suction tip with four tiny holes on the sides of the tip and one larger hole at the end.

Use(s): It is used for suctioning fluids to aid in exposure.
Instrument Insight: This is often used as a retractor at the same time as suctioning. The tip is somewhat malleable.

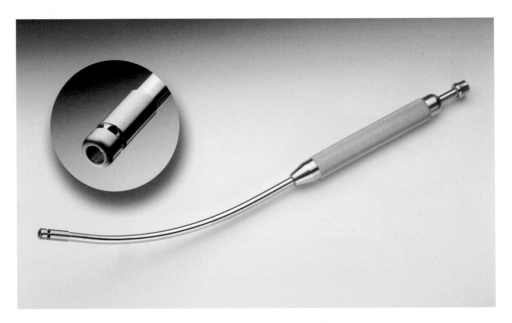

Instrument: VASCULAR SUCTION TIP
Other Names: Cardiac suction tip
Category: Suctioning and Aspirating
Description: This suction tip has a large hole at the distal end and smaller holes on the sides of the tip. This also is manufactured as a single-use disposable tip.

Use(s): This instrument is used to suction fluids to aid in exposure.
Instrument Insight: This suction tip may be a retractor at the same time that it is being used for suctioning.

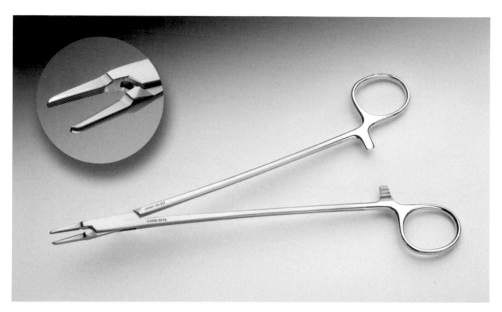

Instrument: RYDER NEEDLE HOLDER
Other Names: Fine Ryder needle holder
Category: Suturing and Stapling
Description: It has finely tapered jaws with carbide inserts.

Use(s): It is used for suturing of purse strings and valve sutures during heart surgery.
Instrument Insight: This is a fine but sturdy instrument. Wipe it clean every time when loading valve sutures.

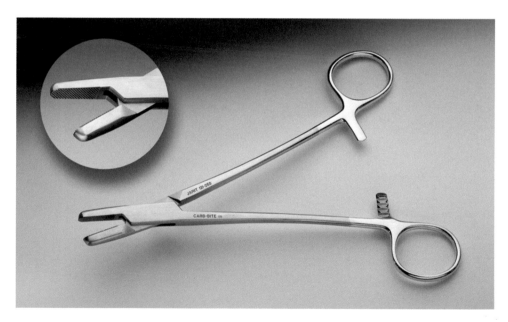

Instrument: STERNAL NEEDLE HOLDER AND WIRE TWISTER
Other Names: Big ugly wire twister, wire twister
Category: Suturing and Stapling
Description: This needle holder–type instrument has rounded heavy jaws with carbide inserts to hold the needle.

Use(s): It is used for placement of sternal wires and as a wire twister.
Instrument Insight: Load heavy sternal wires at the center of the needle so the needle does not bend from the pressure of pushing it through hard bone.

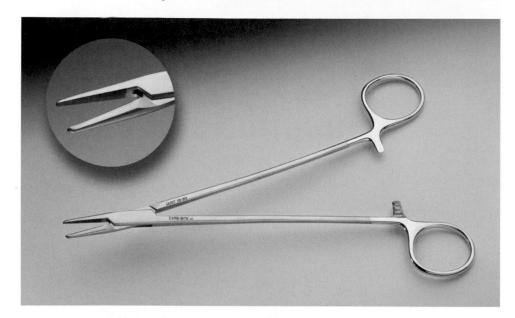

Instrument: COOLEY NEEDLE HOLDER
Category: Suturing and Stapling
Description: This is a needle holder with carbide jaws and fine tips.
Use(s): It is used for placement of purse strings and valve sutures.

Instrument Insight: The carbide jaws hold the needles so there is no slippage while placing the sutures.

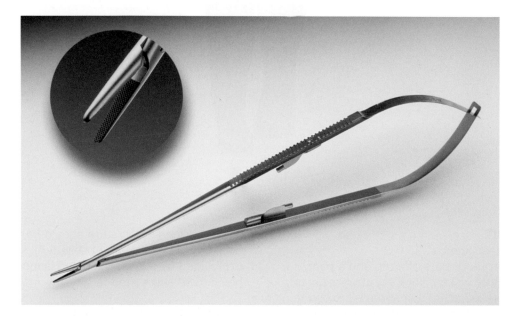

Instrument: CASTROVIEJO NEEDLE HOLDER
Other Names: Castro needle holder
Category: Suturing and Stapling
Description: This needle holder comes in a variety of lengths. It has a flat catch-spring handle.

Use(s): It is used for anastomosis suturing.
Instrument Insight: This is a very delicate instrument and should be protected during sterilization and packaging. It is commonly used for double-armed sutures size 4–0 or smaller.

Basic Operating Room Supplies and Equipment

OPERATING ROOM ATTIRE

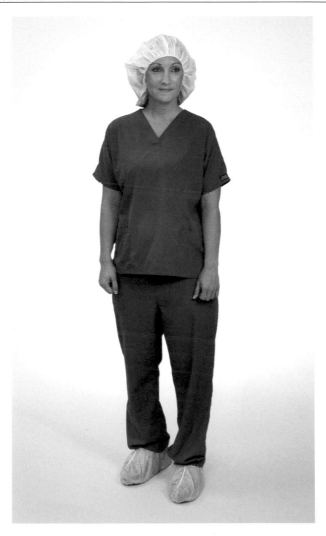

SCRUB SUIT

Other Names: Scrubs

Description: It consists of a top and a pant. Fabric is tightly woven, lint-free, stain-resistant, and resilient. The scrub suit should fit close to the body but not so tight that it would cause the skin to chafe.

Use(s): It replaces street clothes with clean surgical attire in a designated dressing room before entering the semirestricted and restricted areas.

Insight: Clean scrub attire should be donned daily or when it becomes soiled. All scrub attire is provided by the faculties and laundered by a health care accredited facility.

⚠ **CAUTION:** The top should be tucked into the pants to prevent blousing and coming in contact with sterile surfaces. Some pants have drawstrings; these should be tucked inside the waist to prevent the loops from contaminating the sterile field when opening or gowning.

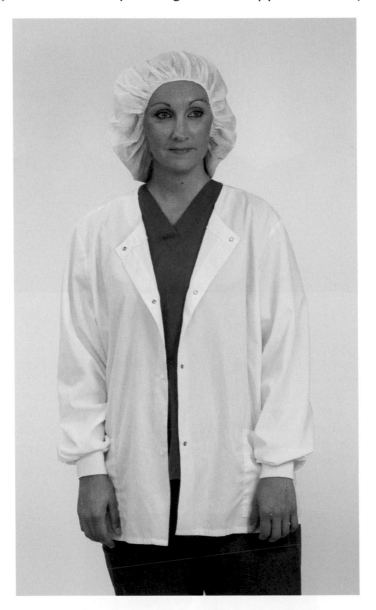

COVER JACKET

Other Names: Warm-up jacket

Description: Long-sleeve jacket with cuffs made of the same material as the scrub suit. The jacket should fit close to the body and be snapped closed.

Use(s): It is used to cover the arms of all unscrubbed personnel entering the restricted area. The jacket prevents contamination by containing shedding skin and bacteria from the arms.

Insight: The jacket should always be snapped, buttoned, or zipped when opening sterile supplies or when approaching the sterile field.

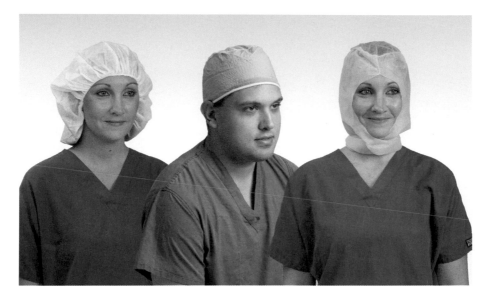

HEADCOVER

Other Names: Bouffant, caps, hoods hat
Description: There are many different styles, each designed for hair type and length. They should be extended over the scalp line from the forehead to cover the sideburns and ear area and around to cover the nape of the neck.
Use(s): Used to cover the head and contain hair, dander, and bacteria when entering the semi-restricted and restricted areas of the OR suite.

Insight: The use of a cloth hat is an intuitional policy.

⚠ **CAUTION:** All hair must be completely contained inside the head cover, to prevent shedding of hair and dander and bacteria. There are high quantities of *Staphylococcus aureus* and other bacteria that are present in the hair and scalp.

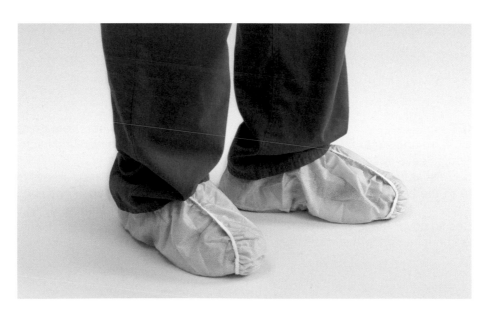

SHOE COVERS

Other Names: Booties
Description: It is a disposable slip-on shoe covering with an elastic band opening. They are water resistant with a nonskid strip on the bottom for traction. The common shoe cover is one-size-fits-most, which fits any shoe up to a man's size 12. Some manufactures do offer an extra-large-to-fit shoes beyond size 12.

Use(s): They help protect the shoes and feet from blood, fluids, and other contaminants.
Insight: These should be changed daily or when they become soiled, wet, or torn. They should not be worn outside of the surgical suite and should be removed before leaving the department.

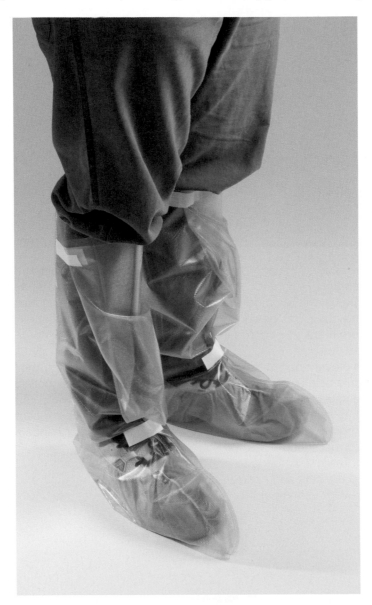

BOOT SHOE COVERS

Other Names: Ortho boots, trauma boots, arthroscopy boots

Description: It is a disposable slip-resistant plastic shoe cover that extends to the knee with adhesive strips that secure them in place at the ankle and the knee. There are many different styles of boots.

Use(s): They are used for complete coverage of the shoes, feet, and lower leg from blood, fluids, and other contaminants.

Insight: These should be disposed of after each procedure and should not be around the department following the case. Boots are commonly worn for procedures where a large amount of fluid, blood, and other contaminates is anticipated. Some examples are arthroscopic repairs, emergency trauma procedures, and C-sections.

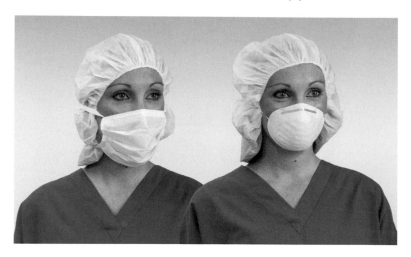

SURGICAL MASKS

Other Names: Face mask

Description: It is a single-use filtration device worn over the mouth and nose. It is designed to prevent infections in the patient. They come in many different types and designs.

Use(s): They are used to prevent microbial contamination of the sterile field by containing the wearers' droplets and aerosols while breathing and talking. It also prevents splashes and spray from entering the ears, mouth, and nose.

Insight: Choosing the correct fitting mask for the wearer is important. The mask needs to conform properly around the chin and nose and must stay in place to prevent venting at the sides and bottom. Masks should be removed and discarded following each procedure. If a mask becomes wet or soiled or is taken down it, should be discarded and replaced.

⚠ **CAUTION:** A mask should be removed and discarded by handling the ties only. The filtration portion of the mask collects bacteria from the nasal and oral airways. Touching the front of the mask will transfer the bacteria to the hands. Always wash your hands after removing your mask.

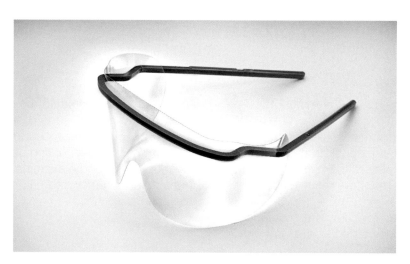

EYE PROTECTION

Other Names: Eyewear, goggles, face shields

Description: There are many different types of eye protection. Eyewear should completely cover the eyes and the eyebrows and wrap around to the temple at the sides. These can be disposable or reusable; following every case, disposables should be discarded and replaced and reusables should be cleaned.

Use(s): It is used to protect the wearer from splashes, sprays, or splatter of blood and bodily fluids.

Insight: Occupational Safety and Health Administration (OSHA) requires eye protection as part of the Bloodborne Pathogens Standard.

Regular eyeglasses do not meet the OSHA requirement unless they have side shields and cover the eyebrow.

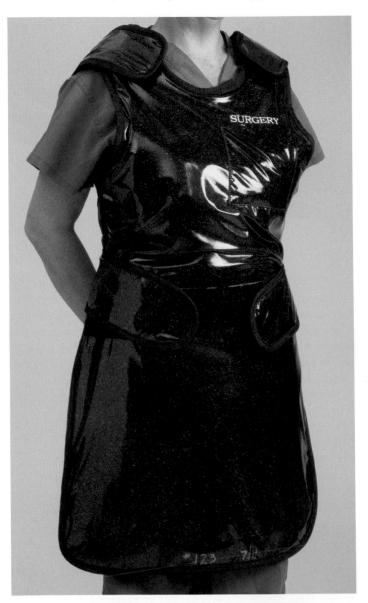

LEAD APRON

Other Names: Lead

Description: It is an apron-style shield that covers the front of the body, with Velcro straps that criss-cross in the back and attach in the front. A two-piece style consists of a vest with Velcro closure in the front and a skirt that wraps around the waist and secures with Velcro at the top. A thyroid shield should be worn in conjunction with the apron. This is a half-circle collar that covers the front of the neck and chest, with a Velcro strap that fasten behind the neck. There are many different styles of aprons available.

Use(s): It is used to protect the wearer from ionizing radiation during procedures in which X-rays and/or fluoroscopy are used. Examples are gallbladders, angiograms, bone, and spine procedures.

Insight: A lead apron is put on before scrubbing and is worn under the sterile gown.

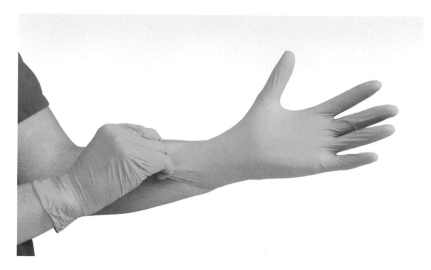

EXAM GLOVES

Other Names: Nonsterile gloves

Description: They are hand coverings that have a separate compartment for each finger and thumb. They cover just above the wrist. They are made of latex or nonlatex material and range in size from extra-small to double extra-large.

Use(s): They are used to protect the hands of a nonsterile team member from coming in contact with blood, body fluids, mucus membranes, tissues, and other potentially infectious items or materials.

Insight: Hand hygiene should be performed immediately following the removal of gloves.

All team members should wear gloves during the postoperative clean-up period.

OSHA requires gloves as part of the Blood-borne Pathogens Standard.

⚠ **CAUTION:** Always check the patient for a latex allergy.

SURGICAL ATTIRE

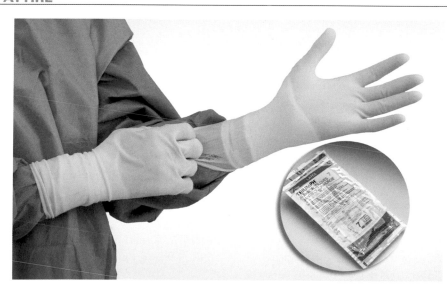

STERILE GLOVES

Other Names: Surgical gloves

Description: They are hand coverings that have a separate compartment for each finger and thumb. They completely cover up to about the mid-portion of the lower arm. Sterile gloves range from size five to nine and go up in half-size increments. They are made of latex and nonlatex material. There are many different types and brands of sterile gloves that differ in composition, strength, thickness, and durability.

Use(s): They are used to protect sterile team members from coming in contact with blood, body fluids, mucus membranes, tissues, and other potentially infectious items or materials.

Insight: Double gloving (wearing two pairs of gloves) is recommended for all invasive procedures.

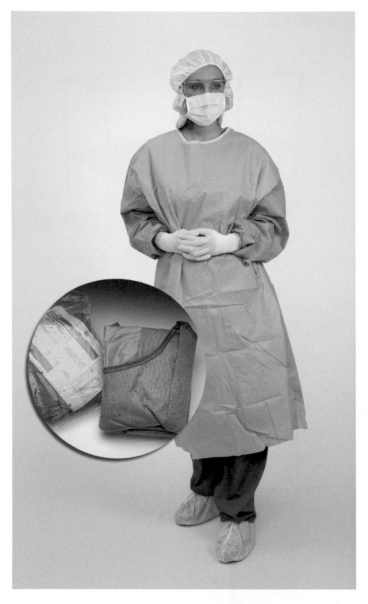

SURGICAL GOWN

Other Names: Sterile gown

Description: This is a long-sleeved dress type barrier that covers the body from the neckline to below the knees. It ties or fastens closed in the back. It may be disposable one-time single-use or nondisposable cloth that is laundered.

Use(s): It is used to create a sterile barrier over the scrub suit when entering the sterile field. A surgical gown is worn by all sterile team members. It protects both the patient and the caregiver.

Insight: Only parts of the gown are considered sterile once donned. The front of the gown is from mid-chest to the waist and the sleeves to just above the elbow. The cuffs of the gown are not impervious and are considered nonsterile after the hands pass through them. These cuffs must be completely covered, and they stay covered with the sterile gloves.

OPERATING ROOM FURNITURE

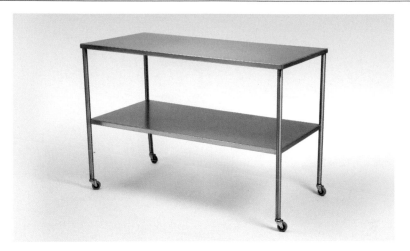

BACK TABLE

Other Names: Instrument table

Description: It is a stainless steel rectangular table with wheels.

Use(s): Once draped, it is used to hold extra supplies and instruments that are not for immediate use.

Insight: The back table cover or custom pack is opened on the back table to create the sterile field.

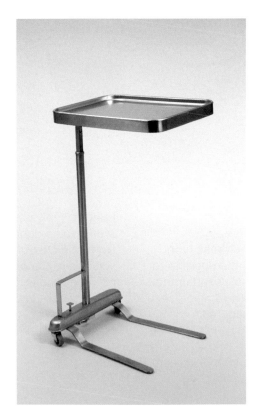

MAYO STAND

Other Names: Mayo tray, instrument tray

Description: It is a small portable stainless steel instrument tray that is open ended on one side so that it can be adjusted in height to fit over the operating room (OR) table.

Use(s): Once draped, it is used for immediate-use instruments and supplies for the procedure.

Insight: The height adjustment is done with the foot control at the bottom of the Mayo stand.

⚠ **CAUTION:** The Mayo stand should never be rested or leaned on. The height adjustment mechanism could give way, collapsing the stand onto the patient.

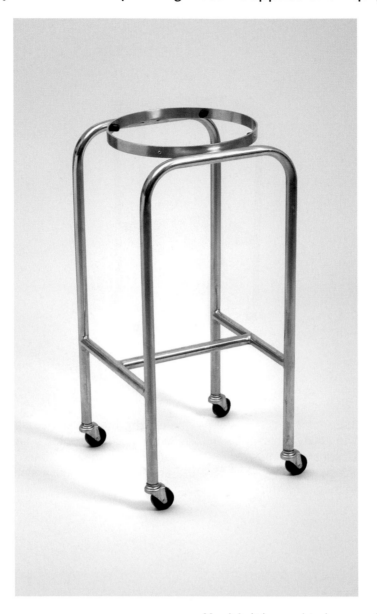

RING STAND
Other Names: Ring, basin stand
Description: It is a stainless steel four-legged rolling stand with a mounted ring at the top. The ring allows a 14 1/2" rimed basin to fit down into it.

Use(s): It is used to house a basin.
Insight: A sterile wrapped basin or basin set is placed in the stand and is opened.

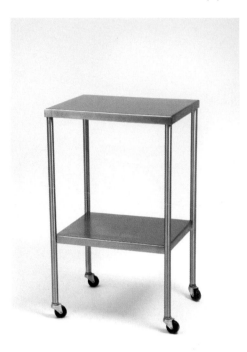

Instrument: PREP TABLE
Other Names: Prep stand, utility table
Description: It is a small square stainless steel table on wheels.
Use(s): It is used to hold surgical skin prep kits and prep supplies.

Insight: It can also be used for small procedures such as a myringotomy and tube placement, or anesthesia may use it for sterile setup when administering spinal anesthetic.

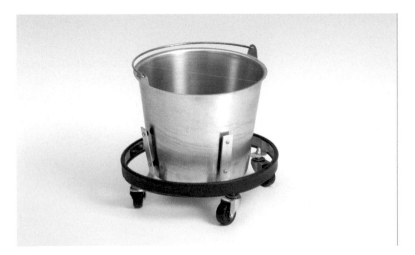

KICK BUCKET
Other Names: Sponge bucket
Description: It is a small round stainless steel frame on wheels that holds a 13-inch stainless steel bucket.

Use(s): It is designated for discarding soiled sponges.
Insight: The kick bucket should be placed close to the sterile field so the sponges can be dropped into it easily.

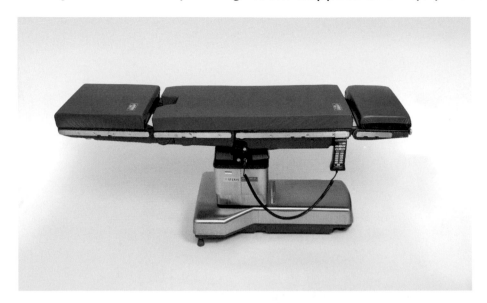

OPERATING ROOM (OR TABLE)

Other Names: OR table, OR bed, operating table

Description: It is a stainless steel hydraulic lift base with a stainless steel frame that houses a radiopaque padded platform or tabletop. The tabletop is jointed at the head, the middle, and foot and can be flexed, rotated, tilted, raised, or lowered. There are a wide variety of attachments used for maintaining the patient in the proper position.

Use(s): It is the table on which the patient is placed for surgery. It is used to manipulate the patient into different positions for the procedure.

Insight: There are many different manufacturers and styles of OR tables.

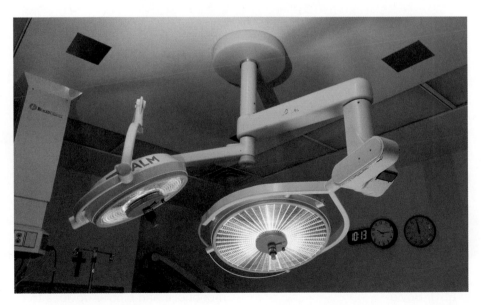

OR LIGHTS

Other Names: Operating room lights, spotlights, overhead lights

Description: It includes two or three light heads that are attached to a boom arm that is mounted to the ceiling.

This allows for the light to be moved around and focused on the surgical area. Most of these lights are either halogen or LED.

Use(s): It is used to illuminate the surgical site.

Insight: Sterile light handle covers are placed on the handles this allows the lights manipulated by the sterile team members during the procedure. These are the only times that sterile team members are allowed to reach above their heads.

⚠ **CAUTION:** Care should be taken when moving these lights to avoid hitting anyone in the head.

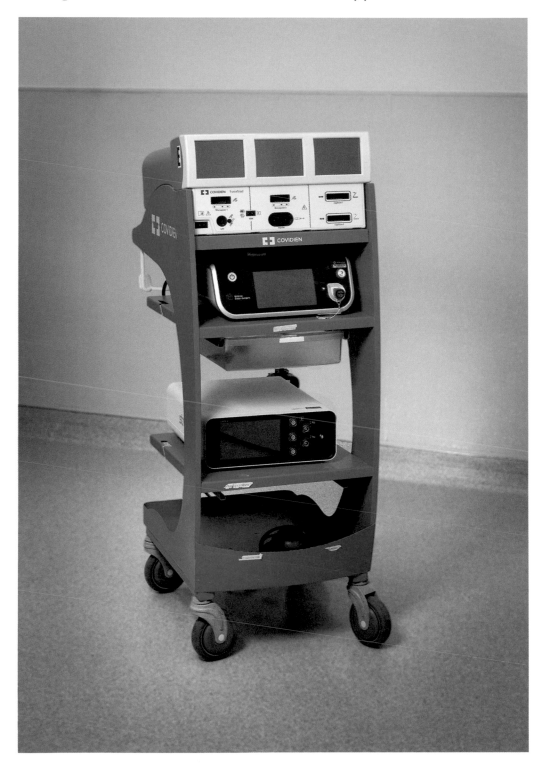

ELECTRICAL SURGICAL UNIT
Other Names: ESU, Bovie
Description: It is a generator box that is activated by a handset or foot control. There are marked receptacles that ensure the correct connection of accessories. A touch screen or buttons allow for power adjustment. The machine has indicator lights and alarm alerts when in use.

Use(s): It generates electrical current to monopolar and bipolar devices to cut, dissect, coagulate, and fulgurate blood vessels and tissues during surgery.
Insight: When using a monopolar, a disbursement pad (grounding pad) should be placed on the patient.

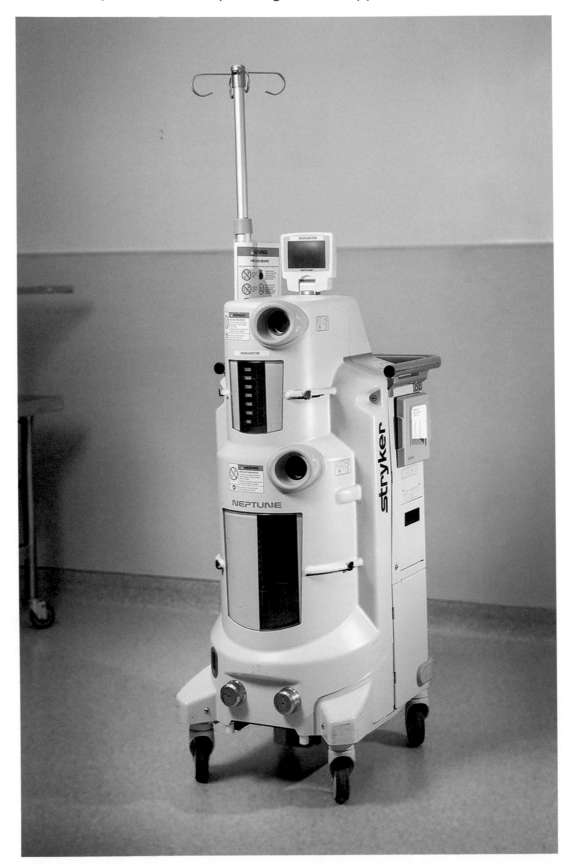

SUCTION

Other Names: Neptune, Dornoch, wall suction
Description: There are many different manufacturers and styles of suction units.

Use(s): It is used in conjunction with suction tubing and tip to suction blood, fluids, and debride from the surgical wound.

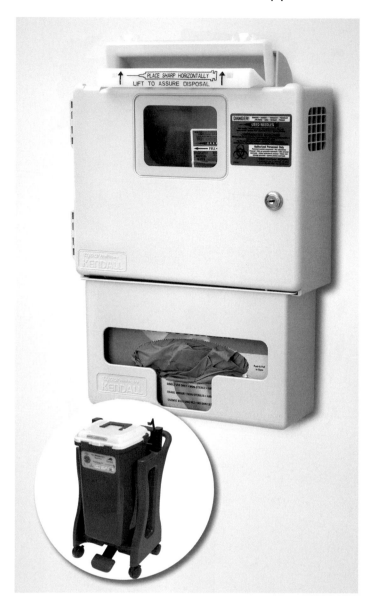

SHARPS CANISTER

Other Names: Sharps Container

Description: It comes in many different styles and sizes. They are made of hard plastic, which prevents sharp items from penetrating through. The containers are often self-locking or self-sealing when full.

Use(s): It is used to dispose of sharp instruments and supplies, such as hypodermic needles, suture needles, scalpel blades, and any sharp disposable instruments.

Insight: Most sharps canisters have a safety locking mechanism that secures the content when the container is full.

⚠ **CAUTION:** Never stick your hand into a sharp canister to retrieve anything.

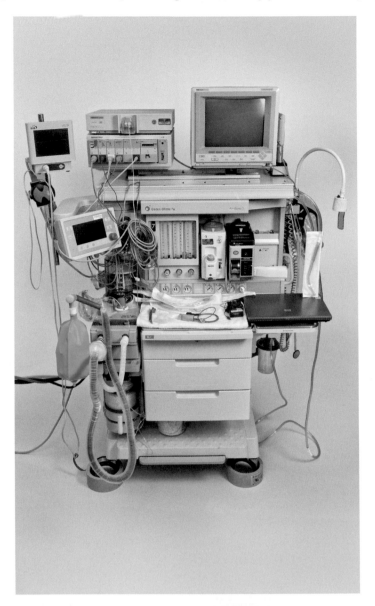

ANESTHESIA MACHINE

Other Names: Anesthesia work station, gas machine

Description: There are many manufacturers and styles of anesthesia machines.

Use(s): It is a complex machine that delivers oxygen and anesthesia gases and ventilates the patient. It also features multiple patient-monitoring systems.

Insight: It is the large piece of equipment at the head of the bed.

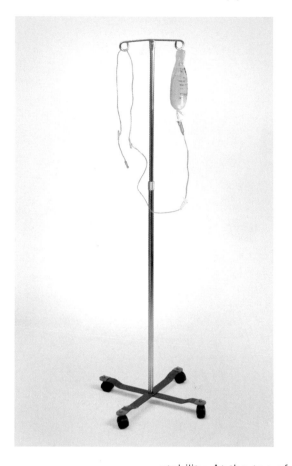

IV POLE

Other Names: Intravenous pole

Description: A tall, slender, adjustable height pole, with a four- or five-wheeled base for stability. At the top of the pole, there are two to four hooks.

Use(s): It is used to hang medication or fluid bags.

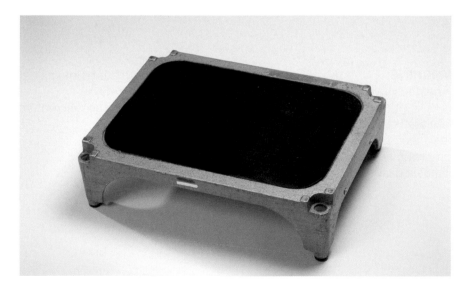

STEP STOOL

Other Names: Standing stool, steps, riser, platform

Description: It is a low platform that can he stacked. Most have an antimicrobial anti-skid mat on the top. There are many different manufacturers and styles.

Use(s): It is used to stand during surgery to better visualize the procedure.

Insight: The manufacturer Platforms should only be stacked one on top of the other and no higher.

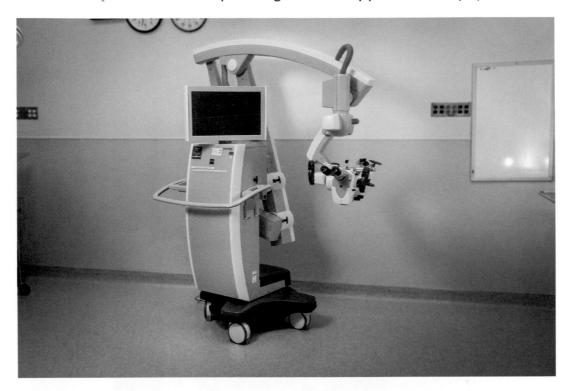

MICROSCOPE

Other Names: Operating microscope

Description: The microscope has a floor base with wheels that can be moved around and fixed into position with brakes. Attached to the base is a suspension arm that allows the movement of the optical system over the operative site and allows for exact positioning of the optics and fixes it into place. The optical system has a binocular eyepiece that often has a splitter beam with a second set of binoculars for the assistant. These eyepieces are attached to a magnification and light source box.

Use(s): This allows the surgeon to illuminate and magnify small structures while performing operative procedures. It is used in microsurgical procedures such as ear, eyes, and neurosurgery.

Insight: The microscope is draped with a clear plastic drape before it is brought into the sterile field.

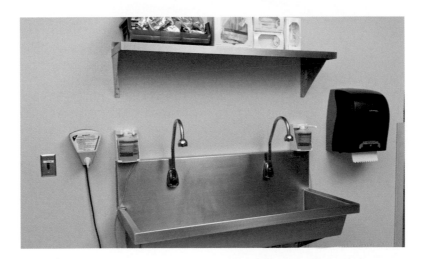

SCRUB SINK

Other Names: surgical sinks, medical sink

Description: Scrub sinks come in many different styles and are made of different materials. The faucet should be high enough for the hands and arms to be rinsed underneath it. The water control can be senor, knee, or foot control.

Use(s): It is used to scrub hands and arms.

Insight: Scrub sinks are located adjacent to the OR in a semirestricted area. Masks should be worn in the scrub area.

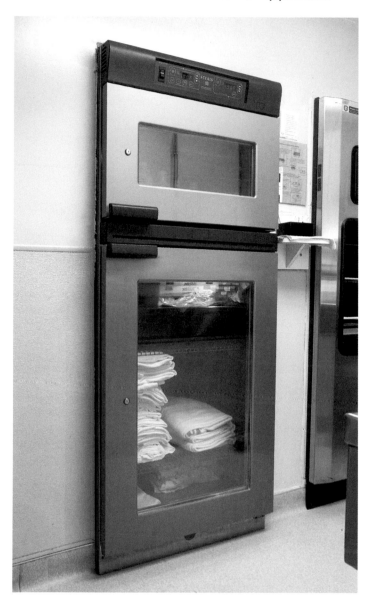

WARMER

Other Names: Blanket warmer, fluid warmer
Description: It is a cabinet that comes in various sizes and may have one, two, or three compartments.
Use(s): It is used to warm and store blankets and fluids to reduce the risk of hypothermia in the surgical patient.

Insight: Sterile fluids and blankets should be stored in separate compartments with separate temperature controls. Fluid should be maintained between 98°F and 99.5°F and blanket should be between 130°F and 150°F. Warmers are located adjacent to the OR in a semirestricted area. Masks should be worn in this area.

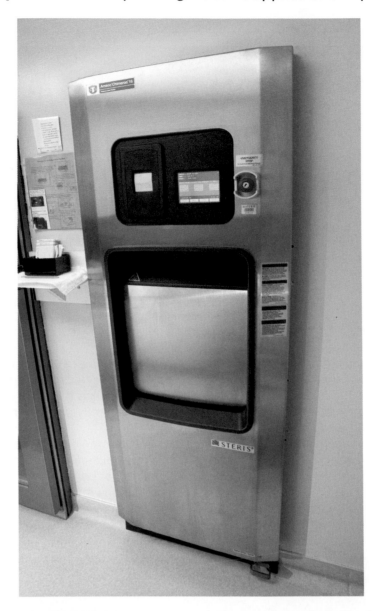

IMMEDIATE USE STEAM STERILIZER

Other Names: Flash sterilizer, flasher

Description: It is a small steam sterilizer that is a rectangular, recessed machine with a vertical sliding door with a foot pedal for hands opening. Inside the door is a stainless steel chamber with metal racks similar to oven racks. Off to the side is a touch control pad for setting and starting the appropriate cycle.

Use(s): It is used to sterilize an unwrapped item that is needed for the procedure, for which there is no conventional sterilized wrapped item to replace it. For example, an instrument is drooped on the floor and there is no package sterile item to replace it.

Insight: Immediate use steam sterilizers are located adjacent to the OR in a semirestricted area. Masks should be worn in this area.

- **For more information, parameters, and guideline, refer to Immediate-Use Steam Sterilizer in Chapter 2, Basic Sterilization**

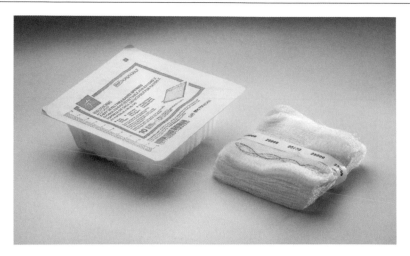

RAYTEC SPONGES

Other Names: Rays

Description: It is a small, loosely woven gauze that is folded to size and has a blue radiopaque strand woven into it. They are banded together in groups of 10 and come in sizes 2 × 2, 4 × 4, and 4 × 8 inches.

Use(s): It is used to blot blood and fluid from a small shallow wound. A Raytec can be loaded on a sponge forceps to blot deep in a wound or for blunt dissection. Also, it can be used to maintain countertraction of the skin while making an incision.

Insight: A sponge stick is created by folding a raytec into third and then in half and clamping the folded edges in the jaws of a ring/sponge forceps. Raytec sponges should be replaced with laparotomy sponges.

⚠ **CAUTION:** The paper or plastic band that is around the Raytecs should be removed and discarded during the initial count so that it does not inadvertently get into the wound.

⚠ **CAUTION:** A 4 × 4 gauze dressing can be easily mistaken for Raytecs; therefore dressings should never be opened onto the sterile field until after the final count. A 4 × 4 gauze dressing does not have a radiopaque strip and could inadvertently get left in a wound.

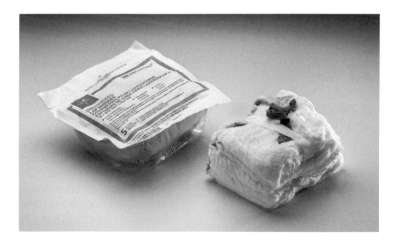

LAPAROTOMY SPONGES

Other Names: Laps, tapes, lap pads

Description: Large prewashed multiple-ply cotton gauze with a blue X-ray detectable loop sewn into one corner. These are banded together in groups of 5 and they come in sizes from 9 × 9 to 36 × 8 inches.

Insight: 18″ × 18″ are the most commonly used size.

Use(s): It is used to absorb blood and body fluids, pack and wall off organs and tissues in the abdominal cavity, or pad retractors.

Insight: Laparotomy sponges that are used to pack or pad are usually moistened with saline before they are placed in the wound.

⚠ **CAUTION:** Always keep track of the number of laparotomy sponges that are placed into the wound. All laps must be removed and accounted for before wound closure.

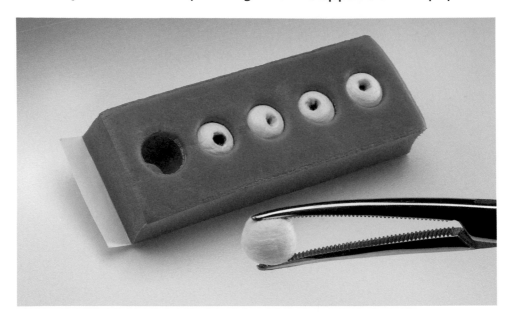

DISSECTOR SPONGES

Other Names: Kitners, cherries, peanuts

Description: It is a small round or oval cotton sponge wrapped in gauze with radiopaque strand woven into it. They come in a package of five mounted on a foam bar that has an individual hole for each dissector. The bottom of the bar has an adhesive strip that adheres it to the Mayo stand to prevent it from being knocked off.

Use(s): They are mounted on forceps and are used to bluntly dissect and separate planes, tissues, and organs.

Insight: These dissectors should always be mounted on the forceps or placed back into their holder.

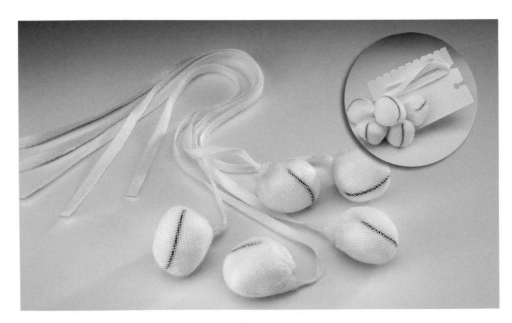

TONSIL SPONGES

Description: It is a cotton ball covered with gauze with a radiopaque strand woven through the gauze and a string attached to the gathered end. Packaged in groups of five.

Use(s): It is used during a tonsillectomy to control bleeding in the tonsillar fossae.

Insight: These are loaded on a clamp for placement, and the string is draped outside of the mouth for easy retrieval.

⚠ **CAUTION:** Always make sure that the retrieval string is attached, or the sponge could drop down into the trachea and cause airway obstruction.

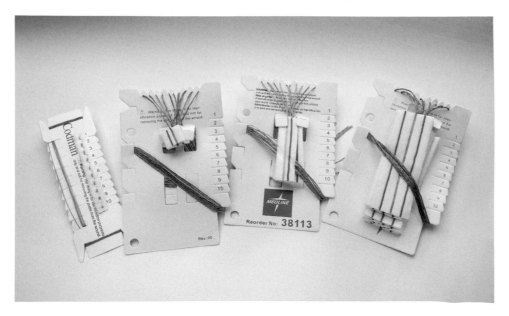

COTTONOID SPONGES

Other Names: Neurosurgical pattie, neuro
pattie, neuro sponge

Description: It is a compressed rayon pledget
with an X-ray-detectable strip down the middle
and a locator string sewn on one end. They
come in various sizes from ¼ × ¼ to 3 × 3
inches and are packaged on a counting card in
groups of 10.

Use(s): They are used for hemostasis and tissue
protection when suctioning.

Insight: They are soaked in saline before use. All
neuro patties must be accounted for before the
closure of the wound.

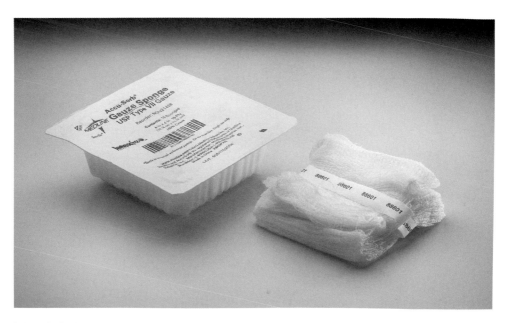

4 × 4 DRESSING SPONGE

Other Names: Gauze sponges

Description: It is a loosely woven gauze folded
to 4″ × 4″.

Use(s): It is used as the intermediate layer of a
dressing.

Insight: Dressing sponges are easily confused
with Raytec sponges; therefore dressings should
never be opened until the final count is
completed.

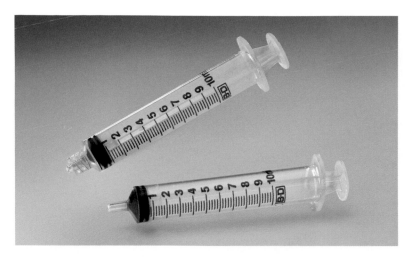

SYRINGE

Other Names: Hypodermic Syringe
Description: It is a hollow calibrated cylinder barrel with a sliding plunger that has a tightly fitting black stopper. Syringes have either a slip or a Luer-Lok tip. A slip tip allows for the plain tip to slide into the hub of the hypodermic needle by simply pushing them together. The Luer-Lok tip has threads that require the hub of the needle to be screwed into it. They are calibrated in milliliters (mL) or cubic centimeters (cc), which is the same measurement. Syringes graduate in size from 1 mL to 60 mL. It is made of plastic or glass; plastic is the most commonly used syringe in the OR.

Use(s): It is used to measure and administer medication, irrigate, and aspirate fluids.
Insight: The Luer-Lok is much more secure and prevents the separation of the needle from the syringe during a high-pressure injection.

⚠ **CAUTION:** An insulin syringe is calibrated in units and is never used to inject anything but insulin. A 1 mL tuberculin is calibrated in hundredths of a milliliter, so pay attention to the calibration.

⚠ **CAUTION:** Anytime medication or fluid is drawn up into a syringe, it should be labeled immediately.

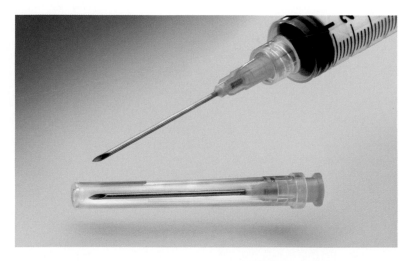

HYPODERMIC NEEDLE

Other Names: Hypo, bore needle
Description: It is a hollow stainless steel cannula with a razor-sharp bevel at the pointed end and a plastic hub on the other end that attaches it to a syringe. The diameter of a hypodermic needle is specified by gauge. The larger the gauge number, the smaller the needle, and vice versa. They range in length from 3/8″ to 5″.

Use(s): It is used to inject medication into the tissues and withdraw body fluids or medication from a vial.

⚠ **CAUTION:** A used needle should never be recapped using both hands. If a needle must be recapped it should be done using the one handed sweep method.

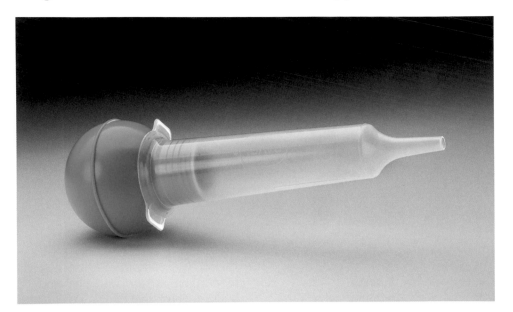

ASEPTO

Other Names: Irrigating syringe
Description: It is an 8-inch-long hollow plastic syringe-like cannula with bulb reservoir that fits in the end barrel.

Compression of the bulb creates a vacuum that pulls fluid into it. When full, it holds approximately 120 mL.
Use(s): It is filled with irrigation fluid to clear away blood and debris from the surgical world.

Insight: Keeping track of the amount of irrigation fluid used during the procedure is the duty of the scrub tech.

⚠ **CAUTION:** An ASEPTO is a syringe that gets filled with fluid, so like any other syringe it needs to be labeled.

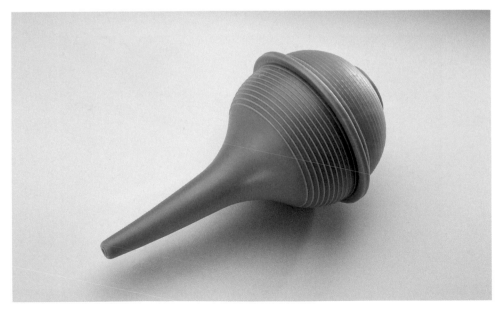

BULB SYRINGE

Other Names: Tonsil syringe, baby sucker
Description: It is a one-piece small cylinder tube that leads to a bulb reservoir. It is about 3½ inches in length.
Use(s): It is used to aspirate and irrigate. Commonly used during C-sections to aspirate mucus and fluid from the newborn's mouth and nose. It is also used during a tonsillectomy to irrigate the mouth and throat.
Insight: During a C-section, always have the empty bulb syringe on your Mayo stand ready to hand to the surgeon when the baby's head is delivered. The bulb syringe should be handed off the field with the baby.

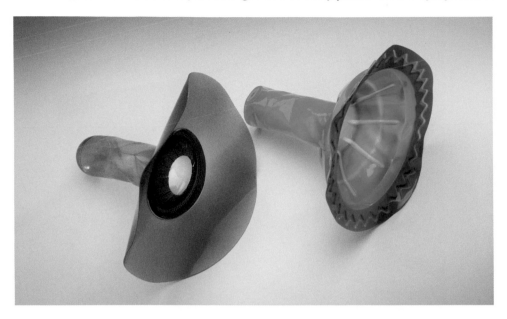

LIGHT HANDLE COVER
Other Names: Light gloves, light cover
Description: A sterile flexible plastic sleeve that fits over the operating room light handles. The cover slides or twists onto the handle.
Use(s): The light handle cover creates a sterile barrier so that the sterile team members can maneuver the lights into the surgical wound. A sterile flexible plastic sleeve that fits over the operating room light handles. The cover slides or twists onto the handle.
Insight: Placing light covers and maneuvering the lights is the only time a sterile team member can raise their hands above their heads.

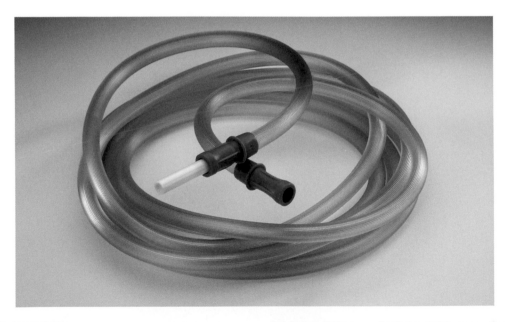

SUCTION TUBING
Other Names: Tubing
Description: It is a clear polyvinyl chloride tubing with a ribbed outer surface and two soft female connectors on each end.
Use(s): Used as a connection between the suction unit and the suction tip to remove fluids and debris from the surgical wound.
Insight: Either end of the tubing can be thrown off the sterile field to be hooked up to the canister. Be sure to keep an appropriate length on your field. Once the tubing is thrown off the field, it cannot be pulled back.

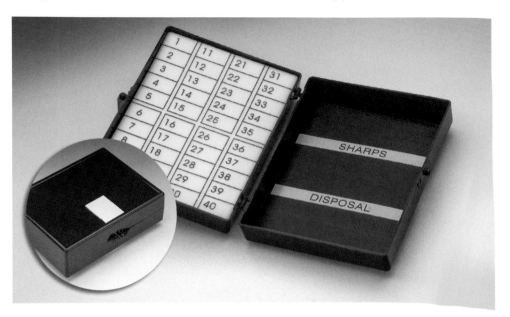

NEEDLE COUNTER

Other Names: Needle mat, sharps holder, needle magnet

Description: These come in a variety of styles and sizes. It is a hard-plastic box that snaps shut and locks. It may be designed with a foam pad on one side and a magnet on the other. The foam side is numbered with a grid in which suture needles are stuck into each slot and can be easily counted. The magnet side is for other sharps such as scalpel blades, hypodermic needles, and safety pins.

Use(s): It is used to contain sharps and needles on the back table.

Insight: After a procedure, all small sharps and needles are placed in the box, it is closed, and the entire box is placed in a larger sharps container.

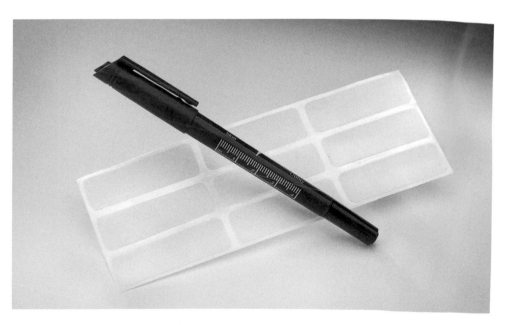

STERILE MARKING PEN AND LABELS

Other Names: sterile marker, marking pen

Description: This is a felt tip maker and adhesive labels.

Use(s): It is used to label all medications and fluids on your sterile field, and/or marking the skin before making the incision.

Insight: All medications and fluids on your sterile field must be labeled, including syringes, basins, and pitchers.

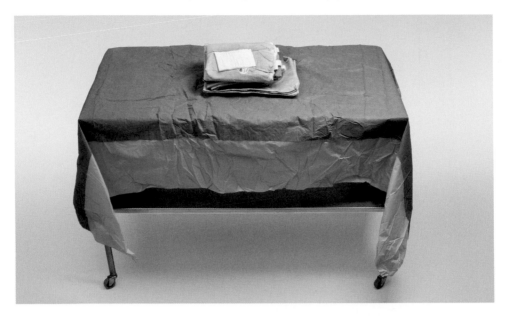

BACK TABLE COVER

Other Names: Table cover
Description: It is a single-use light blue rectangular plastic drape with a darker blue paper covering the middle section.

Use(s): It is used to drape the back table.
Insight: Back table covers are used as the outer wrap of a back table pack or custom pack.

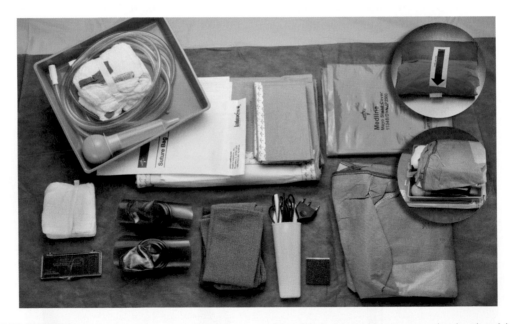

BACK TABLE PACK

Other Names: Custom pack, procedure pack, set-up pack, case packs, trace packs
Description: Single-use preassembled packs are often customized by the facility. It is a back table cover folded around items such as gowns, towels, soft goods, Mayo stand cover, light handles, suction tip and tubing, and other specific items. Many facilities customize these packs to specific types of procedures. A few examples of this are craniotomy packs, total knee packs, Lap Chole packs.

Use(s): It is used to cover the back table and decrease the time spent in opening individual supplies.
Insight: Typically, it is the first item opened and becomes the center of the sterile field.

A covered back table is only sterile on the tabletop.

⚠ **CAUTION:** Always check the outer plastic cover for tears or holes before opening the back table pack.

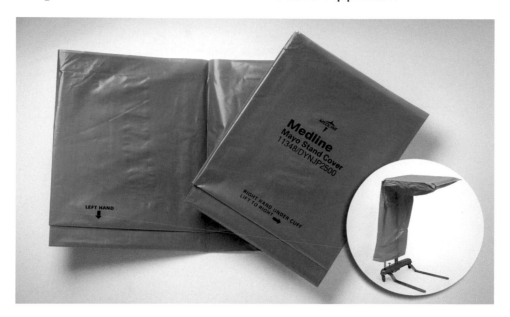

MAYO STAND COVER

Other Names: Mayo cover

Description: It is a single-use pillowcase-like blue plastic slipcover with a darker blue paper covering at the proximal end. This slides around and over the Mayo stand with the paper section covering the tray.

Use(s): A sterile drape covers the Mayo stand.

Insight: The cover is folded unto itself in an accordion style, so as you slide on the Mayo stand it opens to slide around the tray and down the back.

⚠ **CAUTION:** When draping the Mayo stand, it is important to keep your hands completely under the cuff of the cover. While sliding the cover on, it is important to control the proximal end as it is unfolding so that it doesn't flip up and touch the face or fall below the top.

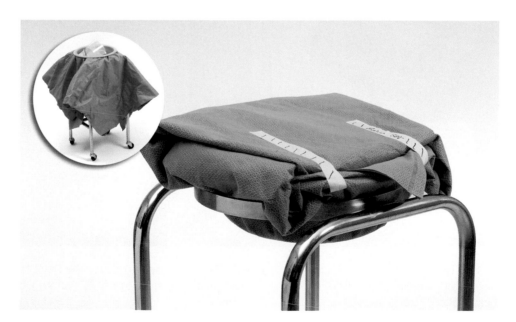

BASIN

Other Names: Basin set, surgical basin

Description: It is a 14 ¼" round bowl that can hold up to 8 ½ quarts of fluid that fits down into a ring stand. These basins can be single-use made of plastic or reusable made of stainless steel.

Use(s): It is often used as a place to open small supplies and can be used to stack patient drapes.

Sometimes surgeons want it filled with water to rinse their hands.

Insight: Some institutions use customized basin sets that may have various items arranged inside the basin. Often a basin set will include a grad pitcher, smaller basins, and med cups.

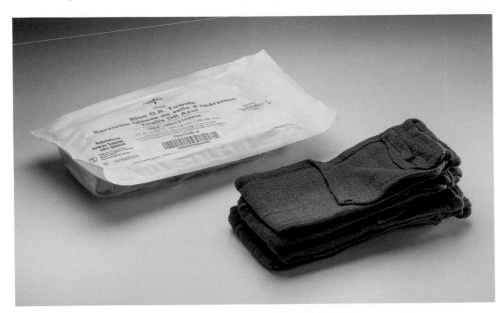

TOWEL PACK

Other Names: Huck towels, towel bundle

Description: A package of rectangular 17 in × 27 in cotton towels. The most common number of towels per pack is four. They are usually blue but may come in other colors such as green or white.

Use(s): These are used for draping the sterile field and drying the hands and arms. Towels are used on the back table and Mayo stand for an extra barrier. Also placed around the incision site before placing the drape.

Insight: Surgical towels can be disposable or reusable. Disposable towels come in sterile packages of even increments from 2 to 10 per package. Reusable towels are lint-free cotton towels that are laundered and reprocessed by the facility.

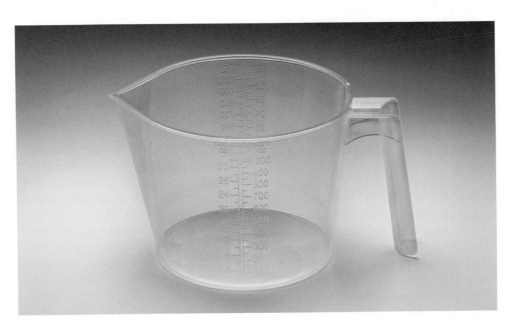

GRADUATED PITCHER

Other Names: Grad pitcher

Description: It is a pouring pitcher that commonly holds a liter (1000 mL) of fluid and is graduated in 100-mL increments. These can be made of plastic for single use or of stainless steel for reusable ones.

These may also come in other sizes such as 250 mL, 500 mL, 1000 mL, 2000 mL, and 3000 mL.

Use(s): It is used to hold and measure irrigation fluid.

Insight: It is important to keep track of how much irrigation is used to estimate patient blood loss.

17

Surgical Setups

PRELIMINARY CONSIDERATIONS

This chapter provides an introduction to procedural setups. It provides an introduction to setting up, photographs of a Mayo stand and back table, a definition of each procedure and the reason that it is performed, and technical tips. The content and illustrations provided are not the only way that these procedures can be set up, but instead give an example of each. There is no right or wrong way to set up. This varies according to the surgeon's preference, the individual who is setting up, and the facility. The importance here is for the learner to have some idea of what the procedure is, what may be needed for the procedure, and why it is performed.

Case Preparation

Case preparation begins with the surgeon's preference card and gathering of extra supplies, instruments, and equipment needed. After this is done, the case cart is brought into the operating room (OR), furniture is properly arranged, and supplies are set around and opened. Sterile supplies should be opened as far away from doors and as close to the incision time as possible. Once the room is open, it should be viewed at all times and not left unattended. Following opening, the surgical technologist will scrub and proceed to gown and glove.

Preparing to Set Up the Sterile Field

Directly after gowning and gloving, the surgical technologist must organize the back table and Mayo stand. This can be overwhelming due to the quantity of instruments and supplies opened. Using a methodical organized approach and creating a routine will decrease anxiety and improve proficiency. The back table provides a large sterile surface area for preparing and storing sterile objects. The back table is arranged with items that are not essential to start, are duplicated, or are infrequently used during the procedure. The Mayo stand is set up with objects that are utilized to initiate the surgery and those frequently used throughout a procedure. Setups are prepared to make a seamless exchange of instruments, supplies, and equipment between the Mayo stand, back table, and surgeon during the operation.

Setup suggestions:
- Leave enough time between opening room and incision to get the setup organized and ready to proceed.
- Create a plan and use the same routine every time you set up.
- Use purposeful movements. Do not move or shift items around. An object should be put in the proper spot and not moved again.
- Avoid doing several things at once; complete one task and then move on to the next.
- Movement in the sterile field should be kept to a minimum.
- Center yourself in the field and use only your upper body and hands to arrange items.
- Divide your back table into thirds and arrange in sections.
    - The first section is the working area. This will be on either the right or left side of the table depending on where you will be standing. This area will be pulled up next to you at the Mayo stand. In this area, arranged items can be quickly retrieved if needed, such as a roll towel with extra instruments, solutions, sutures, needle mat, sponges, and any item that may be used later in the procedure.
    - The second section is where the instrument pan is placed. Some people will place a roll towel with instruments here or even inside the instrument pan.
    - The third section is the area in which extra gowns, gloves, and draping items are placed.
- Emptying your basin set and draping the Mayo stand will give you extra working space if needed. The electrosurgical pencil, light handles, and suction tubing can be placed in the empty basin.
- Towels laid on the flat surface of the table or Mayo stand provide an extra barrier.
- Arrange pitcher, basins, and medicine cups at the edge of the table so that fluids and medications can be easily poured.

- Group like items together, such as sutures, sponges, clips, and syringes. This will help with organization and counts.
- Stack items in order of use; the item on the top would be the one used first. For example, towel on the top, gown in the center, and gloves on the bottom. Draping materials can also be stacked in the same manner.
- When placing the roll towel, leave adequate space from the table's edge to allow the instruments' finger rings to stand up without dropping off the table.
- Ratcheted instruments should be closed only to the first notch. This will prevent them from opening when handing them and will allow for easy opening of the instrument at the field.
- Keep the number of instruments on the Mayo stand to a minimum, choose the same quantity, and place them in the same spot. This will help with organization and keeping track of counts.
- When setting up the Mayo stand, select instruments from each category, such as cutting, clamping, grasping, and retracting. This will help you determine what is needed on the Mayo stand.

PROCEDURES

Dilation and Curettage (D&C)

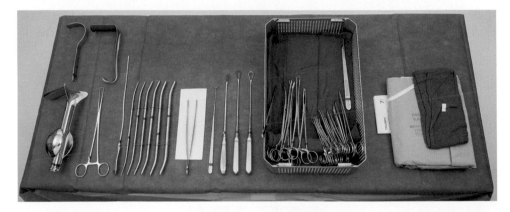

Definition: This is a gradual opening of the cervix and removal (by scraping) of the endocervical and/or endometrial lining of the uterus for pathologic examination.

Reason Performed: It is performed to diagnose and treat uterine conditions such as cancer or abnormal bleeding or to remove uterine content following a miscarriage or abortion.

Tech Tip: The procedure is set up on the back table. There are many different types of tenaculum and dilators, which are determined by the surgeon's preference. Dilators are lined up from smallest to largest and are lubricated before insertion. The surgeon often grabs his or her own instruments so the setup should be placed in the order of use.

Breast Biopsy
MAYO STAND

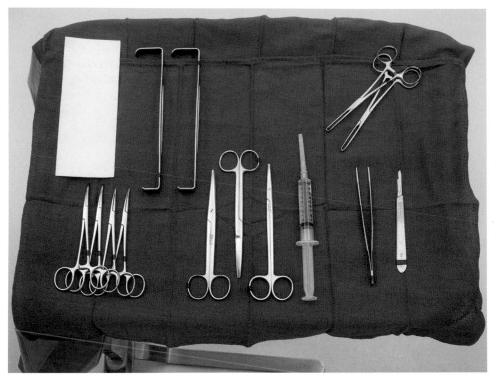

BACK TABLE

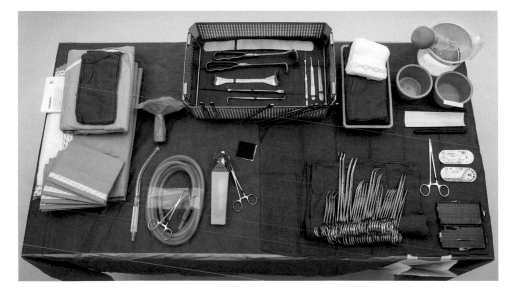

Definition: In this procedure a sample of suspicious breast tissue is removed for pathologic examination.

Reason Performed: It is performed to diagnose or rule out breast cancer.

Tech Tip: Senn or rake retractors may also be added to the Mayo stand. The surgeon may want to mark the specimen with a suture.

Carpal Tunnel Release
MAYO STAND

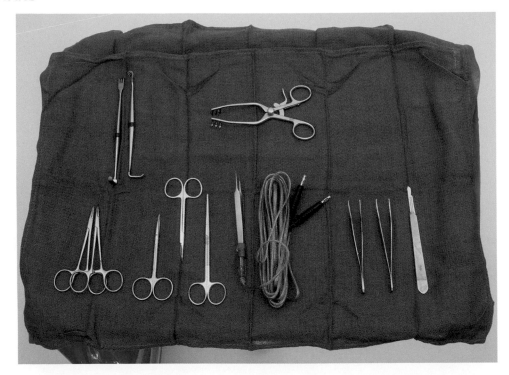

BACK TABLE

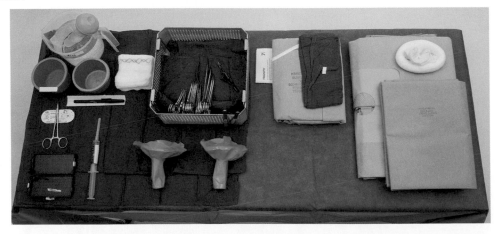

Definition: The transverse carpal ligament is dissected, which decompresses the median nerve.

Reason Performed: It is performed to relieve carpal tunnel syndrome symptoms.

Tech Tip: The setup may be done on the back table. Often the scrub tech will be assisting and the surgeon will be exchanging instruments on his or her own. A carpal tunnel procedure may also be done endoscopically so the setup will change accordingly.

Exploratory Laparotomy
MAYO STAND

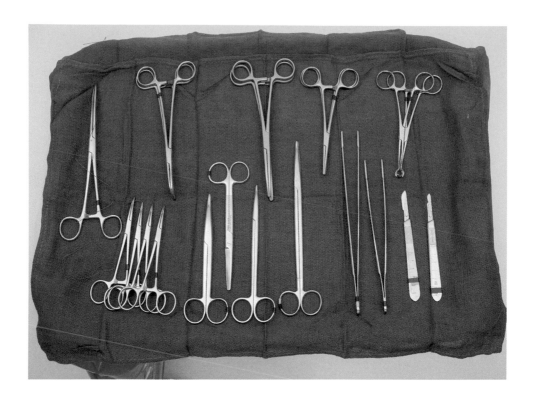

BACK TABLE

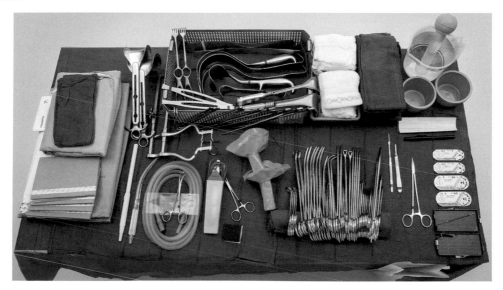

Definition: This is an opening through the peritoneum for examination to diagnose and treat disease that could not be determined via other diagnostic methods.

Reason Performed: It is performed for acute or unexplained abdominal pain, bleeding, or trauma or for staging of malignancy.

Tech Tip: There are many different types of large self-retaining retractors that could be added to this setup. As the surgeon moves deeper into the cavity, exchange shorter instruments for longer instruments on the Mayo stand. Once the abdominal cavity is opened, Raytex sponges should be replaced with laparotomy sponges unless they are loaded on a sponge stick. Initial retractors can be placed on the Mayo stand and exchanged for larger ones as the abdominal cavity is entered. Instruments may also be placed on a roll towel on the Mayo stand.

Inguinal Hernia Repair
MAYO STAND

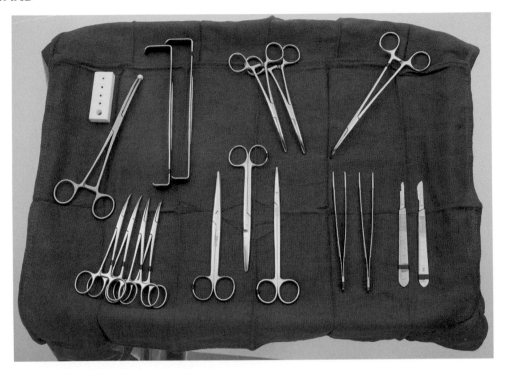

BACK TABLE

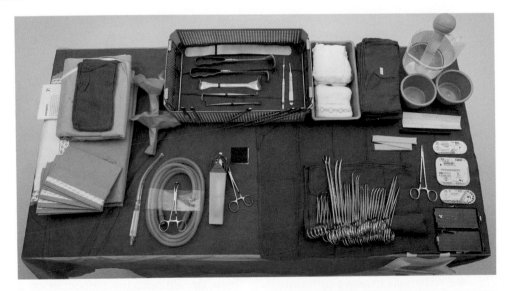

Definition: Also known as a herniorrhaphy, this is the surgical correction of a musculofascial defect in the abdominal wall that results in protrusion of the abdominal contents. The contents are returned to the abdomen, and the defect is sutured, closed, or reinforced with mesh.

Reason Performed: It is performed to return the abdominal viscera back into the abdominal cavity and close or repair the musculofascial defect.
Tech Tip: The Penrose drain is used for retracting the spermatic cord and should be moistened before handing it.

Laparoscopic Appendectomy
MAYO STAND

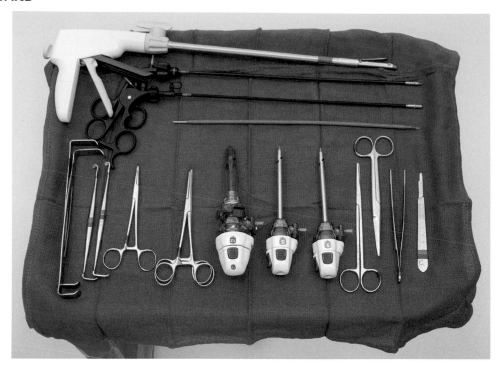

BACK TABLE

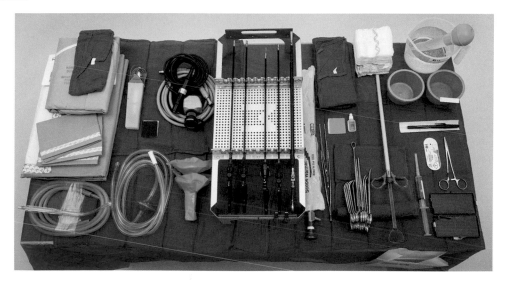

Definition: This is a minimally invasive removal of the appendix. It is performed through several small incisions with the assistance of a video system, laparoscope, and laparoscopic instruments.
Reason Performed: It is performed to treat appendicitis or a ruptured appendix.

Tech Tip: Be sure the stopcocks on the trocars are in the closed position. Make sure the light source is switched to standby when not in use to prevent fire risk. Remember to use bowel technique on the instruments that come into contact with the appendix. Have an endo catch available.

Laparoscopic Cholecystectomy
MAYO STAND

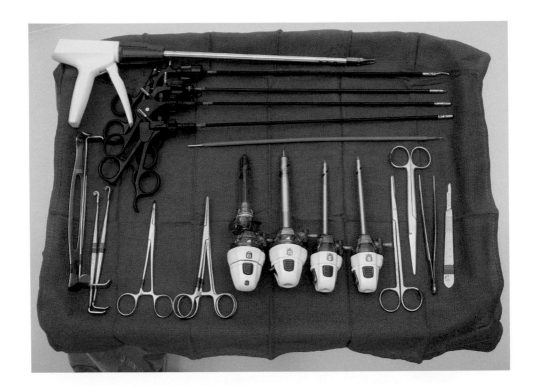

BACK TABLE

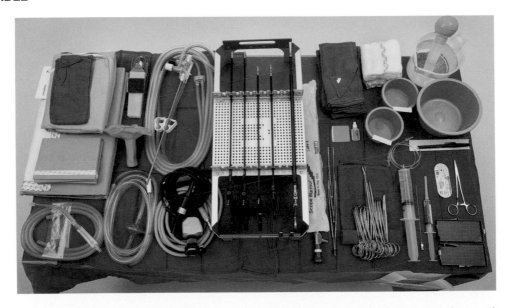

Definition: This is a minimally invasive removal of the gallbladder. It is performed through several small incisions with the assistance of a video system, laparoscope, and laparoscopic instruments.

Reason Performed: It is performed to treat inflammation of the gallbladder (cholecystitis) and gallstones (cholelithiasis).

Tech Tip: Be sure the stopcocks on the trocars are in the closed position. Make sure the light source is switched to standby when not in use to prevent fire risk. Have an endo catch available.

Tonsillectomy and Adenoidectomy (T&A)
MAYO STAND

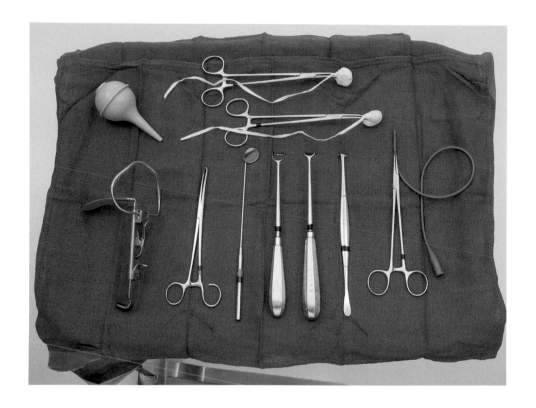

BACK TABLE

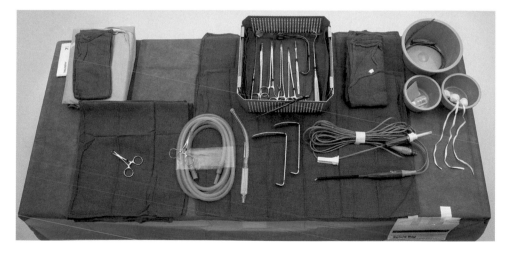

Definition: This is the removal of the tonsils and adenoids.

Reason Performed: It is performed for chronic inflammation and infection of the throat (tonsillitis).

Tech Tip: If the McIvor mouth gag is hooked onto the Mayo stand, do not rest your hands on it; this could cause the mouth gag to be dislodged.

The mouth gag should be handed in the closed position.

Myringotomy and Tube Placement (M&T)
PREP TABLE

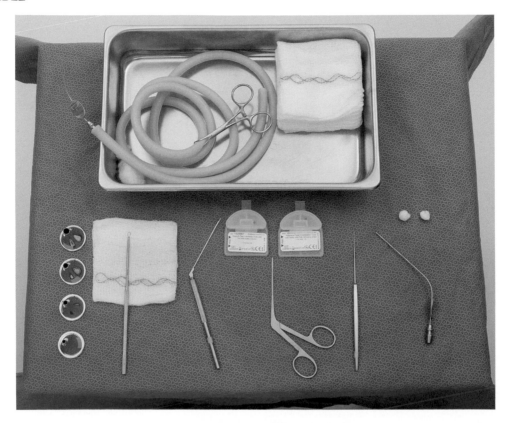

Definition: This is an incision into the tympanic membrane and placement of a ventilation tube (pressure equalization [PE] tube).

Reason Performed: It is performed to relieve pressure and allow drainage of serous or purulent fluid from the middle ear (otitis media).

Tech Tip: May be set up on a prep table or a Mayo stand. The ear speculum size is determined by the size of the patient. When exchanging instruments with the surgeon, they should not have to look away from the microscope. Change the suction tips from a no. 5 to a no. 3 after the surgeon inserts the ear tube. The larger tip can dislodge the tube.

Index

Note: Page numbers followed by "*f*" refer to figures.

A

Abdominal sucker. *See* Poole suction tip
Abdominal wall retractor. *See* Mayo
    abdominal retractor
Ablation wand, 240, 240f
  description of, 240
  insight on, 240
  other names for, 240
  uses of, 240
ACF retractor. *See* Anterior cervical
    fusion retractor
Adson cranial rongeur, 290, 290f
  description of, 290
  insight on, 290
  uses of, 290
Adson forceps, 25. *See also* Adson
    tonsil/Schnidt forceps
  description of, 25
  other names for, 25
  uses of, 25–26
Adson hook, sharp, 305, 305f
  description of, 305
  insight on, 305–306
  uses of, 305
Adson hypophyseal cup tissue forceps,
    302, 302f
  description of, 302
  insight on, 302
  other names for, 302
  uses of, 302
Adson periosteal elevator, 298, 298f
  description of, 298
  other names for, 298
  uses of, 298–299
Adson tissue forceps
  plain, 33, 33f
    description of, 33
    insight on, 33–34
    other names for, 33
    uses of, 33
  toothed, 34, 34f
    caution when using, 34
    description of, 34
    insight on, 34
    other names on, 34
    uses of, 34
Adson tonsil/Schnidt forceps, 200, 200f
  description of, 200
  other names for, 200
  uses of, 200–201
Adson with teeth forceps. *See* Adson
    tissue forceps, toothed
Alexander rasp. *See* Farabeuf rasp

Alligator forceps. *See* Wullstein ear forceps
Allis, big. *See* Allis-Adair forceps
Allis-Adair forceps, 111, 111f
  description of, 111
  insight on, 111
  other names for, 111
  uses of, 111
Allis forceps, 40, 40f
  curved, 203, 203f
    description of, 203
    insight on, 203–204
    other names for, 203
    uses of, 203
  description of, 40
  insight on, 40
  other names for, 40
  uses of, 40
Allison lung retractor, 341, 341f
  category of, 341
  description of, 341
  insight on, 341–342
  other names for, 341
  uses of, 341
Alm retractor, 270, 270f
  description of, 270
  uses of, 270–271
Anderson-Neivert guarded osteotome,
    188, 188f
  description of, 188
  insight on, 188
  uses of, 188
Andrews-Pynchon suction tip, 347, 347f
  category of, 347
  description of, 347
  insight on, 347
  other names for, 347
  uses of, 347
Andrews tongue depressor, 220, 220f
  description of, 220
  other names, 220
  uses of, 220
Anesthesia machine, 365, 365f
  description of, 365
  insight on, 365–366
  other names for, 365
  uses of, 365
Anesthesia work station. *See*
    Anesthesia machine
Aneurysm clip applier and clips, 285, 285f
  caution when using, 285
  description of, 285
  insight on, 285
  uses of, 285

Ankeney retractor, 345, 345f
  category of, 345
  description of, 345
  insight on, 345–346
  other names for, 345
  uses of, 345
Anterior cervical fusion retractor,
    312, 312f
  description of, 312
  other names for, 312
  uses of, 312
Antifog solution, 69, 69f
  description of, 69
  insight on, 69–70
  other names for, 69
  uses of, 69
Antrum rasp. *See* Wiener antrum rasp
Aortic punch, 327, 327f
  category of, 327
  description of, 327
  insight on, 327–328
  other names for, 327
  uses of, 327
Apical elevator, 212, 212f
  description of, 212
  insight on, 212
  other names, 212
  uses of, 212
Appendectomy, laparoscopic, 386,
    386f
Apple needle holder, 87, 87f
  description of, 87
  insight on, 87–88
  uses of, 87
Arch bars, 210, 210f
  description of, 210
  insight on, 210
  uses of, 210
Army-navy retractor, 41, 41f
  description of, 41
  insight on, 41–42
  other names for, 41
  uses of, 41
Army's retractor. *See* Army-navy
    retractor
Arthroscope. *See* 25° 4-mm lens
Arthroscopy boots. *See* Boot shoe
    covers
Arthroscopy probe, 262, 262f
  description of, 262
  insight on, 262–263
  other names for, 262
  uses of, 262

Asepto, 374, 374f
  caution when using, 374
  description of, 374
  insight on, 374
  other names for, 374
  uses of, 374
Atrac grasper, 81, 81f
  description of, 81
  insight on, 81–82
  other names for, 81
  uses of, 81
Atraumatic towel clamp. *See* Towel clip,
  nonpenetrating
Atrial retractor, 99, 99f
  category of, 99
  description of, 99
  insight on, 99
  other names for, 99
  uses of, 99
Aufricht nasal rasp, 180, 180f
  description of, 180
  insight on, 180–181
  uses of, 180
Aufricht nasal retractor, 198, 198f
  description of, 198
  uses of, 198
Automated washer (washer sterilizer),
  10–13
  perp and pack, 11–13
Auvard weighted vaginal speculum,
  116, 116f
  description of, 116
  insight on, 116
  other names for, 116
  uses of, 116

B

Babcock forceps, 40, 40f
  description of, 40
  uses of, 40–41
Baby ribbons. *See* Davis brain spatulas
Baby sucker. *See* Bulb syringe; Delee
  suction
Back table, 358, 358f, 380
  description of, 358
  insight on, 358
  other names for, 358
  uses of, 358
Back table cover, 377, 377f
  description of, 377
  insight on, 377
  other names for, 377
  uses of, 377
Back table pack, 377, 377f
  caution when using, 377–378
  description of, 377
  insight on, 377–378
  other names for, 377
  uses of, 377
Backhaus towel clip. *See* Towel clip,
  penetrating
Bacon cranial rongeur, 289, 289f
  description of, 289
  insight on, 289
  other name for, 289
  uses of, 289
Bailey rib contractor, 340, 340f
  category of, 340
  description of, 340

Bailey rib contractor *(Continued)*
  insight on, 340–341
  other names for, 340
  uses of, 340
Bakes common duct dilators, 57, 57f
  description of, 57
  insight on, 57–58
  other names for, 57
  uses of, 57
Balfour retractor, 61, 61f
  description of, 61
  insight on, 61
  other names for, 61
  uses of, 61
Ball loop electrode, 124, 124f
  description of, 124
  insight on, 124–125
  uses of, 124
Ball tip probe, 303, 303f
  description of, 303
  uses of, 303
Ballenger swivel knife, 183, 183f
  description of, 183
  other names for, 183
  uses of, 183–184
Ballenger V-shaped osteotome, 188, 188f
  description of, 188
  insight on, 188–189
  uses of, 188
Balloon dilator, 132f
  description of, 132
  insight on, 132–133
  uses of, 132
Bandage scissors. *See* Utility scissors
Barbara needle. *See* House-Barbara
  shattering needle
Barnhill adenoid curettes, 203, 203f
  description of, 203
  insight on, 203
  uses of, 203
Baron suction tips, 176, 176f
  description of, 176
  insight on, 176
  other names for, 176
  uses of, 176
Barraquer eye speculum, 156f
  description of, 156
  other names for, 156
  uses of, 156–157
Barraquer iris scissors, 147, 147f
  description of, 147
  insight on, 147
  uses of, 147
Barraquer iris spatula, 143, 143f
  description of, 143
  other names for, 143
  uses of, 143
Barraquer needle holder, 161, 161f
  description of, 161
  uses of, 161
Basin, 378, 378f
  description of, 378
  insight on, 378–379
  other names for, 378
  uses of, 378
Basin set. *See* Basin
Basin stand. *See* Ring stand
Baskin Robin. *See* Adson hypophyseal
  cup tissue forceps

Bayonet. *See* Jansen tissue forceps
B.B. forceps. *See* Cushing bipolar forceps
Bean rongeur. *See* Cushing pituitary
  rongeur
Beaver handle, 33, 33f
  description of, 33
  other names for, 33
  uses of, 33
Beck aortic clamp, 322, 322f
  category of, 322
  description of, 322
  other names for, 322
  uses of, 322–323
Becker septum scissors, 179, 179f
  description of, 179
  uses of, 179–180
Beckman retractor, 264, 264f, 307, 307f
  caution when using, 264, 307–308
  description of, 264, 307
  insight on, 264, 307–308
  uses of, 264, 307
Bellucci scissors, 174, 174f
  description of, 174
  insight on, 174
  other names for, 174
  uses of, 174
Bennett retractor, 263, 263f
  description of, 263
  insight on, 263
  uses of, 263
Bethune rib shears, 335, 335f
  category of, 335
  description of, 335
  insight on, 335–336
  uses of, 335
Beyer rongeur, 289, 298f
  caution when using, 289–290
  description of, 289
  insight on, 289–290
  uses of, 289
Bifurcated prostate retractor. *See* Young
  bifurcated retractor
Big ugly. *See* Sternal needle holder and
  wire twister
Big ugly's forceps. *See* Ferris-Smith
  tissue forceps
Billeau ear loop, 163, 163f
  description of, 163
  insight on, 163–164
  uses of, 163
Biological indicators, 15
Biopsy forceps, 128f. *See also*
  Hysteroscope biopsy forceps
  description of, 128
  insight on, 128–129
  uses of, 128
Bishop-Harmon iris tissue forceps,
  154, 154f
  description of, 154
  uses of, 154–155
Bit block. *See* Mouth prop
Bit edge. *See* Mouth prop
Bivalve speculum. *See* Graves vaginal
  speculum
Blanket warmer. *See* Warmer
Blount knee retractor, 269, 269f
  description of, 269
  insight on, 269–270
  uses of, 269

Blunt curette. *See* Thomas uterine curette
Blunt dissector, 75, 75f
    description of, 75
    insight on, 75–76
    uses of, 75
Blunt grasper, 82, 82f
    description of, 82
    uses of, 82
Blunt hook, 317, 317f
    category of, 317
    description of, 317
    insight on, 317–318
    other names for, 317
    uses of, 317
Blunt tip trocar. *See* Blunt trocar
Blunt trocar, 69, 69f
    description of, 69
    insight on, 69
    other names for, 69
    uses of, 69
Boettcher tonsil scissors, 201, 201f
    description of, 201
    insight on, 201–202
    other names for, 201
    uses of, 201
Boies elevator. *See* Goldman septum
        elevator
Bolt cutter. *See* Large pin cutter
Bone cement injector, 237, 237f
    description of, 237
    insight on, 237
    other names for, 237
    uses of, 237
Bone cement system, 237, 237f
    caution when using, 237–238
    description of, 237
    insight on, 237–238
    uses of, 237
Bone file, 248, 248f
    description of, 248
    insight on, 248–249
    other names for, 248
    uses of, 248
Bone hook, 265, 265f
    caution when using, 265
    description of, 265
    insight on, 265
    uses of, 265
Bone skid. *See* Lever skid humeral head
        retractor
Bone tamp, 236, 236f
    description of, 236
    insight on, 236
    other names for, 236
    uses of, 236
Bonney tissue forceps, 36, 36f
    caution when using, 36–37
    description of, 36
    insight on, 36–37
    other names for, 36
    uses of, 36
Bookwalter, 61, 61f
    description of, 61
    insight on, 61–62
    other names for, 61
    uses of, 61
Boot shoe covers, 353, 353f
    description of, 353
    insight on, 353–354

Boot shoe covers *(Continued)*
    other names for, 353
    uses of, 353
Booties. *See* Shoe covers
Bore needle. *See* Hypodermic needle
Boucheron ear speculum, 176, 176f
    description of, 176
    insight on, 176–177
    uses of, 176
Bouffant. *See* Headcover
Bovie. *See* Electrical surgical unit
Bovie pencil. *See* Electrosurgical pencil
Bovie spatula. *See* Permanent cautery
        spatula
Bowie-Dick test, 16
Bowman lacrimal probe, 155, 155f
    description of, 155
    insight on, 155–156
    other names for, 155
    uses of, 155
Box curette. *See* Kevorkian-Younge
        endocervical curette
Bozeman uterine dressing forceps,
        112, 112f
    description of, 112
    other names for, 112
    uses of, 112
Braun tenaculum. *See* Schroeder
        tenaculum
Breast biopsy, 381–389, 382f
Breast hook. *See* Mammoplasty hook
Bridge. *See* Telescope bridge
Briggs mammoplasty retractor, 232, 232f
    category of, 232
    description of, 232
    uses of, 232
Brown-Adson tissue forceps, 34, 34f
    caution when using, 34–35
    description of, 34
    insight on, 34–35
    other names for, 34
    uses of, 34
Brown forceps. *See* Brown-Adson
        tissue forceps
Browne deltoid retractor, 273, 273f
    description of, 273
    uses of, 273
Bruening septum forceps, 193, 193f
    description of, 193
    uses of, 193–194
Brun curette. *See* Spinal curette
Bruns oval bone curettes, 255, 255f
    description of, 255
    other names for, 255
    uses of, 255–256
Buck ear curette, 170, 170f
    description of, 170
    other names for, 170
    uses of, 170
Buford-Finochietto. *See* Burford rib
        spreader
Bugbee electrode, 125, 125f
    description of, 125
    insight on, 125
    uses of, 125
Bulb retractor. *See* Young bulb retractor
Bulb syringe, 119, 119f, 374, 374f
    description of, 119, 374
    insight on, 119, 374–375

Bulb syringe *(Continued)*
    other names for, 119, 374
    uses of, 119, 374
Bulldog. *See* DeBakey bulldog
Bullet nose dissector. *See* Cone tip
        dissector
Burford rib spreader, 343, 343f
    category of, 343
    description of, 343
    insight on, 343
    other names for, 343
    uses of, 343
Butter knife. *See* Goldman septum
        elevator

C

Caliper. *See* Townley caliper
Canal elevator. *See* House elevator
Canal knife. *See* House joint knife;
        House-Sheehy knife curette
Cannulated pin cutter, 254, 254f
    description of, 254
    insight on, 254
    other names for, 254
    uses of, 254
Caplan scissors, 178, 178f
    description of, 178
    uses of, 178–179
Caps. *See* Headcover
Capsule retractor, 272, 272f
    description of, 272
    other names for, 272
    uses of, 272–273
Capsulorhexis forceps, 153, 153f
    description of, 153
    insight on, 153
    uses of, 153
Cardiac suction. *See* Vascular
        suction tip
Carmalt forceps, 24, 24f
    description of, 24
    other names for, 24
    uses of, 24
Carpal tunnel release, 383, 383f
Carter-Glassman intestinal clamp,
        53, 53f
    description of, 53
    other names for, 53
    uses of, 53
Case packs. *See* Back table pack
Castro. *See* Castroviejo corneal
        scissors; Castroviejo needle holder
Castroviejo caliper, 142, 142f
    description of, 142
    uses of, 142
Castroviejo corneal scissors, 147f
    description of, 147
    other names for, 147
    uses of, 147–148
Castroviejo eye speculum, 157f
    description of, 157
    uses of, 157
Castroviejo needle holder, 160, 160f,
        349, 349f
    category of, 349
    description of, 160, 349
    insight on, 349
    other names for, 349
    uses of, 153, 349

Castroviejo suturing tissue forceps, 153f
    description of, 154
    insight on, 153–154
    uses of, 153
Cat paw. *See* Mathieu retractor
Cat paw retractor. *See* Senn retractor
Cath element. *See* Catheter deflecting
    element
Catheter deflecting element, 123, 123f
    description of, 123
    insight on, 123
    other names for, 123
    uses of, 123
Cautery pencil. *See* Electrosurgical
    pencil
Cautery spatula. *See* Permanent
    cautery spatula
Cawood retractor. *See* Minnesota
    cheek retractor
CD4 power system. *See* Cordless driver 4
CEEA stapler. *See* Intraluminal stapler
Cement gun. *See* Bone cement injector
Cerebellar retractor, 308, 308f
    caution when using, 308
    description of, 308
    insight on, 308
    uses of, 308
Cervical dilators. *See* Hank dilators;
    Hegar dilators; Pratt uterine dilators
Chandler elevator. *See* Chandler
    retractor
Chandler retractor, 265, 265f
    description of, 265
    insight on, 265–266
    other names for, 265
    uses of, 265
Channel locks. *See* Pliers
Charnley retractor, 267, 267f
    description of, 267
    insight on, 267–268
    other names for, 267
    uses of, 267
Cheek retractor. *See* Minnesota cheek
    retractor
Chemical indicators, 14
Cherries. *See* Dissector sponges
Chest spreader. *See* Ankeney retractor;
    Burford rib spreader; Finochietto rib
    spreader
Cholecystectomy, laparoscopic, 387, 387f
Cicherelli mastoid rongeur, 167, 167f
    description of, 167
    insight on, 167
    other names for, 167
    uses of, 167
Cinelli guarded osteotome, 190, 190f
    description of, 190
    insight on, 190
    uses of, 190
Circular stapler. *See* Intraluminal stapler
Clamp. *See* Crile forceps; Kelly forceps
    angled. *See* Cooley clamp; DeBakey
        peripheral vascular clamp
Claw grasper, 82f
    caution when using, 82–83
    description of, 82
    insight on, 82–83
    other names for, 82
    uses of, 82

Clayman lens forceps. *See* Lens
    insertion forceps
Clip applier. *See* Endo clip applier;
    Hemoclip applier
Cloward cervical retractor, 313, 313f
    description of, 313
    uses of, 313
Cloward vertebra spreader, 312, 312f
    description of, 312
    uses of, 312–313
Coag scissors. *See* Endoscopic
    scissors
Coakley antrum curettes, 187, 187f
    description of, 187
    other names for, 187
    uses of, 187–188
Cobb curettes, 297, 297f
    description of, 297
    uses of, 297–298
Cobb elevator, 297, 297f
    description of, 297
    insight on, 297
    uses of, 297
Cobb ring curettes, 298, 298f
    description of, 298
    uses of, 298
Coblation wand, 200, 200f
    description of, 200
    insight on, 200
    uses of, 200
Cobra. *See* Cobra grasper
Cobra grasper, 97, 97f
    category of, 97
    description of, 97
    other names for, 97
    uses of, 97
Cobra retractor, 269, 269f
    description of, 269
    insight on, 269
    uses of, 269
Cold cone knife. *See* Long angled #3
    knife handle
Colibri tissue forceps, 152, 152f
    description of, 152
    insight on, 152–153
    uses of, 152
Columella retractor. *See* Cottle
    columella forceps
Common duct dilators. *See* Bakes
    common duct dilators
Cone tip dissector, 76f
    description of, 76
    insight on, 76–77
    other names for, 76
    uses of, 76
Cookie cutter. *See* Areola marker
Cool cut. *See* Ablation wand
Cooley arterial retractor, 342, 342f
    category of, 342
    description of, 342
    insight on, 342
    other names for, 342
    uses of, 342
Cooley clamp, 321, 321f
    category of, 321
    description of, 321
    insight on, 321
    other names for, 321
    uses of, 321

Cooley coarctation clamp, 326, 326f
    category of, 326
    description of, 326
    other names for, 326
    uses of, 326–327
Cooley needle holder, 349, 349f
    category of, 349
    description of, 349
    insight on, 349
    uses of, 349
Cooley scissors, 330, 330f
    category of, 330
    description of, 330
    uses of, 330–331
Cord clamp, 104, 104f
    description of, 104
    insight on, 104
    uses of, 104
Cordless driver
    insight on, 246–247
Cordless driver 4, 246, 246f
    description of, 246
    other names for, 246
    uses of, 246
Cottle angular scissors, 179, 179f
    description of, 179
    insight on, 179
    other names for, 179
    uses of, 179
Cottle bone crusher, 177, 177f
    description of, 177
    insight on, 177–178
    uses of, 177
Cottle chisel, 189, 189f
    description of, 189
    insight on, 189–190
    other names for, 189
    uses of, 189
Cottle columella forceps, 195, 195f
    description of, 195
    insight on, 195
    other names for, 195
    uses of, 195
Cottle double hook retractor, 197, 197f
    description of, 197
    insight on, 197–198
    uses of, 197
Cottle knife guide and retractor, 197
    description of, 197
    uses of, 197
Cottle mallet, 178, 178f
    description of, 178
    insight on, 178
    other names for, 178
    uses of, 178
Cottle nasal knife, 185, 185f
    description of, 185
    insight on, 185
    uses of, 185
Cottle nasal speculum, 195, 195f
    uses of, 195–196
Cottle osteotome, 189, 189f
    description of, 189
    insight on, 189
    uses of, 189
Cottle septal elevator, 186, 186f
    description of, 186
    insight on, 186–187
    uses of, 186

Cottle tenaculum
  double, 229, 229f
    category of, 229
    caution when using, 229–230
    description of, 229
    insight on, 229
    other names for, 229
    uses of, 229
  single, 229, 229f
    category of, 229
    caution when using, 229
    description of, 229
    insight on, 229
    uses of, 229
Cottonoid sponges, 372, 372f
  description of, 372
  insight on, 372
  other names for, 372
  uses of, 372
Cover jacket, 351, 351f
  description of, 351
  insight on, 351–352
  other names for, 351
  uses of, 351
Crabtree dissector, 172, 172f
  description of, 172
  insight on, 172
  other names for, 172
  uses of, 172
Crane elevator, 211, 211f
  description of, 211
  other names, 211
  uses of, 211
Crane pick. *See* Crane elevator
Crego elevator, 250, 250f
  description of, 250
  insight on, 250–251
  uses of, 250
Cricket retractor. *See* Holzheimer
    retractor
Crile forceps, 23, 23f. *See also* Kelly
    forceps
  description of, 23
  insight on, 23
  other names for, 23
  uses of, 23
Crile-Wood needle holder, 31–32, 48f
  description of, 48
  insight on, 48
  other names for, 48
  uses of, 48
Crimper. *See* McGee wire crimping
    forceps
Cryer elevator, 211, 211f
  description of, 211
  insight on, 211–212
  other names, 211
  uses of, 211
Cryer forceps. *See* Lower anterior
    extraction forceps (151); Upper
    anterior extraction forceps (150)
Cup forceps. *See* Adson hypophyseal
    cup tissue forceps
Curettes. *See* Bruns oval bone curettes
  angled. *See* Lucas bone curette
Curved needle driver. *See* Heaney
    needle holder
Curved needle holder. *See* Heaney
    needle holder

Curved rings. *See* Thoracic ring forceps
Curved scissors, 95, 95f
  category of, 95
  description of, 95
  other names for, 95
  uses of, 95–96
Cushing bayonet tissue forceps, 302, 302f
  description of, 302
  insight on, 302–303
  uses of, 302
Cushing bipolar forceps, 286, 286f
  description of, 286
  insight on, 286
  other names for, 286
  uses of, 286
Cushing pituitary rongeur, 291, 291f
  caution when using, 291–292
  description of, 291
  insight on, 291–292
  other names for, 291
  uses of, 291
Cushing rongeur, 257, 257f
  description of, 257
  insight on, 257
  uses of, 257
Cushing vein retractor, 342, 342f
  category of, 342
  description of, 342
  insight on, 342–343
  uses of, 342
Custom pack. *See* Back table pack
CV suction tip. *See* Andrews-Pynchon
    suction tip
Cystoscope sheath and obturator,
    136, 136f
  description of, 136
  insight on, 136
  uses of, 136

D

da Vinci endoscope, 101, 101f
  category of, 101
  description of, 101
  insight on, 101
  uses of, 101
da Vinci robotic ports, 99, 99f
  category of, 99
  description of, 99
  insight on, 99–100
  other names for, 99
  uses of, 99
da Vinci system, 93, 93f
Dandy forceps, 286, 286f
  description of, 286
  other names for, 286
  uses of, 286–287
Dandy nerve hook, 306, 306f
  description of, 306
  uses of, 306
Davidson scapula retractor, 344, 344f
  category of, 344
  description of, 344
  insight on, 344–345
  uses of, 344
Davis brain spatulas, 303, 303f
  description of, 303
  insight on, 303–304
  other names for, 303
  uses of, 303

Davis scalp retractor, 310, 310f
  description of, 310
  uses of, 310–311
Dean rongeur, 167, 167f
  description of, 167
  insight on, 167–168
  uses of, 167
Dean scissors, 215, 215f
  description of, 215
  insight on, 215
  other names, 215
  uses of, 215
Deaver, small. *See* Deaver retractor, baby
Deaver retractor, 59, 59f
  baby, 118, 118f
    description of, 118
    other names for, 118
    uses of, 118–119
  description of, 59
  insight on, 59–60
  uses of, 59
DeBakes forceps. *See* DeBakey tissue
    forceps
DeBakey aortic clamp, 324, 324f
  category of, 324
  description of, 324
  uses of, 324
DeBakey bulldog, 319, 319f
  category of, 319
  description of, 319
  insight on, 319
  other names for, 319
  uses of, 319
DeBakey coarctation clamp, 325, 325f
  category of, 325
  description of, 325
  insight on, 325–326
  other names for, 325
  uses of, 325
DeBakey-Diethrich tissue forceps,
    338, 338f
  category of, 338
  description of, 338
  insight on, 338
  other names for, 338
  uses of, 338
DeBakey forceps, 97, 97f. *See also*
    DeBakey tissue forceps
  category of, 97
  description of, 97
  insight on, 97–98
  uses of, 97
DeBakey peripheral vascular clamp,
    324, 324f
  category of, 324
  description of, 324
  insight on, 324–325
  other names for, 324
  uses of, 324
DeBakey sidewinder aorta clamp,
    326, 326f
  category of, 326
  description of, 326
  insight on, 326
  other names for, 326
  uses of, 326
DeBakey tissue forceps, 36, 36f
  description of, 36
  insight on, 36

DeBakey tissue forceps *(Continued)*
    other names for, 36
    uses of, 36
DeBakey vascular tissue forceps, 339,
        339f
    category of, 339
    description of, 339
    insight on, 339
    uses of, 339
Deflecting bridge. *See* Catheter
        deflecting element
Deflecting mechanism. *See* Catheter
        deflecting element
Deflector. *See* Catheter deflecting
        element
Delee suction, 119, 119f
    caution when using, 119–120
    description of, 119
    insight on, 119–120
    other names for, 119
    uses of, 119
Delicate grasper. *See* Prograsp forceps
Dental mirror. *See* Mouth mirror
Dental pick. *See* Root tip pick
Depth gauge, 234, 234f. *See also* Sims
        uterine sound
    description of, 234
    insight on, 234–235
    other names for, 234
    uses of, 234
Dermamesher, 222, 222f
    category of, 222
    description of, 222
    insight on, 222–223
    other names for, 222
    uses of, 222
Dermatome, 223, 223f
    category of, 223
    caution when using, 223
    description of, 223
    insight on, 223
    other names for, 223
    uses of, 223
Dermatome blade, 223, 223f
    category of, 223
    caution when using, 223–224
    description of, 223
    insight on, 223–224
    other names for, 223
    uses of, 223
Desjardin gallstone forceps, 56, 56f
    description of, 56
    other names for, 56
    uses of, 56–57
Desmarres chalazion clamp, 151, 151f
    description of, 151
    insight on, 151
    other names for, 151
    uses of, 151
Desmarres lid retractor, 158f
    description of, 158
    uses of, 158–159
Diamond-flex retractor. *See* Endoflex
        retractor
Diamond pin cutter, 254, 254f
    description of, 254
    insight on, 254–255
    other names for, 254
    uses of, 254

Diathermy pencil. *See* Electrosurgical
        pencil
Diethrich bulldog, 319, 319f
    category of, 319
    description of, 319
    insight on, 319–320
    uses of, 319
Diethrich scissors, 328, 328f
    category of, 328
    description of, 328
    insight on, 328
    other names for, 328
    uses of, 328
Dilation and curettage (D & C), 381, 381f
Dissector. *See* Endo kittner
Dissector sponges, 371, 371f
    description of, 371
    insight on, 371
    other names for, 371
    uses of, 371
Ditto. *See* House strut hook
Dolphin nose dissector, 76, 76f
    description of, 76
    insight on, 76
    uses of, 76
Dornoch. *See* Suction
Double-ended Rich. *See* Richardson-
        Eastman retractor
Double-tooth tenaculum. *See* Schroeder
        vulsellum
Doyen clamp. *See* Doyen intestinal clamp
Doyen elevator and stripper. *See* Doyen
        rib raspatories
Doyen intestinal clamp, 53, 53f
    description of, 53
    insight on, 53–54
    other names for, 53
    uses of, 53
Doyen rib raspatories, 334, 334f
    category of, 334
    description of, 334
    insight on, 334–335
    other names for, 334
    uses of, 334
Dr. Fog. *See* Antifog solution
Dressing forceps. *See* Bozeman uterine
        dressing forceps
Drill bit guide. *See* Drill guide
Drill bit set, 247, 247f
    description of, 247
    other names for, 247
    uses of, 247
Drill box. *See* Drill bit set
Drill chuck. *See* Chuck and key
Drill guide, 238, 238f
    description of, 238
    insight on, 238
    other names for, 238
    uses of, 238
Drill sleeve. *See* Drill guide
Duckbill right and left biter, 257, 257f
    description of, 257
    insight on, 257–258
    uses of, 257
Duckbill speculum. *See* Graves vaginal
        speculum
Duckbill straight biter, 258
    description of, 258
    uses of, 258

Ducks scissors. *See* Diethrich scissors
Duct probes. *See* Bowman lacrimal
        probe
Dura hook, 304, 304f
    description of, 304
    insight on, 304–305
    uses of, 304
Dura scissors, angled. *See* Taylor dural
        scissors
Duval forceps. *See* Pennington forceps
Duval lung forceps, 339, 339f
    category of, 339
    description of, 339
    insight on, 339–340
    other names for, 339
    uses of, 339

E

Ear cup forceps. *See* Oval cup forceps,
        straight, right, left
Ear curettes. *See* Billeau ear loop;
        House double-ended curette;
        Spratt mastoid curettes
Ear knife. *See* House sickle knife;
        Myringotomy knife
Ear suction. *See* Baron suction tips
Ear syringe. *See* Bulb syringe
Eastman retractor, 118, 118f. *See also*
        Richardson-Eastman retractor
    description of, 118
    insight on, 118
    other names for, 118
    uses of, 118
EEA stapler. *See* Intraluminal stapler
Electrical surgical unit, 362, 362f
    description of, 362
    insight on, 362–363
    other names for, 362
    uses of, 362
Electrosurgical pencil, 21, 21f
    caution when using, 21–22
    description of, 21
    insight on, 21–22
    other names for, 21
    uses of, 21
Elevator, angular. *See* Crane elevator
Ellik evacuator, 134, 134f
    description of, 134
    insight on, 134–135
    uses of, 134
Endo catch, 74, 74f
    description of, 74
    insight on, 74
    other names for, 74
    uses of, 74
Endo clip applier, 88, 88f
    description of, 88
    other names for, 88
    uses of, 88–89
Endo fan retractor, 84, 84f
    description of, 84
    insight on, 84–85
    other names for, 84
    uses of, 84
Endo-fog. *See* Antifog solution
Endo GIA stapler, 89, 89f
    description of, 89
    insight on, 89
    uses of, 89

Endo harmonic scalpel, 73, 73f
    description of, 73
    insight on, 73–74
    other names for, 73
    uses of, 73
Endo KD. *See* Endo kittner
Endo kit. *See* Endo kittner
Endo kittner, 70, 70f
    description of, 70
    insight on, 70–71
    other names for, 70
    uses of, 70
Endo paddle retractor, 85, 85f
    description of, 85
    insight on, 85
    uses of, 85
Endo peanut. *See* Endo kittner
Endo pouch. *See* Endo catch
Endo right-angle forceps, 75, 75f
    description of, 75
    insight on, 75
    other names for, 75
    uses of, 75
Endo scrub. *See* Endo-scrub lens
    cleaning sheath
Endo-scrub lens cleaning sheath, 198,
    198f
    description of, 198
    insight on, 198
    other names for, 198
    uses of, 198
Endo shears. *See* Endoscopic scissors
Endocervical curette. *See* Kevorkian-
    Younge endocervical curette
Endoeye, 92f
    description of, 92
    insight on, 92
    other names for, 92
    uses of, 92
Endoflex retractor, 85, 85f
    description of, 85
    insight on, 85–86
    other names for, 85
    uses of, 85
Endopath thoracic trocar, 317, 317f
    category of, 317
    description of, 317
    insight on, 317
    other names for, 317
    uses of, 317
Endosac. *See* Endo catch
Endoscopic allis forceps, 80f
    description of, 80
    uses of, 80–81
Endoscopic aspirating needle, 87, 87f
    caution when using, 87
    description of, 87
    uses of, 87
Endoscopic babcock forceps, 81, 81f
    description of, 81
    uses of, 81
Endoscopic biopsy forceps, 78, 78f
    description of, 78
    insight on, 78–79
    uses of, 78
Endoscopic biopsy punch, 79, 79f
    description of, 79
    insight on, 79
    uses of, 79

Endoscopic camera, 89, 89f, 137, 137f,
    275, 275f
    description of, 89, 137, 275
    insight on, 89–90, 137, 275
    uses of, 89, 137, 275
Endoscopic cholangiogram forceps, 79, 79f
    description of, 79
    insight on, 79–80
    other names for, 79
    uses of, 79
Endoscopic Debakey forceps, 80, 80f
    description of, 80
    uses of, 80
Endoscopic hook scissors, 78, 78f
    description of, 78
    insight on, 78
    uses of, 78
Endoscopic scissors, 77, 77f
    description of, 77
    insight on, 77–78
    other names for, 77
    uses of, 77
EndoWrist, 94, 94f
    description of, 94
    insight on, 94
    uses of, 94
Enucleation scissors, 149, 149f
    description of, 149
    uses of, 149–150
ESU. *See* Electrical surgical unit
Ethylene oxide gas (EtO), 20
Evacuator, disposable. *See* Microvasive
    evacuator
Exam gloves, 356, 356f
    caution when using, 356
    description of, 356
    insight on, 356
    other names for, 356
    uses of, 356
Exploratory laparotomy, 384, 384f
Eye bipolar forceps. *See* Jeweler's
    bipolar forceps
Eye cautery forceps. *See* Jeweler's
    bipolar forceps
Eye protection, 354, 354f
    description of, 354
    insight on, 354–355
    other names for, 354
    uses of, 354
Eye suture scissors, 149f
    description of, 149
    insight on, 149
    uses of, 149
Eyewear. *See* Eye protection

F

Face mask. *See* Surgical masks
Face shields. *See* Eye protection
Fan finger retractor. *See* Endo fan
    retractor
Fan retractor. *See* Atrial retractor
Fancy clamp. *See* Adson forceps;
    Adson tonsil/Schnidt forceps
Farabeuf rasp, 332, 332f
    category of, 332
    description of, 332
    insight on, 332
    other names for, 332
    uses of, 332

Farrior ear speculum, 177, 177f
    description of, 177
    insight on, 177
    uses of, 177
Favaloro. *See* Internal mammary
    retractor
Female dilators. *See* Walther female
    urethral sounds
Female sounds. *See* Walther female
    urethral sounds
Fenestrated grasper. *See* Prograsp
    forceps
Fenestrated rongeur. *See* Wilde rongeur
Ferguson gallstone scoop, 52, 52f
    description of, 52
    insight on, 52–53
    other names for, 52
    uses of, 52
Ferris-Smith tissue forceps, 37, 37f
    caution when using, 37
    description of, 37
    insight on, 37
    other names for, 37
    uses of, 37
Fiberoptic light cord, 90f, 137, 137f, 275,
    275f
    caution when using, 90, 137–138,
        275
    description of, 90, 137, 275
    insight on, 90, 137–138, 275
    other names for, 90, 137, 275
    uses of, 90, 137, 275
Filiforms and followers, 132, 132f
    description of, 132
    insight on, 132
    uses of, 132
Fine needle driver. *See* Crile-Wood
    needle holder
Fine needle holder. *See* Crile-Wood
    needle holder
Finger-control suction. *See* Baron
    suction tips
Finger retractor. *See* Atrial retractor;
    Holzheimer retractor
Finochietto rib spreader, 343, 343f
    category of, 343
    description of, 343
    other names for, 343
    uses of, 343–344
5-mm 0-degree endoscope, 91, 91f
    caution when using, 91–92
    description of, 91
    insight on, 91–92
    other names for, 91
    uses of, 91
Flag elevators. *See* Cryer elevator
Flap knife. *See* House joint knife
Flash sterilizer, 18–19. *See also*
    Immediate use steam sterilizer
Flasher. *See* Immediate use steam
    sterilizer
Fletcher forceps. *See* Foerster sponge
    forceps
Flexible ureteroscope, 139, 139f
    description of, 139
    insight on, 139
    uses of, 139
Flexipath. *See* Endopath thoracic trocar
Fluid warmer. *See* Warmer

Foerster sponge forceps, 39, 39f
    description of, 39
    insight on, 39–40
    other names for, 39
    uses of, 39
Fogarty clamp with jaw inserts, 323, 323f
    category of, 323
    description of, 323
    insight on, 323–324
    other names for, 323
    uses of, 323
Forceps. *See* Simpson obstetrical
        forceps
Fork. *See* Capsule retractor
45 clamp. *See* DeBakey peripheral
        vascular clamp
4 × 4 dressing sponge, 372, 372f
    description of, 372
    insight on, 372–373
    other names for, 372
    uses of, 372
4-mm sheath and sharp obturator,
        239, 239f
    description of, 239
    insight on, 239–240
    uses of, 239
4-mm sheath with blunt obturator,
        239, 239f
    description of, 239
    insight on, 239
    uses of, 239
Fox eye shield, 141f
    description of, 141
    insight on, 141
    uses of, 141
Frazier suction tip, 46, 46f
    description of, 46
    insight on, 46–47
    uses of, 46
Fred. *See* Antifog solution
Freeman areola marker, 221, 221f
    category of, 221
    description of, 221
    insight on, 221–222
    other names for, 221
    uses of, 221
Freer elevator, 251, 251f. *See also* Freer
        septum elevator
    description of, 251
    insight on, 251
    uses of, 251
Freer septum elevator, 186, 186f
    description of, 186
    other names for, 186
    uses of, 186
Freer septum knife, 184, 184f
    description of, 184
    insight on, 184
    other names for, 184
    uses of, 184
Fukuda. *See* Fukuda humeral head
        retractor
Fukuda humeral head retractor,
        271, 271f
    description of, 271
    other names for, 271
    uses of, 271–272
Fukushima. *See* Leyla retractor;
        Teardrop suction tip

G

Gallbladder trocar, 55, 55f
    description of, 55
    insight on, 55–56
    uses of, 55
Garrett vascular dilators, 341, 341f
    category of, 341
    description of, 341
    insight on, 341
    uses of, 341
Gas machine. *See* Anesthesia machine
Gauze sponges. *See* 4 × 4 dressing
        sponge
Gaylor punch. *See* Thomas-Gaylor
        uterine biopsy forceps
Gelfoam masher. *See* House gelfoam
        press
Gelpi retractor, 46, 46f
    caution when using, 46
    description of, 46
    insight on, 46
    uses of, 46
Gemini forceps, 54, 54f. *See also*
        Lahey gall duct forceps;
        Mixter forceps
    description of, 54
    insight on, 54
    other names for, 54
    uses of, 54
Geobacillus stearothermophilus
        biological indicators, 15
Gerald tissue forceps, 337, 337f
    category of, 337
    description of, 337
    insight on, 337–338
    other names for, 337
    uses of, 337
GIA stapler. *See* Linear cutter-stapler
Gigli saw, 244, 244f
    caution when using, 244–245
    description of, 244
    uses of, 244–245
Gillies hook. *See* Skin hook
Gimmick. *See* House elevator
Glassman clamp. *See* Carter-Glassman
        intestinal clamp
Glidewire. *See* Guidewire
Glover bulldog, 320, 320f
    category of, 320
    description of, 320
    insight on, 320
    uses of, 320
Glover patent ductus, 322, 322f
    category of, 322
    description of, 322
    insight on, 322
    uses of, 322
Gluck rib shear, 332, 332f
    category of, 332
    description of, 332
    insight on, 332–333
    other names for, 332
    uses of, 332
Goelet retractor, 42, 42f
    description of, 42
    insight on, 42
    other names for, 42
    uses of, 42
Goggles. *See* Eye protection

Goldies. *See* Potts-Smith tissue forceps
Goldman septum elevator, 187, 187f
    description of, 187
    other names for, 187
    uses of, 187
Grad pitcher. *See* Graduated pitcher
Graduated pitcher, 379, 379f
    description of, 379
    insight on, 379
    other names for, 379
    uses of, 379
Graether collar button, 143, 143f
    description of, 143–144
    other names for, 143
    uses of, 143
Graspers. *See* Hysteroscope grasping
        forceps
Graves vaginal speculum, 116, 116f
    description of, 116
    insight on, 116–117
    other names for, 116
    uses of, 116
Gravity displacement, 17
Green retractor, 207, 207f
    description of, 207
    other names for, 207
    uses of, 207–208
Grunwald suture ring, 318, 318f
    category of, 318
    caution when using, 318
    description of, 318
    insight on, 318
    other names for, 318
    uses of, 318
Guidewire, 125, 125f
    description of, 125
    insight on, 125–126
    other names for, 125
    uses of, 125

H

Halsey needle holder, 233, 233f
    category of, 233
    description of, 233
    uses of, 233
Halstead forceps, 22, 22f
    description of, 22
    other names for, 22
    uses of, 22
Hammer. *See* Mallet
Hank dilators, 114, 114f
    description of, 114
    insight on, 114
    other names for, 114
    uses of, 114
Harmonic scalpel, 22, 22f
    description of, 22
    insight on, 22
    other names for, 22
    uses of, 22
Harrington heart retractor. *See*
        Harrington retractor
Harrington retractor, 60, 60f
    description of, 60
    other names for, 60
    uses of, 60
Hartman forceps. *See* Halstead
        forceps
Hasson trocar. *See* Blunt trocar

Headcover, 352, 352f
  caution when using, 352
  description of, 352
  insight on, 352
  other names for, 352
  uses of, 352
Heaney-Ballentine hysterectomy
      forceps, 103, 103f
  description of, 103
  insight on, 103–104
  other names for, 103
  uses of, 103
Heaney clamp. *See* Heaney-Ballentine
      hysterectomy forceps
Heaney hysterectomy forceps, 103, 103f
  description of, 103
  insight on, 103
  other names for, 103
  uses of, 103
Heaney needle driver. *See* Heaney
      needle holder
Heaney needle holder, 120, 120f
  description of, 120
  insight on, 120
  other names for, 120
  uses of, 120
Heaney retractor, 117, 117f
  description of, 117
  insight on, 117–118
  other names for, 117
  uses of, 117
Heaney uterine biopsy curette, 106, 106f
  caution when using, 106
  description of, 106
  uses of, 106
Heavy tissue scissors. *See* Mayo
      scissors, curved
Heavy wire cutter, 336, 336f
  category of, 336
  description of, 336
  insight on, 336
  other names for, 336
  uses of, 336
Hegar dilators, 114, 114f
  description of, 114
  insight on, 114–115
  other names for, 114
  uses of, 114
Heiss retractor. *See* Holzheimer
      retractor
Hemoclip applier, 51, 51f, 320, 320f.
      See also Endo clip applier; Surgiclip
      applier
  category of, 320
  description of, 51, 320
  insight on, 51, 320–321
  other names for, 51, 320
  uses of, 51, 320
Hemostat forceps. *See* Crile forceps;
      Kelly forceps
Herrick kidney clamp, 126, 126f
  description of, 126
  other names for, 126
  uses of, 126–127
Heymann-Knight angular scissors. *See*
      Knight angular scissors
Hibbs retractor, 263, 263f
  description of, 263
  uses of, 263–264

Hoen periosteal elevator, 299, 299f
  description of, 299
  uses of, 299
Hohmann. *See* Hohmann retractor, sharp
Hohmann retractor
  blunt, 267, 267f
    description of, 267
    uses of, 267
  mini, 266, 266f
    description of, 266
    insight on, 266
    uses of, 266
  sharp, 266, 266f
    description of, 266
    insight on, 266–267
    other names for, 266
    uses of, 266
Holzheimer retractor, 231, 231f. *See
      also* Jarit cross action retractor
  category of, 231
  description of, 231
  other names of, 231
  uses of, 231–232
Hoods hat. *See* Headcover
Hooks. *See* Cottle tenaculum, double
House-Barbara shattering needle, 171, 171f
  description of, 171
  insight on, 171
  other names for, 171
  uses of, 171
House-Dieter malleus nipper, 173, 173f
  description of, 173
  other names for, 173
  uses of, 173–174
House double-ended curette, 169, 169f
  description of, 169
  insight on, 169–170
  other names for, 169
  uses of, 169
House elevator, 166, 166f
  description of, 166
  insight on, 166
  other names for, 166
  uses of, 166
House gelfoam press, 163, 163f
  description of, 163
  other names for, 163
  uses of, 163
House hough, 171, 171f
  description of, 171
  insight on, 171–172
  uses of, 171
House joint knife, 165, 165f
  description of, 165
  insight on, 165–166
  other names for, 165
  uses of, 165
House oval window pick, 168, 168f
  description of, 168
  insight on, 168–169
  other names for, 168
  uses of, 168
House pick, 168, 168f
  description of, 168
  insight on, 168
  uses of, 168
House-Sheehy knife curette, 165, 165f
  description of, 165
  insight on, 165

House-Sheehy knife curette *(Continued)*
  other names for, 165
  uses of, 165
House sickle knife, 164, 164f
  description of, 164
  insight on, 164–165
  other names for, 164
  uses of, 164
House strut caliper, 162–208, 162f
  description of, 162
  other names for, 162
  uses of, 162–163
House strut hook, 172, 172f
  description of, 172
  insight on, 172–173
  other names for, 172
  uses of, 172
Huck towels. *See* Towel pack
Hudson brace. *See* Hudson handheld drill
Hudson handheld drill, 301, 301f
  description of, 301
  insight on, 301–302
  other names for, 301
  uses of, 301
Hulka tenaculum, 110, 110f
  caution when using, 110–111
  description of, 110
  other names for, 110
  uses of, 110–111
Humby. *See* Watson skin graft knife
Humeral head. *See* Fukuda humeral
      head retractor
Humeral head retractor, 271, 271f
  description of, 271
  uses of, 271
Hunt chalazion clamp, 151, 151f
  description of, 151
  insight on, 151–152
  other names for, 151
  uses of, 151
Hunter bowel grasper, 83, 83f
  description of, 83
  uses of, 83
Hupp tracheal hook, 204, 204f
  description of, 204
  insight on, 204
  other names for, 204
  uses of, 204
Hurd dissector, 207, 207f
  description of, 207
  other names for, 207
  uses of, 207
Hurd elevator. *See* Hurd dissector
Hydragrip. *See* Fogarty clamp with jaw
      inserts
Hydrogen peroxide gas plasma
      (HPGP), 19–20
Hypo. *See* Hypodermic needle
Hypodermic needle, 373, 373f
  caution when using, 373–374
  description of, 373
  insight on, 373–374
  other names for, 373
  uses of, 373
Hyster clamps. *See* Heaney hysterectomy
      forceps
Hysteroscope biopsy forceps, 108, 108f
  description of, 108
  insight on, 108–109

Hysteroscope biopsy forceps *(Continued)*
  other names for, 108
  uses of, 108
Hysteroscope grasping forceps, 113f
  description of, 113
  insight on, 113–114
  other names for, 113
  uses of, 113
Hysteroscope scissors, 108, 108f
  description of, 108
  insight on, 108
  other names for, 108
  uses of, 108
Hysteroscopic scissors. *See*
    Hysteroscope scissors

I

Iglesias. *See* Working element
Immediate use steam sterilizer, 18–19, 369f
  description of, 369
  insight on, 369
  other names for, 369
  uses of, 369
Inguinal hernia repair, 385, 385f
Instrument table. *See* Back table
Instrument tray. *See* Mayo stand
Insufflation needle. *See* Verres needle
Insufflation tubing, 71, 71f
  description of, 71
  insight on, 71
  uses of, 71
Internal mammary retractor, 346, 346f
  category of, 346
  description of, 346
  insight on, 346–347
  other names for, 346
  uses of, 346
Intraluminal stapler, 65, 65f
  description of, 65
  insight on, 65
  other names for, 65
  uses of, 65
Intravenous pole. *See* IV pole
Iris scissors, 224, 224f
  category of, 224
  caution when using, 224–225
  description of, 224
  insight on, 224–225
  uses of, 224
Iris spatula. *See* Barraquer eye
    speculum
Irish retractor. *See* O'Sullivan-O'Connor
    retractor
Irrigating cannula. *See* Irrigating needle
Irrigating needle, 144, 144f
  description of, 144
  insight on, 144–145
  other names for, 144
  uses of, 144
Irrigating syringe. *See* Asepto
Irrigation tubing, 121, 121f
  description of, 121
  insight on, 121–122
  other names for, 121
  uses of, 121
Israel rake retractor, 268, 268f
  description of, 268
  insight on, 268–269
  uses of, 268

Israelli retractor. *See* Volkman retractor
IV pole, 366f
  description of, 366
  other names for, 366
  uses of, 366

J

J hook, 72, 72f
  description of, 72
  insight on, 72–73
  uses of, 72
Jacobs Chuck and key, 242, 242f
  description of, 242
  other names for, 242
  uses of, 242
Jacobs tenaculum. *See* Jacobs vulsellum
Jacobs uterine forceps. *See* Jacobs
    vulsellum
Jacobs vulsellum, 109, 109f
  caution when using, 109
  description of, 109
  insight on, 109
  other names for, 109
  uses of, 109
Jacobsen needle holder, 315, 315f
  description of, 315
  uses of, 315
Jameson forceps, 155, 155f
  description of, 155
  other names for, 155
  uses of, 155
Jameson muscle hook, 159, 159f
  description of, 159
  uses of, 159–160
Jameson scissors. *See* Reynolds scissors
Jamison scissors, 226, 226f, 329, 329f
  category of, 226, 329
  description of, 226, 329
  insight on, 329
  other names for, 329
  uses of, 226–227, 329
Jansen mastoid retractor, 175, 175f
  description of, 175
  uses of, 175–176
Jansen-Middleton septum forceps,
    190, 190f
  description of, 190
  insight on, 190–191
  uses of, 190
Jansen scalp retractor, 311, 311f
  description of, 311
  uses of, 311
Jansen tissue forceps, 194, 194f
  description of, 194
  insight on, 194
  other names for, 194
  uses of, 194
Jaritrack retractor. *See* Bookwalter
Javid carotid artery clamp, 323, 323f
  category of, 323
  description of, 323
  insight on, 323
  other names for, 323
  uses of, 323
Javid carotid shunt clamp. *See* Javid
    carotid artery clamp
Jennings mouth gag, 206, 206f
  description of, 206
  uses of, 206–207

Jeweler's bipolar forceps, 141, 141f
  description of, 141
  insight on, 141–142
  other names for, 141
  uses of, 141
Jeweler's forceps, 152, 152f
  description of, 152
  insight on, 152
  uses of, 152
Jimmy. *See* Crabtree dissector
Joker. *See* Adson periosteal elevator
Jones towel clip. *See* Towel clip,
    penetrating
Joplin. *See* Lewin bone holding
    forceps
Joseph button-end knife, 184, 184f
  description of, 184
  uses of, 184–185
Joseph double skin hook, 228, 228f
  category of, 228
  caution when using, 228
  description of, 228
  insight on, 228–229
  uses of, 228
Joseph hook. *See* Skin hook
Joseph scissors, 201, 201f
  description of, 201
  insight on, 201
  uses of, 201
Joseph single skin hook, 228, 228f
  category of, 228
  caution when using, 228
  description of, 228
  insight on, 228
  uses of, 228
Joseph skin hooks, 204, 204f
  description of, 204
  other names for, 204
  uses of, 204–205

K

K wires. *See* Kirschner wires
Kaye facelift scissors, 225, 225f
  category of, 225
  description of, 225
  other names for, 225
  uses of, 225
Kelly forceps, 23, 23f. *See also* Crile
    forceps
  description of, 23
  other names for, 23
  uses of, 23–24
Kelly retractor, 59, 59f
  description of, 59
  insight on, 59
  uses of, 59
Kelly scissors, 214, 214f
  description of, 214
  insight on, 214–215
  other names, 214
  uses of, 214
Kern bone holding forceps, 260, 260f
  description of, 260
  insight on, 260
  uses of, 260
Kerrison-Costen rongeur, 183, 183f
  description of, 183
  insight on, 183
  uses of, 183

Kerrison rongeur, 182, 182f, 291, 291f
  caution when using, 291
  description of, 182, 291
  insight on, 182–183, 291
  other names for, 182, 291
  uses of, 182, 291
Kevorkian curette. *See* Kevorkian-
    Younge endocervical curette
Kevorkian-Younge endocervical curette,
    105, 105f
  description of, 105
  other names for, 105
  uses of, 105–106
Key elevator. *See* Key periosteal elevator
Key periosteal elevator, 250, 250f
  description of, 250
  insight on, 250
  uses of, 250
Kick bucket, 360, 360f
  description of, 360
  insight on, 360–361
  other names for, 360
  uses of, 360
Killian nasal speculum, 196, 196f
  description of, 196
  uses of, 196–197
Kirschner wires, 240, 240f
  description of, 240
  insight on, 240–241
  other names for, 240
  uses of, 240
Kitners. *See* Dissector sponges
Kleppinger bipolar forceps, 73, 73f
  description of, 73
  insight on, 73
  uses of, 73
Knapp iris scissors, 146, 146f
  description of, 146
  uses of, 146–147
Knapp strabismus scissors, 146, 146f
  description of, 146
  uses of, 146
Knee arthroplasty set. *See* Total knee
    instruments
Knight angular scissors, 180, 180f
  description of, 180
  other names for, 180
  uses of, 180
Knot pusher, 88, 88f
  description of, 88
  insight on, 88
  uses of, 88
Koch forceps. *See* Kocher forceps
Kocher forceps, 41, 41f
  caution when using, 41
  curved. *See* Ochsner forceps, curved
  description of, 41
  insight on, 41
  other names for, 41
  uses of, 41
Kolbel self-retaining glenoid retractor,
    273, 273f
  description of, 273
  uses of, 273–274

L

L hook, 72, 72f
  description of, 72
  insight on, 72
  uses of, 72

Lacrimal dilators. *See* Bowman lacrimal
    probe
Lahey forceps. *See* Gemini forceps;
    Mixter forceps
Lahey gall duct forceps, 54, 54f
  description of, 54
  insight on, 54–55
  other names for, 54
  uses of, 54
Lambert-Kay aorta clamp, 325, 325f
  category of, 325
  description of, 325
  insight on, 325
  other names for, 325
  uses of, 325
Lambotte osteotome, 253, 253f
  description of, 253
  insight on, 253–254
  uses of, 253
Langenbeck periosteal elevator, 299, 299f
  description of, 299
  uses of, 299–300
Lap pads. *See* Laparotomy sponges
Laparoscopic appendectomy, 386, 386f
Laparoscopic cart, 66, 66f
  description of, 66
  insight on, 66
  other names for, 66
  trocars, 66–67
  uses of, 66
Laparoscopic cholecystectomy, 387
Laparoscopic tolly. *See* Laparoscopic cart
Laparoscopic tower. *See* Laparoscopic cart
Laparotomy, exploratory, 384, 384f
Laparotomy sponges, 370, 370f
  caution when using, 370–371
  description of, 370
  insight on, 370–371
  other names for, 370
  uses of, 370
Laps. *See* Laparotomy sponges
Large bone cutters. *See* Liston bone
    cutting forceps
Large frag set. *See* Large fragment set
Large fragment set, 276, 276f
  description of, 276
  insight on, 276–277
  other names for, 276
  uses of, 276
Large mouth rongeur. *See* Stille-Luer
    rongeur
Large needle driver, 100, 100f
  category of, 100
  description of, 100
  insight on, 100–101
  other names for, 100
  uses of, 100
Large needle holder. *See* Large needle
    driver
Large pin cutter, 255, 255f
  caution when using, 255
  description of, 255
  insight on, 255
  other names for, 255
  uses of, 255
Laryngeal mirror, 199, 199f. *See also*
    Mouth mirror
  description of, 199
  insight on, 199
  uses of, 199

Lateral retractor. *See* Eastman retractor;
    Heaney retractor
LDS stapler. *See* Ligating and dividing
    stapler
Lead. *See* Lead apron
Lead apron, 355, 355f
  description of, 355
  insight on, 355–356
  other names for, 355
  uses of, 355
Lead hand, 243, 243f
  description of, 243
  insight on, 243–244
  uses of, 243
Lebsche knife, 331, 331f
  category of, 331
  description of, 331
  insight on, 331–332
  other names for, 331
  uses of, 331
Lee bronchus clamp, 327, 327f
  category of, 327
  description of, 327
  insight on, 327
  uses of, 327
Leep loop electrode, 102, 102f
  description of, 102
  insight on, 102–103
  other names for, 102
  uses of, 102
Left upper molar extraction forceps
    (88L), 216, 216f
  description of, 216
  insight on, 216
  other names, 216
  uses of, 216
Leiberman eye speculum, 158f
  description of, 158
  uses of, 158
Leksell rongeur, 290, 290f
  caution when using, 290–291
  description of, 290
  insight on, 290–291
  uses of, 290
Lempert elevator, 166, 166f
  description of, 166
  insight on, 166–167
  uses of, 166
Lens endoscope. *See* 10-mm 0°
    endoscope; 10-mm 30° endoscope
Lens inserter. *See* Lens insertion
    forceps
Lens insertion forceps, 150, 150f
  description of, 150
  other names for, 150
  uses of, 150–151
Lens rigid endoscope. *See* 5-mm 0°
    endoscope
Lens warmer, 70, 70f
  description of, 70
  insight on, 70
  uses of, 70
Lever skid humeral head retractor,
    272, 272f
  description of, 237
  other names for, 272
  uses of, 272
Lewin bone holding forceps, 261, 261f
  description of, 261
  insight on, 261

Lewin bone holding forceps *(Continued)*
  other names for, 261
  uses of, 261
Lewis rasp, 181, 181f
  description of, 181
  insight on, 181
  uses of, 181
Leyla retractor, 308, 308f
  caution when using, 308–309
  description of, 308
  other names for, 308
  uses of, 308–309
Leyla-Yasargil. *See* Leyla retractor
Lift scissors. *See* Kaye facelift scissors
Ligaclip. *See* Surgiclip applier
Ligaclip applier. *See* Hemoclip applier
Ligasure, 71, 71f
  description of, 71
  insight on, 71–72
  uses of, 71
Ligating and dividing stapler, 64, 64f
  description of, 64
  insight on, 64–65
  other names for, 64
  uses of, 64
Light cord. *See* Fiberoptic light cord
Light cover. *See* Light handle cover
Light gloves. *See* Light handle cover
Light handle cover, 375, 375f
  description of, 375
  insight on, 375
  other names for, 375
  uses of, 375
Lilly scissors, 331, 331f
  category of, 331
  description of, 331
  insight on, 331
  uses of, 331
Linear cutter-stapler, 63, 63f
  description of, 63
  insight on, 63–64
  other names for, 63
  uses of, 63
Linear stapler, 64, 64f
  description of, 64
  insight on, 64
  other names for, 64
  uses of, 64
Liposuction cannula, 232, 232f
  category of, 232
  description of, 232
  insight on, 232–233
  uses of, 232
Lister bandage scissors, 27, 27f
  caution when using, 27–28
  description of, 27
  insight on, 27–28
  other names for, 27
  uses of, 27
Liston bone cutting forceps, 251, 251f
  description of, 251
  insight on, 251–252
  other names for, 251
  uses of, 251
Littler plastic surgery scissors, 225, 225f
  category of, 225
  description of, 225
  insight on, 225–226
  other names for, 225
  uses of, 225

Littler scissors, 247, 247f
  description of, 247
  insight on, 247–248
  uses of, 247
Littler's. *See* Littler plastic surgery
    scissors
Long angled #3 knife handle, 107, 107f
  description of, 107
  insight on, 107–108
  other names for, 107
  uses of, 107
Long curved forceps. *See* Sarot forceps
Long handle. *See* #3 long knife handle
Long knife. *See* #3 long knife handle
Long scalpel. *See* #3 long knife handle
Loop. *See* Leep loop electrode; Loop
    electrode
Loop electrode, 124, 124f
  description of, 124
  insight on, 124
  other names for, 124
  uses of, 124
Lothrop uvula retractor, 205, 205f
  description of, 205
  uses of, 205–206
Love nerve root retractor (angled), 306,
    306f
  description of, 306
  insight on, 306–307
  uses of, 306
Low-heat sterilizers, 19
Lower anterior extraction forceps (151),
    218, 218f
  description of, 218
  insight on, 218
  other names, 218
  uses of, 218
Lower molar extraction forceps (17),
    217, 217f
  description of, 217
  insight on, 217
  other names, 217
  uses of, 217
Lowman bone clamp, 260, 260f
  description of, 260
  insight on, 260–261
  uses of, 260
Lowsley prostatic tractor, 129, 129f
  description of, 129
  insight on, 129–130
  uses of, 129
Lucas bone curette, 213, 213f
  description of, 213
  other names, 213
  uses of, 213–214
Lung clamp. *See* Duval lung forceps;
    Pennington forceps
Luxating elevator. *See* Apical elevator

M

Male sounds. *See* Van Buren urethral
    sounds
Malleable retractor. *See* Ribbon
    retractor
Mallet, 235, 235f, 285, 285f. *See also*
    Cottle mallet
  description of, 235, 285
  insight on, 235–236, 285–286
  other names for, 235
  uses of, 235, 285

Maltz-Lipsett. *See* Maltz rasp
Maltz rasp, 181, 181f
  description of, 181
  insight on, 181–182
  other names for, 181
  uses of, 181
Mammary forceps. *See* Gerald tissue
    forceps
Mammary retractor. *See* Internal
    mammary retractor
Mammoplasty hook, 227, 227f
  category of, 227
  caution when using, 227–228
  description of, 227
  insight on, 227–228
  other names for, 227
  uses of, 227
Mandibular forceps (17), #17. *See* Lower
    molar extraction forceps (17)
Mandibular universal forceps. *See*
    Lower anterior extraction forceps
    (151)
Manual cleaning, 7–8
Marking pen. *See* Sterile marking pen
    and labels
Martin cartilage clamp, 259, 259f
  description of, 259
  other names for, 259
  uses of, 259
Maryland bipolar forceps, 95, 95f
  category of, 95
  description of, 95
  insight on, 95
  other names for, 95
  uses of, 95
Maryland dissector, 77, 77f
  description of, 77
  insight on, 77
  uses of, 77
Maryland forceps. *See* Maryland bipolar
    forceps
Masterson clamp. *See* Heaney-Ballentine
    hysterectomy forceps
Mastoid rongeur. *See* Cicherelli mastoid
    rongeur
Mathieu retractor, 230, 230f
  category of, 230
  caution when using, 230
  description of, 230
  insight on, 230
  other names for, 230
  uses of, 230
Matson rib stripper, 335, 335f
  category of, 335
  description of, 335
  insight on, 335
  other names for, 335
  uses of, 335
Maxillary left forceps, #88L. *See*
    Left upper molar extraction
    `forceps (88L)
Maxillary right forceps, #88R. *See* Right
    upper molar extraction forceps
    (88R)
Maxillary universal forceps. *See* Upper
    anterior extraction forceps (150)
Mayo abdominal retractor, 60, 60f
  description of, 60
  other names for, 60
  uses of, 60–61

Mayo cover. *See* Mayo stand cover
Mayo forceps. *See* Rochester-Péan
    forceps
Mayo-guyon vessel clamp, 128f
    description of, 128
    uses of, 128
Mayo-Hegar needle holder, 48, 48f
    description of, 48
    insight on, 48–49
    other names for, 48
    uses of, 48
Mayo scissors
    curved, 26, 26f
        caution when using, 26–27
        description of, 26
        insight on, 26–27
        other names for, 26
    straight, 26, 26f,
        caution when using, 26
        description of, 26
        insight on, 26
        other names for, 26
Mayo stand, 358, 358f, 380
    caution when using, 358–359
    description of, 358
    insight on, 358–359
    other names for, 358
    uses of, 358
Mayo stand cover, 378, 378f
    caution when using, 378
    description of, 378
    insight on, 378
    other names for, 378
    uses of, 378
Mayo tray. *See* Mayo stand
Mayo uterine scissors, 106, 106f
    description of, 106
    other names for, 106
    uses of, 106–107
McGee wire crimping forceps, 174, 174f
    description of, 174
    insight on, 174–175
    other names for, 174
    uses of, 174
McIvor mouth gag, 206, 206f
    description of, 206
    insight on, 206
    uses of, 206
McKissock keyhole, 222, 222f
    category of, 222
    description of, 222
    insight on, 222
    other names for, 222
    uses of, 222
McPherson needle holder, 160, 160f
    description of, 160
    uses of, 160–161
McPherson tying forceps, 154f
    description of, 154
    insight on, 154
    uses of, 154
Measuring stick. *See* Ruler
Measuring tool. *See* House strut caliper
Medical sink. *See* Scrub sink
Meltzer adenoid punch, 202, 202f
    description of, 202
    insight on, 202
    other names for, 202
    uses of, 202

Meniscus clamp. *See* Martin cartilage
    clamp
Metacarpal pins. *See* Kirschner wires
Metzenbaum scissors, curved, 27, 27f
    caution when using, 27
    description of, 27
    insight on, 27
    other names for, 27
    uses of, 27
Meyerding finger retractor, 230, 230f
    category of, 230
    description of, 230
    uses of, 230–231
Meyerding handheld retractor, 310, 310f
    description of, 310
    uses of, 310
Meyerding hemilaminectomy retractor.
    See Williams hemilaminectomy
    retractors
Meyerding laminectomy retractor,
    309, 309f
    description of, 309
    insight on, 309
    uses of, 309
Meyhoeffer chalazion curettes, 145, 145f
    description of, 145
    insight on, 145–146
    uses of, 145
Micro cups. *See* Oval cup forceps,
    straight, right, left
Micro knife, 296, 296f
    description of, 296
    uses of, 296–297
Micro scissors. *See* Rhoton micro scissors
Microscope, 367, 367f
    description of, 367
    insight on, 367
    other names for, 367
    uses of, 367
Microsurgical instruments, handling, 2
Microvasive evacuator, 135, 135f
    description of, 135
    insight on, 135
    other names for, 135
    uses of, 135
Midas rex drill, 301, 301f
    description of, 301
    insight on, 301
    other names for, 301
    uses of, 301
Middle ear scissors. *See* Bellucci
    scissors
Miller rasp, 249, 249f
    description of, 249
    insight on, 249
    other names for, 249
    uses of, 249
Mills/Dennis micro ring tissue forceps,
    337, 337f
    category of, 337
    description of, 337
    insight on, 337
    uses of, 337
Minnesota cheek retractor, 218, 218f
    description of, 218
    other names, 218
    uses of, 218–219
Mitral valve retractor. *See* Cooley
    arterial retractor

Mixter forceps, 25, 25f. *See also*
    Endo right angle forceps; Gemini
    forceps; Lahey gall duct forceps
    description of, 25
    other names for, 25
    uses of, 25
Molt bone curette, 214, 214f
    description of, 214
    other names, 214
    uses of, 214
Molt mouth gag, 219, 219f
    description of, 219
    other names, 219
    uses of, 219
Monopolar pencil. *See* Electrosurgical
    pencil
Mosquito forceps. *See* Halstead forceps
Mother-in-law grasper. *See* Claw
    grasper
Mouth gag. *See* Molt mouth gag
Mouth mirror, 209, 209f
    description of, 209
    insight on, 209–210
    other names, 209
    uses of, 209
Mouth prop, 219, 219f
    description of, 219
    insight on, 219–220
    other names, 219
    uses of, 219
Mucous trap. *See* Delee suction
Murphy-Lane bone skid, 264, 264f
    description of, 264
    insight on, 264–265
    uses of, 264
Murphy retractor, 43, 43f
    caution when using, 43
    description of, 43
    insight on, 43
    other names for, 43
    uses of, 43
Muscle clamp. *See* Jameson forceps
Muscle hook. *See* Von Graefe
    strabismus hook
Myringotomy and tube placement
    (M & T), 389, 389f
Myringotomy knife, 164, 164f
    description of, 164
    insight on, 164
    uses of, 164

N

Nasal chisel. *See* Cottle chisel
Nasal curettes. *See* Coakley antrum
    curettes
Navy's retractor. *See* Army-navy
    retractor
Needle counter, 376, 376f
    description of, 376
    insight on, 376
    other names for, 376
    uses of, 376
Needle magnet. *See* Needle counter
Needle mat. *See* Needle counter
Needlenose pliers, 261, 261f
    description of, 261
    uses of, 261–262
Neptune. *See* Suction
Nerve hook. *See* Blunt hook

Nested right angle retractor. *See* Parker retractor
Neuro pattie. *See* Cottonoid sponges
Neuro sponge. *See* Cottonoid sponges
Neurocautery suction. *See* Suction coagulator tip
Neurosurgical pattie. *See* Cottonoid sponges
Nezhat-Dorsey suction tips, 86f
  description of, 86
  uses of, 86–87
Nipper. *See* House-Dieter malleus nipper
Nipple washer. *See* Areola marker
Nonsterile gloves. *See* Exam gloves
Notched retractor. *See* Young bulb retractor
#1 penfield dissector, 293, 293f
  description of, 293
  uses of, 293–294
#2 penfield dissector, 294, 294f
  description of, 294
  uses of, 294
#3 knife handle, 28, 28f
  caution when using, 28–29
  description of, 28
  insight on, 28–29
  long angled, 107, 107f
    description of, 107
    insight on, 107–108
    other names for, 107
    uses of, 107
  other names for, 28
  uses of, 28
#3 long knife handle, 29, 29f
  caution when using, 29
  description of, 29
  other names for, 29
  uses of, 29
#3 penfield dissector, 294, 294f
  description of, 294
  uses of, 294–295
#4 knife handle, 32, 32f
  caution when using, 32
  description of, 32
  insight on, 32
  other names for, 32
  uses of, 32
#4 penfield dissector, 295, 295f
  description of, 295
  insight on, 295
  uses of, 295
#5 penfield dissector, 295, 295f
  description of, 295
  uses of, 295–296
#7 knife handle, 29, 29f
  caution when using, 29–30
  description of, 29
  other names for, 29
  uses of, 29–30
#10 blade, 30, 30f
  caution when using, 30
  description of, 30
  insight on, 30
  uses of, 30
#11 blade, 30, 30f
  caution when using, 30–31
  description of, 30
  insight on, 30–31
  uses of, 30

#12 blade, 31, 31f
  caution when using, 31
  description of, 31
  insight on, 31
  other name for, 31
  uses of, 31
#15 blade, 31, 31f
  caution when using, 31–32
  description of, 31
  insight on, 31–32
  uses of, 31
#20 blade, 32, 32f
  description of, 32
  insight on, 32–33
  uses of, 32

O

Obtuse clamp. *See* Mixter forceps
Ochsner forceps. *See also* Kocher forceps
  curved, 111, 111f
    caution when using, 111–112
    description of, 111
    other names for, 111
    uses of, 111–112
O'Connor retractor. *See* O'Sullivan-O'Connor retractor
Olsen clamp. *See* Endoscopic cholangiogram forceps
Omni retractor, 62, 62f
  description of, 62
  insight on, 62
  other names for, 62
  uses of, 62
Omni tract. *See* Omni retractor
150. *See* Upper anterior extraction forceps (150)
151. *See* Lower anterior extraction forceps (151)
Operating microscope. *See* Microscope
Operating room, 361, 361f
  description of, 361
  insight on, 361
  other names for, 361
  uses of, 361
Operating room lights. *See* OR lights
Operating table. *See* Operating room
Optical trocar. *See* Visiport
OR bed. *See* Operating room
OR lights, 361, 361f
  caution when using, 361–362
  description of, 361
  insight on, 361–362
  other names for, 361
  uses of, 361
OR table. *See* Operating room
Oral suction. *See* Yankauer suction tip, nondisposable
Oral suction tip. *See* Yankauer suction tip
Oral tip. *See* Yankauer suction tip, nondisposable
Ortho Balfour. *See* Charnley retractor
Ortho boots. *See* Boot shoe covers
O'Sullivan-O'Connor retractor, 117, 117f
  description of, 117
  insight on, 117
  other names for, 117
  uses of, 117
O'Sullivan retractor. *See* O'Sullivan-O'Connor retractor

Otis urethrotome, 129f
  caution when using, 129
  description of, 129
  insight on, 129
  uses of, 129
Oval chalazion clamp. *See* Desmarres chalazion clamp
Oval cup forceps, straight, right, left, 173, 173f
  description of, 173
  insight on, 173
  other names for, 173
  uses of, 173
Oval pick window pick. *See* House oval window pick
Overhead lights. *See* OR lights
Overstreet endometrial polyp forceps, 112
  description of, 112
  other names for, 112
  uses of, 112–113
Ozone, 20
  storage and holding of sterile instruments, 20

P

Packing forceps. *See* Bozeman uterine dressing forceps
Paget blade. *See* Dermatome blade
Paget dermatome. *See* Dermatome
Paper clip. *See* Barraquer eye speculum
Park bench retractor. *See* Parker retractor
Parker retractor, 44, 44f
  description of, 44
  insight on, 44–45
  other names for, 44
  uses of, 44
Parsonnet epicardial, 344f
Parsonnet epicardial retractor, 344
  category of, 344
  description of, 344
  insight on, 344
  uses of, 344
Patent ductus. *See* DeBakey coarctation clamp
Peacock retractor. *See* Endo fan retractor
Péan forceps. *See* Rochester-Péan forceps
Peanuts. *See* Dissector sponges
Peapod rongeur, 292, 292f
  caution when using, 292–293
  description of, 292
  insight on, 292–293
  uses of, 292
Pedicle clamp. *See* Beck aortic clamp; Herrick kidney clamp; Wertheim-Cullen pedicle clamp
Pennington forceps, 56, 56f
  description of, 56
  other names for, 56
  uses of, 56
Periosteal elevator. *See* West periosteal elevator
Permanent cautery spatula, 94, 94f
  category of, 94
  description of, 94
  insight on, 94–95
  other names for, 94
  uses of, 94
Personal protective equipment (PPE), 7

Pick, angle. *See* Root tip pick
Pierce double ended elevator, 185, 185f
  description of, 185
  insight on, 185–186
  uses of, 185
Pillar retractor. *See* Hurd dissector
Pin cutter. *See* Cannulated pin cutter;
    Diamond pin cutter; Heavy wire cutter
PK dissecting forceps, 96, 96f
  category of, 96
  description of, 96
  insight on, 96–97
  other names for, 96
  uses of, 96
PK forceps. *See* PK dissecting forceps
Plain tissue forceps, 35, 35f
  description of, 35
  other names for, 35
  uses of, 35
Plate bender. *See* Plate bending pliers
Plate bending pliers, 243, 243f
  description of, 243
  insight on, 243
  other names for, 243
  uses of, 243
Plate clamp. *See* Plate forceps
Plate forceps, 259, 259f
  description of, 259
  other names for, 259
  uses of, 259–260
Plate holders. *See* Plate forceps
Plate holding forceps. *See* Plate forceps
Platform. *See* Step stool
Pliers, 262, 262f
  description of, 262
  other names for, 262
  uses of, 262
Point of use decontamination, 6–7
Pole retractor, 83, 83f
  description of, 83
  other names for, 83
  uses of, 83–84
Polyp forceps. *See* Overstreet
    endometrial
Poole suction tip, 47, 47f
  description of, 47
  insight on, 47
  other names for, 47
  uses of, 47
Poppen suction tip, 314, 314f
  description of, 314
  insight on, 314
  uses of, 314
Posterior scissors. *See* Cottle angular
    scissors
Potts. *See* Potts-Smith scissors
Potts elevator, 210, 210f
  description of, 210
  insight on, 210–211
  other names, 210
  uses of, 210
Potts scissors, 96, 96f
  category of, 96
  description of, 96
  uses of, 96
Potts-Smith scissors, 328, 328f
  category of, 328
  description of, 328
  insight on, 328–329

Potts-Smith scissors *(Continued)*
  other names for, 328
  uses of, 328
Potts-Smith tissue forceps, 338, 338f
  category of, 338
  description of, 338
  insight on, 338–339
  other names for, 338
  uses of, 338
Powered instruments, handling of, 2
Pratt rectal speculum, 62, 62f
  description of, 62
  insight on, 62–63
  uses of, 62
Pratt uterine dilators, 115, 115f
  description of, 115
  insight on, 115
  other names for, 115
  uses of, 115
Prep stand. *See* Prep table
Prep table, 360, 360f
  description of, 360
  insight on, 360
  other names for, 360
  uses of, 360
Prevacuum sterilization, 17
Probe and grooved director, 57, 57f
  description of, 57
  uses of, 57
Procedure pack. *See* Back table pack
Prograsp forceps, 98, 98f
  category of, 98
  description of, 98
  other names for, 98
  uses of, 98–99
Prop. *See* Molt mouth gag
Prostate retractor, anterior. *See* Young
    anterior retractor
Pulsavac, 274, 274f
  description of, 274
  other names for, 274
  uses of, 274
Pulse lavage. *See* Pulsavac
Pump tubing, 238, 238f
  description of, 238
  uses of, 238–239
Punch. *See* Aortic punch; Meltzer
    adenoid punch
Punctal lacrimal dilator. *See* Wilder
    lacrimal dilator
Pusher. *See* Endo kittner
Putti bone rasp, 249, 249f
  caution when using, 249–250
  description of, 249
  insight on, 249–250
  other names for, 249
  uses of, 249
Putti Platte. *See* Putti bone rasp

Q

Quality assurance of sterilization
    process, 13

R

Ragnell retractor, 231, 231f, 268, 268f
  category of, 231
  description of, 231, 268
  uses of, 231, 268
Rake retractor. *See* Volkman retractor

Randall stone forceps. *See also*
    Desjardin gallstone forceps
  description of, 130
  uses of, 130–131
Raney clip appliers, 283, 283f
  description of, 283
  insight on, 283–284
  other names for, 283
  uses of, 283
Raney clips, 284, 284f
  description of, 284
  insight on, 284
  uses of, 284
Rasp. *See* Bone file
Rat tail. *See* Putti bone rasp
Rat tooth forceps. *See* Adson tissue
    forceps, toothed; Toothed tissue
    forceps
Rays. *See* Raytec sponges
Raytec sponges, 370, 370f
  caution when using, 370
  description of, 370
  insight on, 370
  other names for, 370
  uses of, 370
Reducer caps, 122, 122f
  description of, 122
  insight on, 122
  other names for, 122
  uses of, 122
Reduction marker. *See* McKissock
    keyhole
Resano forceps, 98, 98f
  category of, 98
  description of, 98
  other names for, 98
  uses of, 98
Resectoscope sheath and obturator,
    136, 136f
  description of, 136
  insight on, 136–137
  uses of, 136
Retractors, 3, 4f
Reynolds scissors, 227, 227f, 329, 329f
  category of, 227, 329
  description of, 227, 329
  insight on, 329–330
  other names for, 329
  uses of, 227, 329
Rhoton dissector extended set, 296, 296f
  description of, 296
  insight on, 296
  uses of, 296
Rhoton micro bayonet, 288, 288f
  description of, 288
  insight on, 288–289
  uses of, 288
Rhoton micro needle holders, 315, 315f
  description of, 315
  insight on, 315
  uses of, 315
Rhoton micro scissors, 288, 288f
  description of, 288
  other names for, 288
  uses of, 288
Rib approximator. *See* Bailey rib
    contractor
Rib cutter. *See* Gluck rib shear;
    Sauer-bruch rib rongeur

Rib spreader. *See* Finochietto rib spreader
Ribbon retractor, 44
    description of, 44
    insight on, 44
    other names for, 44
    uses of, 44
Rich retractor. *See* Richardson retractor
    big. *See* Richardson-Eastman
        retractor
    double-ended. *See* Richardson-
        Eastman retractor
Richardson-Eastman retractor, 58, 58f
    description of, 58
    insight on, 58
    other names for, 58
    uses of, 58
Richardson retractor, 58, 58f
    description of, 58
    insight on, 57
    other names for, 58
    uses of, 58
Right angle forceps. *See* Gemini
        forceps; Lahey gall duct forceps;
        Mixter forceps
Right angle retractor. *See* Heaney
    retractor
Right-angle scissors. *See* Dean scissors
Right upper molar extraction forceps
        (88R), 216, 216f
    description of, 216
    insight on, 216–217
    other names, 216
    uses of, 216
Rigid endoscope. *See* 10-mm
        0° endoscope; 10-mm 30°
        endoscope
Ring. *See* Ring stand
Ring curette. *See* Buck ear curette
Ring forceps. *See* Foerster sponge
        forceps
Ring stand, 359, 359f
    description of, 359
    insight on, 359–360
    other names for, 359
    uses of, 359
Riser. *See* Step stool
Robotic instruments, 93f
Rochester-Péan forceps, 24, 24f
    description of, 24
    other names for, 24
    uses of, 24
Rod cutter. *See* Large pin cutter
Roeder towel clip. *See* Towel clip,
    penetrating
Root elevators. *See* Cryer elevator
Root tip pick, 212, 212f. *See also* Crane
        elevator
    description of, 212
    other names, 212
    uses of, 212–213
Rosen knife. *See* House-Sheehy knife
    curette
Rosen needle, 170, 170f
    description of, 170
    insight on, 170–171
    uses of, 170
Round chalazion clamp. *See* Hunt
    chalazion clamp
Round handle. *See* Beaver handle

Rubin morselizer, 193, 193f
    description of, 193
    uses of, 193
Ruler, 235, 235f
    description of, 235
    insight on, 235
    other names for, 235
    uses of, 235
Rumel tourniquet hook (stylet), 316, 316f
    category of, 316
    description of, 316
    insight on, 316–317
    uses of, 316
Russian star forceps. *See* Russian
        tissue forceps
Russian tissue forceps, 38, 38f
    description of, 38
    insight on, 38
    other names for, 38
    uses of, 38
Russians forceps. *See* Russian tissue
    forceps
Ryder needle holder, 49, 49f, 348, 348f
    category of, 348
    description of, 49, 348
    fine. *See* Ryder needle holder
    insight on, 49, 348
    other names for, 49, 348
    uses of, 49, 348

S

S retractor, 84, 84f
    description of, 84
    other names for, 84
    uses of, 84
Sarot bronchus clamp, 336, 336f
    category of, 336
    description of, 336
    insight on, 336–337
    uses of, 336
Sarot forceps, 55, 55f
    description of, 55
    insight on, 55
    other names for, 55
    uses of, 55
Satinksy partial occlusion clamp. *See*
        Satinsky vena cava clamp
Satinsky vena cava clamp, 321, 321f
    category of, 321
    description of, 321
    insight on, 321–322
    other names for, 321
    uses of, 321
Sauerbruch rib rongeur, 333, 333f
    category of, 333
    description of, 333
    insight on, 318
    other names for, 333
    uses of, 333
Sawyer rectal retractor, 63, 63f
    description of, 63
    insight on, 63
    uses of, 63
Scalp clip applier. *See* Raney clip
        appliers
Scalp clip gun, 284, 284f
    description of, 284
    insight on, 284–285
    uses of, 284

Scalpel handle. *See* #3 knife handle
Schiotz tonometer. *See* Tonometer
Schmidt forceps. *See* Adson tonsil/
        Schnidt forceps
Schroeder tenaculum, 109, 109f
    caution when using, 109–110
    description of, 109
    insight on, 109–110
    other names for, 109
    uses of, 109
Schroeder vulsellum, 110, 110f
    caution when using, 110
    description of, 110
    insight on, 110
    other names for, 110
    uses of, 110
Scofield/Meyerding self-retaining
        retractor. *See* Scoville retractor
Scoop. *See* Ferguson gallstone scoop
Scoop forceps. *See* Adson hypophyseal
        cup tissue forceps
Scoville brain spatula, 304, 304f
    description of, 304
    insight on, 304
    uses of, 304
Scoville nerve root retractor (angled),
        307, 307f
    description of, 307
    insight on, 307
    uses of, 307
Scoville retractor, 311, 311f
    description of, 311
    other names for, 311
    uses of, 311–312
Screw depth gauge. *See* Depth gauge
Screwdriver kit. *See* Universal
        screwdriver set
Scrub sink, 367, 367f
    description of, 367
    insight on, 367–368
    other names for, 367
    uses of, 367
Scrub suit, 350, 350f
    caution when using, 350–351
    description of, 350
    insight on, 350–351
    other names for, 350
    uses of, 350
Scrubs. *See* Scrub suit
Seals. *See* Reducer caps
Self-retaining retractor. *See* Balfour
    retractor
Semken tissue forceps. *See* Toothed
        tissue forceps
Senn retractor, 42, 42f
    caution when using, 42–43
    description of, 42
    insight on, 42–43
    other names for, 42
    uses of, 42
Septal knife. *See* Freer septum knife
Serrefine clamps, 145f
    description of, 145
    insight on, 145
    other names for, 145
    uses of, 145
Set-up pack. *See* Back table pack
70-degree telescope, 138, 138f
    caution when using, 138–139

70-degree telescope *(Continued)*
   description of, 138
   insight on, 138–139
   other names for, 138
   uses of, 138
70° endoscope. *See* 70° telescope
70° lens. *See* 70° telescope
Shark forceps. *See* Resano forceps
Sharp curette. *See* Sims uterine curette
Sharps canister, 364, 364f
   caution when using, 364–365
   description of, 364
   insight on, 364–365
   other names for, 364
   uses of, 364
Sharps holder. *See* Needle counter
Shattering needle. *See* House-Barbara
   shattering needle
Shaver, 258, 258f
   description of, 258
   insight on, 258–259
   uses of, 258
Shears. *See* Curved scissors
Shoe covers, 352, 352f
   description of, 352
   insight on, 352–353
   other names for, 352
   uses of, 352
Shoemaker rib shear. *See* Stille-Giertz
   rib shear
Shoulder skid. *See* Lever skid humeral
   head retractor
Sickle knife. *See* #12 blade
Side biter. *See* Lambert-Kay aorta clamp
Simpson obstetrical forceps, 113, 113f
   description of, 113
   other names for, 113
   uses of, 113
Sims uterine curette, 105, 105f
   description of, 105
   insight on, 105
   other names for, 105
   uses of, 105
Sims uterine sound, 115, 115f
   description of, 115
   other names for, 115
   uses of, 115–116
Single-tooth tenaculum. *See* Schroeder
   tenaculum
Singley tissue forceps, 37, 37f
   description of, 37
   other names for, 37
   uses of, 37–38
Sinskey hook, 144, 144f
   description of, 144
   uses of, 144
Sinus shaver. *See* Straightshot
   microdebrider
Skin hook, 45, 45f
   caution when using, 45
   description of, 45
   insight on, 45
   other names for, 45
   single. *See* Joseph skin hooks
   uses of, 45
Skin mesher. *See* Dermamesher
Skin stapler, 49f
   description of, 49
   insight on, 49–50
   uses of, 49

Small bone curette. *See* House double-
   ended curette
Small frag. *See* Small fragment set
Small fragment set, 277, 277f
   description of, 277
   insight on, 277–279
   other names for, 277
   uses of, 277
Small-mouthed rongeur. *See* Zaufel-
   Jansen rongeur
Small rasp. *See* Miller rasp
Smooth forceps. *See* Plain tissue forceps
Smooth pins. *See* Steinman pins, smooth
Snake retractor. *See* Endoflex retractor
Snap forceps. *See* Crile forceps
Softjaw. *See* Fogarty clamp with jaw
   inserts
Sound. *See* Sims uterine sound
Spencer suture scissors, 215, 215f
   description of, 215
   insight on, 215–216
   other names, 215
   uses of, 215
Spinal curette, 300, 300f
   description of, 300
   other names for, 300
   uses of, 300–301
Sponge bucket. *See* Kick bucket
Sponge stick forceps. *See* Foerster
   sponge forceps
Spoon. *See* Ferguson gallstone scoop
Spotlights. *See* OR lights
Spratt mastoid curettes, 169, 169f
   description of, 169
   other names for, 169
   uses of, 169
Spurling rongeur (straight), 292, 292f
   caution when using, 292
   description of, 292
   insight on, 292
   uses of, 292
Standing stool. *See* Step stool
Staple remover, 50, 50f
   caution when using, 50–51
   description of, 50
   insight on, 50–51
   other names for, 50
   uses of, 50
Star forceps. *See* Russian tissue
   forceps
Stat forceps. *See* Crile forceps
Steam sterilization (high heat), 17–20
   gravity displacement, 17
   hydrogen peroxide gas plasma
    (HPGP), 19–20
   immediate use steam sterilizer (flash
    sterilizer), 18–19
   low-heat sterilizers, 19
   prevacuum sterilization, 17
Steinman pins
   smooth, 241, 241f
    description of, 241
    insight on, 241
    other names for, 241
    uses of, 241
   threaded, 241, 241f
    description of, 241
    insight on, 241–242
    other names for, 241
    uses of, 241

Step stool, 366, 366f
   description of, 366
   insight on, 366–367
   other names for, 366
   uses of, 366
Steps. *See* Step stool
Sterile gloves, 356, 356f
   description of, 356
   insight on, 356–357
   other names for, 356
   uses of, 356
Sterile gown. *See* Surgical gown
Sterile marker. *See* Sterile marking pen
   and labels
Sterile marking pen and labels, 376, 376f
   description of, 376
   insight on, 376–377
   other names for, 376
   uses of, 376
Sterile processing department, 7–9
   manual cleaning, 7–8
   ultrasonic cleaner, 9
Sterilization
   automated washer (washer sterilizer),
    10–13
    perp and pack, 11–13
   ethylene oxide gas (EtO), 20
   ozone, 20
    storage and holding of sterile
     instruments, 20
   point of use decontamination, 6–7
   steam sterilization (high heat), 17–20
    gravity displacement, 17
    hydrogen peroxide gas plasma
     (HPGP), 19–20
    immediate use steam sterilizer
     (flash sterilizer), 18–19
    low-heat sterilizers, 19
    prevacuum sterilization, 17
   sterile processing department, 7–9
    manual cleaning, 7–8
    ultrasonic cleaner, 9
   sterilization of the instruments, 13–16
    biological indicators, 15
    Bowie-Dick test, 16
    chemical indicators, 14
    quality assurance of the
     sterilization process, 13
Sternal knife. *See* Lebsche knife
Sternal needle holder and wire twister,
   348, 348f
   category of, 348
   description of, 348
   insight on, 348–349
   other names for, 348
   uses of, 348
Sternal saw, 334, 334f
   category of, 334
   description of, 334
   insight on, 334
   other names for, 334
   uses of, 334
Stevens tenotomy scissors, 148f, 226,
   226f
   category of, 226
   description of, 148, 226
   other names for, 148
   uses of, 148–149, 226
Stille bone chisel, 252, 252f
   description of, 252

Stille bone chisel *(Continued)*
    insight on, 252–253
    uses of, 252
Stille bone gouge, 252, 252f
    description of, 252
    insight on, 252
    uses of, 252
Stille bone osteotome, 253, 253f
    description of, 253
    insight on, 253
    uses of, 253
Stille-Giertz rib shear, 333, 333f
    category of, 333
    description of, 333
    insight on, 333
    other names for, 333
    uses of, 333
Stille-Luer rongeur, 256, 256f
    caution when using, 256
    description of, 256
    insight on, 256
    other names for, 256
    uses of, 256
Stone basket, 130, 130f
    description of, 130
    insight on, 130
    uses of, 130
Straight clamp. *See* Cooley coarctation
    clamp
Straight curette. *See* Molt bone
    curette
Straight elevator. *See* Apical elevator
Straight rongeur. *See* Stille-Luer
    rongeur
Straightshot microdebrider, 192, 192f
    description of, 192
    other names for, 192
    uses of, 192
Straightshotshaver. *See* Straightshot
    microdebrider
Stripper. *See* Matson rib stripper
Strully scissors, 287, 287f
    caution when using, 287
    description of, 287
    insight on, 287
    uses of, 287
Strut. *See* House strut caliper
Stryker core system, 246, 246f
    description of, 246
    insight on, 246
    other names for, 246
    uses of, 246
Stryker sternal saw. *See* Sternal saw
Stryker system 6 power, 245, 245f
    description of, 245
    insight on, 245–246
    uses of, 245
Subramanian. *See* DeBakey sidewinder
    aorta clamp
Suction, 363, 363f
    description of, 363
    other names for, 363
    uses of, 363–364
Suction coagulator. *See* Suction
    coagulator tip
Suction coagulator tip, 199, 199f
    description of, 199
    insight on, 199–200
    other names for, 199
    uses of, 199

Suction irrigator, 86f
    description of, 86
    insight on, 86
    uses of, 86
Suction tubing, 375, 375f
    description of, 375
    insight on, 375–376
    other names for, 375
    uses of, 375
Surgical basin. *See* Basin
Surgical curette. *See* Molt bone curette
Surgical gloves. *See* Sterile gloves
Surgical gown, 357, 357f
    description of, 357
    insight on, 357
    other names for, 357
    uses of, 357
Surgical instruments
    care and handling of, 1–2
    categorization of, 3–5
        accessory, 3
        clamping and occluding, 4
        cutting and dissecting, 4
        grasping and holding, 4
        probing and dilating, 4
        retracting and exposing, 4–5
        sets, 5
        suctioning and aspirating, 5
        suturing and stapling, 5
        viewing, 5
    history of, 1
    parts of, 2–3, 3f, 4f
Surgical masks, 354, 354f
    caution when using, 354
    description of, 354
    insight on, 354
    other names for, 354
    uses of, 354
Surgical sinks. *See* Scrub sink
Surgiclip applier, 51, 51f
    description of, 51
    other names for, 51
    uses of, 51
Suture guide holder. *See* Grunwald
    suture ring
Suture ring. *See* Grunwald suture ring
Suture scissors. *See* Mayo scissors,
    straight; Spencer suture scissors
Suturecut needle driver, 100, 100f
    category of, 100
    description of, 100
    insight on, 100
    uses of, 100
Sweetheart retractor. *See* Harrington
    retractor
Swivel knife. *See* Ballenger swivel knife
Syringe
    hypodermic syringe, 373, 373f
        caution when using, 373
        description of, 373
        insight on, 373
        other names for, 373
        uses of, 373

T

T-bar Potts elevator. *See* Potts elevator
TA stapler. *See* Linear stapler
Table cover. *See* Back table cover
Takahashi nasal forceps, 191, 191f
    description of, 191

Takahashi nasal forceps *(Continued)*
    insight on, 191
    uses of, 191
Tamp. *See* Bone tamp
Tapes. *See* Laparotomy sponges
Taylor dural scissors, 287, 287f
    caution when using, 287–288
    description of, 287
    other names for, 287
    uses of, 287–288
Taylor hip retractor, 270, 270f
    description of, 270
    insight on, 270
    uses of, 270
Taylor spinal retractor, 313, 313f
    description of, 313
    uses of, 313–314
Teardrop suction tip, 314, 314f
    description of, 314
    insight on, 314–315
    other names for, 314
    uses of, 314
Telescope bridge, 122, 122f
    description of, 122
    insight on, 122–123
    other names for, 122
    uses of, 122
10-mm 0-degree endoscope, 90f
    description of, 90
    insight on, 90–91
    other names for, 90
    uses of, 90
10-mm 30-degree endoscope, 91, 91f
    caution when using, 91
    description of, 91
    insight on, 91
    other names for, 91
    uses of, 91
Tenaculums. *See* Cottle tenaculum,
    double
    double-tooth. *See* Schroeder
        vulsellum
    single-tooth. *See* Schroeder
        tenaculum
Tenotomy. *See* Jamison scissors
30-degree telescope, 138, 138f
    caution when using, 138
    description of, 138
    insight on, 138
    other names for, 138
    uses of, 138
30° endoscope. *See* 30° telescope
30° lens. *See* 30° telescope
35 clamp. *See* DeBakey peripheral
    vascular clamp
Thomas-Gaylor uterine biopsy forceps,
    107, 107f
    description of, 107
    other names for, 107
    uses of, 107
Thomas uterine curette, 104, 104f
    description of, 104
    other names for, 104
    uses of, 104–105
Thoracic ring forceps, 340, 340f
    category of, 340
    description of, 340
    other names for, 340
    uses of, 340
Thoracoport. *See* Endopath thoracic trocar

Threaded pins. *See* Steinman pins, threaded
Thyroid retractor. *See* Green retractor
Tissue forceps
  with teeth. *See* Toothed tissue forceps
  without teeth. *See* Plain tissue forceps
Tissue scissors. *See* Kelly scissors; Metzenbaum scissors, curved
Titaniums. *See* DeBakey-Diethrich tissue forceps
Tongs. *See* Simpson obstetrical forceps
Tongue blade. *See* Andrews tongue depressor
Tongue depressor. *See* Wieder tongue blade
Tonometer, 140, 140f
  description of, 140
  other names for, 140
  uses of, 140–141
Tonsil blade. *See* #12 blade
Tonsil forceps. *See* Allis forceps, curved
Tonsil grasper. *See* Allis forceps, curved
Tonsil scissors. *See* Boettcher tonsil scissors
Tonsil snare, 202, 202f
  description of, 202
  insight on, 202–203
  uses of, 202
Tonsil sponges, 371, 371f
  caution when using, 371–372
  description of, 371
  insight on, 371–372
  other names for, 371
  uses of, 371
Tonsil suction tip. *See* Yankauer suction tip
Tonsil syringe. *See* Bulb syringe
Tonsillectomy and adenoidectomy (T & A), 388, 388f
Toomey syringe, 135, 135f
  description of, 135
  insight on, 135–136
  uses of, 135
Toothed grasper. *See* Cobra grasper
Toothed tissue forceps, 35, 35f
  caution when using, 35–36
  description of, 35
  insight on, 35–36
  other names for, 35
  uses of, 35
Total arthroplasty set. *See* Total hip instruments
Total hip instruments, 280f, 281f, 282
  description of, 282
  insight on, 282
  other names for, 282
  uses of, 282
Total knee instruments, 279, 279f
  description of, 279
  insight on, 279–281
  other names for, 279
  uses of, 279
Towel bundle. *See* Towel pack
Towel clip
  nonpenetrating, 39, 39f
    caution when using, 39
    description of, 39
    other names for, 39
    uses of, 39

Towel clip *(Continued)*
  penetrating, 38, 38f
    caution when using, 38–39
    description of, 38
    insight on, 38–39
    other names for, 38
    uses of, 38
Towel pack, 379, 379f
  description of, 379
  insight on, 379
  other names for, 379
  uses of, 379
Townley caliper, 236, 236f
  description of, 236
  other names for, 236
  uses of, 236–237
TPS system. *See* Stryker core system
Trace packs. *See* Back table pack
Trach hook. *See* Hupp tracheal hook
Tracheal spreader. *See* Trousseau tracheal dilator
Trauma boots. *See* Boot shoe covers
Triangle forceps. *See* Pennington forceps
Trousseau tracheal dilator, 208, 208f
  description of, 208
  other names for, 208
  uses of, 208
Tube clamp. *See* Vorse tubing occluding clamp
Tubing. *See* Suction tubing
Turbinate scissors. *See* Cottle angular scissors
25° 4-mm lens, 274, 274f
  description of, 274
  insight on, 274–275
  other names for, 274
  uses of, 274
Tympanostomy knife. *See* Myringotomy knife

U
Ultrasonic cleaner, 9
Ultrasonic scalpel. *See* Endo harmonic scalpel; Harmonic scalpel
Universal screwdriver set, 242, 242f
  description of, 242
  insight on, 242–243
  other names for, 242
  uses of, 242
University of Minnesota retractor. *See* Minnesota cheek retractor
Up-biter. *See* Kerrison rongeur
Upper anterior extraction forceps (150), 217, 217f
  description of, 217
  insight on, 217–218
  other names, 217
  uses of, 217
Ureter clamp. *See* Mixter forceps
Urethral dilators. *See* Van Buren urethral sounds; Walther female urethral sounds
U.S. retractor. *See* Army-navy retractor
Uterine dilators. *See* Hank dilators; Hegar dilators; Pratt uterine dilators
Uterine manipulator. *See* Hulka tenaculum
Uterine scissors. *See* Mayo uterine scissors

Utility scissors, 248, 248f
  description of, 248
  insight on, 248
  other names for, 248
  uses of, 248
Utility table. *See* Prep table

V
Van Buren. *See* Van Buren urethral sounds
Van buren urethral sounds, 131, 131f
  description of, 131
  insight on, 131–132
  other names for, 131
  uses of, 131
Vannas. *See* Vannas capsulotomy scissors
Vannas capsulotomy scissors, 150, 150f
  description of, 150
  other names for, 150
  uses of, 150
Vascular suction tip, 347
  category of, 347
  description of, 347
  insight on, 347–348
  other names for, 347
  uses of, 347
Veress needle, 74, 74f
  description of, 74
  insight on, 74–75
  other names for, 74
  uses of, 74
Versa port trocars, 67, 67f
  description of, 67
  insight on, 67
  uses of, 67
Versa step trocars, 68, 68f
  description of, 68
  insight on, 68–69
  uses of, 68
Video cart. *See* Laparoscopic cart
Vienna nasal speculum, 196, 196f
  description of, 196
  uses of, 196
Visiport, 67, 67f
  description of, 67
  insight on, 67–68
  other names for, 67
  uses of, 67
Volkman retractor, 43, 43f
  caution when using, 43–44
  description of, 43
  insight on, 43–44
  other names for, 43
  uses of, 43
Von Graefe Strabismus hook, 159, 159f
  description of, 159
  uses of, 159
Vorse tubing occluding clamp, 318, 318f
  category of, 318
  description of, 318
  insight on, 318–319
  other names for, 318
  uses of, 318
Vulsellum. *See* Jacobs vulsellum

W
Wall suction. *See* Suction
Walsham septum straightener, 192, 192f
  description of, 192
  insight on, 192–193
  uses of, 192

Walter forceps. *See* Potts-Smith tissue forceps
Walther female urethral sounds, 131, 131f
description of, 131
insight on, 131
other names for, 131
uses of, 131
Warm-up jacket. *See* Cover jacket
Warmer, 368, 368f
description of, 368
insight on, 368–369
other names for, 368
uses of, 368
Water tubing. *See* Irrigation tubing
Watson skin graft knife, 224, 224f
category of, 224
description of, 224
insight on, 224
other names for, 224
uses of, 224
Webster needle holder, 233, 233f
category of, 233
description of, 233
uses of, 233
Weighted speculum. *See* Auvard weighted vaginal speculum
Weitlaner retractor, 45, 45f
caution when using, 46
description of, 45
insight on, 45–46
other names for, 45
uses of, 45–46
Wells enucleation spoon, 142, 142f
description of, 142
uses of, 142–143
Wertheim clamp, 127, 127f
description of, 127
uses of, 127–128
Wertheim-cullen pedicle clamp, 127, 127f
description of, 127
other names for, 127
uses of, 127
West periosteal elevator, 213, 213f
description of, 213
other names, 213
uses of, 213
Westcott tenotomy scissors, 148, 148f
description of, 148
uses of, 148
Whisk. *See* Allison lung retractor
Wieder tongue blade, 205, 205f
description of, 205
other names for, 205
uses of, 205
Wiener antrum rasp, 182, 182f
description of, 182

Wiener antrum rasp *(Continued)*
other names for, 182
uses of, 182
Wilde dressing forceps. *See* Wilde tissue forceps
Wilde ethmoid forceps, 191, 191f
description of, 191
insight on, 192
uses of, 191
Wilde rongeur, 293, 293f
caution when using, 293
description of, 293
insight on, 293
other names for, 293
uses of, 293
Wilde tissue forceps, 194, 194f
description of, 194
other names for, 194
uses of, 194–195
Wilder lacrimal dilator, 156, 156f
description of, 156
other names for, 156
uses of, 156
Williams eye speculum, 157f
description of, 157
uses of, 157–158
Williams hemilaminectomy retractors, 309, 309f
description of, 309
insight on, 309–310
other names for, 309
uses of, 309
Wire cutters. *See* Wire scissors
Wire scissors, 28, 28f
caution when using, 28
description of, 28
insight on, 28
other names for, 28
uses of, 28
Wire speculum. *See* Barraquer eye speculum
Wire twister. *See* Sternal needle holder and wire twister
Woodson dura separator, 305, 305f
description of, 305
uses of, 305
Woodson elevator, 300, 300f
description of, 300
uses of, 300
Working element, 123, 123f
description of, 123
insight on, 123–124
other names for, 123
uses of, 123
Wullstein ear forceps, 175, 175f
description of, 175

Wullstein ear forceps *(Continued)*
other names for, 175
uses of, 175

X
Xcel blunt port. *See* Blunt trocar
Xcel trocars, 68, 68f
description of, 68
insight on, 68
uses of, 68

Y
Yankauer, baby. *See* Andrews-Pynchon suction tip
Yankauer suction tip, 47, 47f
description of, 47
insight on, 47–48
nondisposable, 208, 208f
description of, 208
insight on, 208
other names for, 208
uses of, 208
other names for, 47
uses of, 47
Yasar scissors. *See* Yasargil scissors
Yasargil scissors, 330, 330f
category of, 330
description of, 330
insight on, 330
other names for, 330
uses of, 330
Young anterior retractor, 133, 133f
description of, 133
other names for, 133
uses of, 133
Young bifurcated retractor, 134
description of, 134
insight on, 134
other names for, 134
uses of, 134
Young bulb retractor, 133, 133f
description of, 133
insight on, 133–134
other names for, 133
uses of, 133
Young renal clamp, 126, 126f
description of, 126
uses of, 126

Z
Zaufel-Jansen rongeur, 256, 256f
caution when using, 256–257
description of, 256
insight on, 256–257
other names for, 256
uses of, 256